The Survival of Colon and Rectal Cancer

The Survival of Colon and Rectal Cancer

Editor

Susanne Merkel

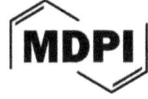

Basel • Beijing • Wuhan • Barcelona • Belgrade • Novi Sad • Cluj • Manchester

Editor
Susanne Merkel
Friedrich-Alexander-Universität
Erlangen-Nürnberg
Erlangen
Germany

Editorial Office
MDPI AG
Grosspeteranlage 5
4052 Basel, Switzerland

This is a reprint of articles from the Special Issue published online in the open access journal *Cancers* (ISSN 2072-6694) (available at: https://www.mdpi.com/journal/cancers/special_issues/76E53X0TTV).

For citation purposes, cite each article independently as indicated on the article page online and as indicated below:

Lastname, A.A.; Lastname, B.B. Article Title. *Journal Name* **Year**, *Volume Number*, Page Range.

ISBN 978-3-7258-1679-8 (Hbk)
ISBN 978-3-7258-1680-4 (PDF)
doi.org/10.3390/books978-3-7258-1680-4

Cover image courtesy of Susanne Merkel

© 2024 by the authors. Articles in this book are Open Access and distributed under the Creative Commons Attribution (CC BY) license. The book as a whole is distributed by MDPI under the terms and conditions of the Creative Commons Attribution-NonCommercial-NoDerivs (CC BY-NC-ND) license.

Contents

Ross Jarrett and Nicholas P. West
Macroscopic Evaluation of Colon Cancer Resection Specimens
Reprinted from: *Cancers* 2023, *15*, 4116, doi:10.3390/cancers15164116 1

Masoud Karimi, Pia Osterlund, Klara Hammarström, Israa Imam, Jan-Erik Frodin
and Bengt Glimelius
Associations between Response to Commonly Used Neo-Adjuvant Schedules in Rectal Cancer
and Routinely Collected Clinical and Imaging Parameters
Reprinted from: *Cancers* 2022, *14*, 6238, doi:10.3390/cancers14246238 13

Sigmar Stelzner, Thomas Kittner, Michael Schneider, Fred Schuster, Markus Grebe,
Erik Puffer, et al.
Beyond Total Mesorectal Excision (TME)—Results of MRI-Guided Multivisceral Resections in T4
Rectal Carcinoma and Local Recurrence
Reprinted from: *Cancers* 2023, *15*, 5328, doi:10.3390/cancers15225328 27

Susanne Merkel, Maximilian Brunner, Carol-Immanuel Geppert, Robert Grützmann,
Klaus Weber and Abbas Agaimy
Proposal of a T3 Subclassification for Colon Carcinoma
Reprinted from: *Cancers* 2022, *14*, 6186, doi:10.3390/cancers14246186 41

Paweł Mroczkowski, Samuel Kim, Ronny Otto, Hans Lippert, Radosław Zajdel,
Karolina Zajdel and Anna Merecz-Sadowska
Prognostic Value of Metastatic Lymph Node Ratio and Identification of Factors Influencing the
Lymph Node Yield in Patients Undergoing Curative Colon Cancer Resection
Reprinted from: *Cancers* 2024, *16*, 218, doi:10.3390/cancers16010218 54

Anne Jacobsen, Jürgen Siebler, Robert Grützmann, Michael Stürzl and Elisabeth Naschberger
Blood Vessel-Targeted Therapy in Colorectal Cancer: Current Strategies and Future Perspectives
Reprinted from: *Cancers* 2024, *16*, 890, doi:10.3390/cancers16050890 68

Jing Chen, Yi-Wen Song, Guan-Zhan Liang, Zong-Jin Zhang, Xiao-Feng Wen,
Rui-Bing Li, et al.
A Novel m7G-Related Gene Signature Predicts the Prognosis of Colon Cancer
Reprinted from: *Cancers* 2022, *14*, 5527, doi:10.3390/cancers14225527 86

Stefi Nordkamp, Davy M. J. Creemers, Sofie Glazemakers, Stijn H. J. Ketelaers,
Harm J. Scholten, Silvie van de Calseijde, et al.
Implementation of an Enhanced Recovery after Surgery Protocol in Advanced and Recurrent
Rectal Cancer Patients after beyond Total Mesorectal Excision Surgery: A Feasibility Study
Reprinted from: *Cancers* 2023, *15*, 4523, doi:10.3390/cancers15184523 105

Vinzenz Völkel, Michael Gerken, Kees Kleihues-van Tol, Olaf Schoffer, Veronika Bierbaum,
Christoph Bobeth, et al.
Treatment of Colorectal Cancer in Certified Centers: Results of a Large German Registry Study
Focusing on Long-Term Survival
Reprinted from: *Cancers* 2023, *15*, 4568, doi:10.3390/cancers15184568 117

Mihailo Andric, Jessica Stockheim, Mirhasan Rahimli, Sara Al-Madhi, Sara Acciuffi,
Maximilian Dölling, et al.
Influence of Certification Program on Treatment Quality and Survival for Rectal Cancer Patients
in Germany: Results of 13 Certified Centers in Collaboration with AN Institute
Reprinted from: *Cancers* 2024, *16*, 1496, doi:10.3390/cancers16081496 130

Michael K. Rooney, Melisa Pasli, George J. Chang, Prajnan Das, Eugene J. Koay,
Albert C. Koong, et al.
Patient-Reported Sexual Function, Bladder Function and Quality of Life for Patients with
Low Rectal Cancers with or without a Permanent Ostomy
Reprinted from: *Cancers* 2024, *16*, 153, doi:10.3390/cancers16010153 147

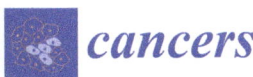

Review

Macroscopic Evaluation of Colon Cancer Resection Specimens

Ross Jarrett and Nicholas P. West *

Pathology & Data Analytics, Leeds Institute of Medical Research, St. James's University Hospital, School of Medicine, University of Leeds, Leeds LS9 7TF, UK
* Correspondence: n.p.west@leeds.ac.uk

Simple Summary: Colon cancer is a common disease that is primarily treated by surgically removing the affected bowel, but the quality of surgery is variable internationally, leading to suboptimal patient outcomes. Pathologists should provide feedback to surgeons and can help to improve long-term patient outcomes. This review summarises the key aspects of pathological quality control that should be adopted internationally to improve the chances of survival from this deadly disease.

Abstract: Colon cancer is a common disease internationally. Outcomes have not improved to the same degree as in rectal cancer, where the focus on total mesorectal excision and pathological feedback has significantly contributed to improved survival and reduced local recurrence. Colon cancer surgery shows significant variation around the world, with differences in mesocolic integrity, height of the vascular ligation and length of the bowel resected. This leads to variation in well-recognised quality measures like lymph node yield. Pathologists are able to assess all of these variables and are ideally placed to provide feedback to surgeons and the wider multidisciplinary team to improve surgical quality over time. With a move towards complete mesocolic excision with central vascular ligation to remove the primary tumour and all mechanisms of spread within an intact package, pathological feedback will be central to improving outcomes for patients with operable colon cancer. This review focusses on the key quality measures and the evidence that underpins them.

Keywords: colon cancer; pathology; quality of surgery; feedback; macroscopic assessment

1. Introduction

With global diagnoses of more than 1.8 million new cases per year, colorectal cancer is the third most frequent malignant disease seen in male and female populations [1]. When magnified further, the data show an uneven split between colon and rectal cancers of approximately 70% and 30%, respectively [2]. Colorectal cancer is a good candidate for surgical intervention with a curative aim [3], and the way in which the resection specimen is evaluated is fundamental within this context. Indeed, the evaluation by pathologists can facilitate changes to standardised surgical procedures, resulting in superior patient outcomes.

Initially described by Heald, total mesorectal excision (TME) is now the international standard approach for surgically resecting rectal cancers [4]. The paradigm shift that TME created has not only vastly improved oncological outcomes via a standardised surgical approach, but also, importantly, utilised pathological evaluation and feedback [5,6]. An identical principle for the resection of colon cancer is the recently described complete mesocolic excision (CME) with central vascular ligation (CVL) [7]. Pioneered by Hohenberger and colleagues in Erlangen, Germany, this approach has also led to significant improvements in oncological outcomes. These outcomes have been replicated in other centres utilising the technique [8–11]. Although CME with CVL provides many of the same oncological benefits of TME, it is still yet to be adopted as an international surgical standard, with many centres still favouring 'conventional' approaches largely due to concerns over morbidity with high-tie surgery [12–14].

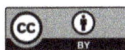

2. Paving the Way: Jamieson and Dobson

As far back as 1909, well before CME was described, Jamieson and Dobson first described the lymphatic drainage of colon cancer and the optimal principles for surgical resection [15]. Their proposal relied on the fundamental principle that colon cancer lymphatic drainage follows the arterial supply. Thus, to prevent any remaining cancer from being left in situ and disease recuring locally or distally post-surgery, 'whole-package' resection is required, including the tumour and associated lymphatics, which brings benefits by reducing the risk of spread as well as preventing tumour spillage. This is exactly the same principle that TME is built upon [4,7].

Anatomically speaking, the mesocolon and mesorectum are continuous structures [16–18]. Similarly, the embryological tissue planes of these structures are analogous. Each is contained within a peritoneum and visceral fascia; 'whole-package' resection in both CME and TME is made possible due to the presence of these planes [4,7]. One important difference is the marked variability in the vasculature of the colon compared to the rectum [7,19]. This poses idiosyncratic surgical challenges, which three-dimensional computed tomography (CT) angiography has been suggested to overcome [20,21].

Whilst Jamieson and Dobson diligently charted the lymphatic drainage of colon cancer over one hundred years ago, more recently, the Japanese Society for Cancer of the Colon and Rectum (JSCCR) published a system to more thoroughly classify colon lymph node anatomy based on their proximity to the wall of the bowel [15,22]. Initially, a cancer will drain to the paracolic (D1) nodes, which are closest to the bowel wall and follow the path of the marginal arteries. Intermediate (D2) nodes represent the next drainage layer, and these follow the path of the branches of the superior and inferior mesenteric arteries. Finally, the highest level of drainage potentially included in standard specimens is provided by the central (D3) nodes. These nodes are found on both the right and left sides of the colon. On the right, they reside at the origin of the ileocolic, right colic and middle colic arteries, and on the left side, they run along the inferior mesenteric artery from the origin at the aorta to the branch of the left colic artery [22].

3. Contemporary CME with CVL

According to Hohenberger, there are three key components to CME with CVL. Sharp dissection should be achieved along the embryological tissue planes, whereby the visceral and parietal fascia are separated, resulting in an intact surgical specimen lined by peritoneum and fascia, as applicable. The primary aim is to ensure this lining remains intact, thus reducing the risk of tumour spillage. Next, to facilitate the removal of the D3 lymph nodes and maximise the lymph node harvest, CVL should be performed on the supplying colonic arteries. This may also be referred to as "high-tie" and involves ligation of the vessels close to their root. The level of venous ligation generally does not receive the same attention in the literature as the arterial tie, but Hohenberger confirms that the veins should also be ligated centrally. The scientific rationale for this is less clear. Hohenberger finally specifies that by resecting an adequate length of bowel, more longitudinal paracolic nodes will be removed [7,23]. A lack of randomised trials means the relative significance of each of these components is not yet fully understood.

In Japan, the JSCCR also recognises the importance of operating within the embryological plane, although they do not undertake CVL on all patients. The decision on the level of vascular ligation is made inter-operatively and largely depends on the depth of primary tumour invasion [22]. More specifically, they advise that T1 tumours undergo D2 resection with intermediate vascular ligation, while T2-4 undergo D3 resection with CVL [22,24].

What is deemed an adequate length of longitudinal bowel resection from the primary tumour is also a point of difference between Hohenberger and the JSCCR. The latter advocate a more conservative length (rarely more than 10 cm), while the former is more radical, going at least one vascular arcade beyond the tumour, which results in a longer length of bowel resected [24,25]. There are several Japanese studies that support a more conservative approach. Longitudinal lymphatic spread beyond the paracolic area in left-

and right-sided tumours was found to be as low as 0% and 1–4%, respectively [26,27]. In contradiction to this, another study found that in 16% of cases, the first metastatic lymph node was found in the paracolic region, in excess of 5 cm from the primary tumour [28]. Despite this, West et al. found that while the length of resection was variable, there was a high rate of mesocolic plane excision in both Japanese and Hohenberger cases. The long-term outcomes for both were also analogous, leading to the suggestion that the operating plane is likely to be of greatest significance, with the height of the ligation having a smaller influence in some cases [24]. A comparison of CME, D3 and conventional surgery is shown in Figure 1.

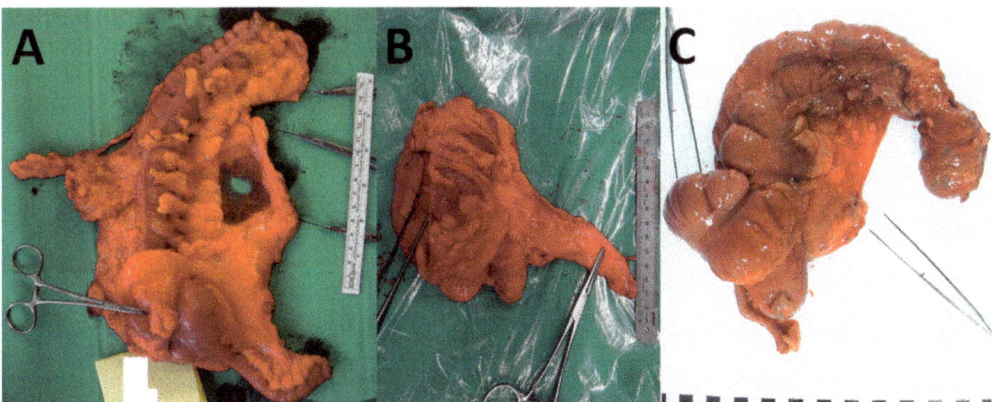

Figure 1. A comparison of CME, D3 and conventional surgery, showing a right hemicolectomy resected through CME with CVL (**A**), D3 resection (**B**) and conventional D2 resection (**C**). Note the increased length of the vascular pedicle with both CME and D3 surgery compared to conventional D2 surgery. Also note the significantly longer length of the colon removed with the CME approach compared to D3.

A further development is the expanded use of laparoscopic and robotic-assisted techniques [29]. Concerning CME, several retrospective comparative studies and a randomised controlled trial have been conducted to compare open versus laparoscopic techniques [30–36]. Findings were consistent across these studies; operating times, oncological benefit, safety profile and specimen quality were similar between the two groups. For D3 resection, a Japanese randomised controlled trial was conducted to compare open versus laparoscopic techniques; oncological outcomes were equivalent, but lower complications and shorter hospitalisation were apparent [31,36]. Other retrospective comparative studies also concur with this [29,32,33,35]. While robotic-assisted CME has predominantly been utilised for right-sided procedures, studies conducted show that despite a laparoscopic or open environment, the oncological benefit and safety profile results are similar [37,38]. However, although robotic CME increased operating time, it also increased lymph node yield and was associated with low conversion rates [37–40]. Initial findings show encouraging results in this area.

4. Oncological Outcomes and Benefits

Hohenberger et al. reported a series of cases performed over 24 years, during which there were defined periods of analysis: pre-CME (1978–1984), development of CME (1985–1994) and implementation of CME (1995–2002). Between the pre-CME and implementation periods, 5-year cancer related survival after surgery increased by 6% (82.1% to 89.1%) and 5-year recurrence rates decreased by 2.9% (6.5% to 3.6%) [7]. Notwithstanding these significant results, there are some limitations with the series; the duration over which the study was conducted carries potential confounders, and as it was a non-randomised study, exactly how patients were selected is unclear. However, significantly increased disease-free or disease-specific survival as a result of CME has been shown in several subsequent studies [8,9]. Decreased rates of local and distal recurrence have also been shown [10,11]. However, this is not a universal picture, as other studies have shown no significant difference in overall survival with the use of CME; however, pathological quality control is not uniform [9,41–43]. In addition, increased morbidity has been associated with CME use, especially in right-sided tumours [22,24], although this has been disputed by a recent meta-analysis [44].

To date, there have been only retrospective studies published that compare CME with non-CME and, importantly, no randomised controlled trials. With evidence increasingly suggesting that CME is largely effective due to an integral mesocolic plane, it is essential that independent pathological analysis take place on resected specimens. Indeed, it is notable that many studies conducted in this area do not consider this an essential component. However, two important randomised controlled trials are ongoing. COLD compares D2 and D3 lymph node dissection in colon cancer [45], and RELARC compares D2 dissection with CME for laparoscopic right hemicolectomy in colon cancer [46].

Some studies looking at CME have reported results that encourage its use. Two studies reported that surgeons employing the technique regularly are more likely to produce a high-quality specimen compared to those that do not [25,47]. Another study found that 88.5% of specimens were judged to be in the mesocolic plane following CME, whereas conventional surgery was found to be 47.4% [25]. In addition, Ng et al. found that at a large referral centre, two-thirds of all colon cancer resections were performed in the mesocolic plane [14]. It is therefore all the more pertinent that West et al. found a 15% improvement in 5-year overall survival for patients with resections in the mesocolic plane versus those in the muscularis propria [48]. This benefit increased to 27% for stage III disease. A large review considering 18,989 patients from 27 studies also found significant positive impacts on 3-year and 5-year overall survival as well as 3-year disease-free survival [49].

One can argue that simple standardisation of a surgical procedure provides further rationale to adopt CME as the convention; studies have elicited better quality resections via standardisation [50,51], which can facilitate better patient outcomes [52,53]. Further significant results from a Danish study were found in which one hospital underwent a CME education programme and was compared to five others that did not; in the CME educated group versus the conventional group, mesocolic plane excision was 75% vs. 48%, distance between tumour and ligation point was 105 mm vs. 84 mm, mean lymph node yield was 28 vs. 18 and improved 4-year disease-free survival was 85.8% [95% CI 81.4–90.1] vs. 73.4% [66.2–80.6] [9,50]. When the original programme was rolled out across the other five sites, mesocolic plane excision increased from 58% to 70% ($p < 0.001$) [54]. It is also apparent that through such education programmes, CME can be relatively quickly learned and adopted [50,55].

5. The Pathologist, a Gatekeeper to Quality Control

The pathologist is uniquely suited to the role of assessing the quality of colon cancer resection specimens. Not only are they independent of the surgery, but they are also exposed to specimens from multiple surgeons. When harnessed by the MDT, this essential experience facilitates a rich feedback loop, wherein the pathologist is able to supply direct feedback to the MDT, including photographic records. The role has already been exemplified in TME and is now considered standard of care following rectal cancer surgery. The Medical Research Council CR07 trial demonstrated an improvement in the quality of resected specimens over time when assessing how the plane of surgery affected local recurrence in rectal cancer. Between 1998 and 2005, mesorectal plane excisions increased from less than 50% to more than 60%, muscularis propria excision decreased from over 20% to 10%, and circumferential resection margin involvement decreased from 21% to 10% [6]. Pathological quality control and direct feedback to the MDT during the trial are likely to have contributed to improving the quality of the resected surgical specimen over time.

Although other factors, such as the introduction of MRI for surgical planning and adjuvant chemotherapy, have played their part in the sustained improvements in long-term rectal cancer survival, the improvement in specimen quality should not be understated [30].

6. Pathological Assessment of Mesocolic Integrity

In CME, the integrity of the resected mesocolon should not be breached. This is described as surgery in the mesocolic plane. This results in the cancer and potential mechanisms of spread (tumour deposits, lymphatics, lymph nodes, nerves and blood vessels), being contained within a package lined by the peritoneum and fascia [7,15]. The requirement to be scrupulous concerning mesocolic integrity is founded in studies that show improved patient outcomes resulting from CME [7,36]. The integral package brings significant benefits by reducing the risk of intra-abdominal recurrence in two ways. Firstly, it prevents spillage of tumour cells into the peritoneal cavity, and secondly, it increases surgical radicality [48]. In a single-centre retrospective study, mesocolic versus muscularis propria plane surgery conferred a 15% overall survival advantage at 5 years for mesocolic plane patients [48]. In addition, the advantage increased to 27% in stage III patients, showing that it is even more crucial to remove the mesocolon intact at the later stages of disease.

Largely based on the CR07 trial [5,56] and subsequently developed for the MRC CLASICC trial [57], a three-tier system is used to grade the plane of surgery (see Table 1 and Figure 2). This provides an objective specimen quality assessment and facilitates the evaluation of patient prognosis. The assessment should first be performed on the intact, fresh specimen. Then, a secondary assessment should commence on the intact and cross-sectionally sliced formalin-fixed specimen to establish the presence of any defects as well as their respective depths. The optimal plane of surgery is represented by the mesocolic plane, whereby the peritoneal and fascial linings are intact. Only defects that are less than 5 mm in depth are permitted at this grade. Intermediate quality is represented by the intramesocolic plane. At this grade, the depth of any single defect must be in excess of 5 mm but must not extend down to the muscularis propria. A poor-quality specimen is represented by the muscularis propria plane, in which a defect is found that extends on to the muscularis propria or deeper, e.g., surgical perforation. Importantly, a final grading is governed by considering the poorest quality area, even if it is limited in size [48].

Table 1. Pathological assessment of the mesocolic plane.

Plane	Description
Mesocolic plane	Mesocolon intact and covered by peritoneum and fascia (where relevant). Defects measure no more than 5 mm in maximum size.
Intramesocolic plane	Mesocolic defects greater than 5 mm in size that do not extend down to the muscularis propria.
Muscularis propria plane	Substantial mesocolic defects that extend down on to the muscularis propria or beyond, e.g., perforation.

The process of mesocolic grading is prone to a degree of intra- and inter-observer variation. Munkedal et al. found that inter-observer agreement was poor (k < 0.4), while intra-observer agreement was fair to good (k 0.4–0.7) [58]. They proposed several refinements to the grading system to improve reproducibility, one of which drew on the Japanese classification of lymphatic drainage: only the mesocolon in the tumour lymphatic drainage field should be assessed. However, they suggest excluding from evaluation the area within 10 mm of the longitudinal margins, regardless of inclusion in the drainage area. This is due to consistent irregularity at the margins, which risks unreliability. Finally, on some specimens there are 'peritoneal windows' (fused serosal layers devoid of intervening fat), which if damaged in isolation should also not be a cause for downgrading [58]. Identifying and minimising inter-observer variation is essential to avoiding bias; thus, it is paramount to centrally moderate specimen grading within a clinical trial setting. The UK FOxTROT trial is an exemplar of this; locally across 80 centres, pathologists graded specimens, and these will be compared centrally to facilitate calculation of inter-observer variation [59].

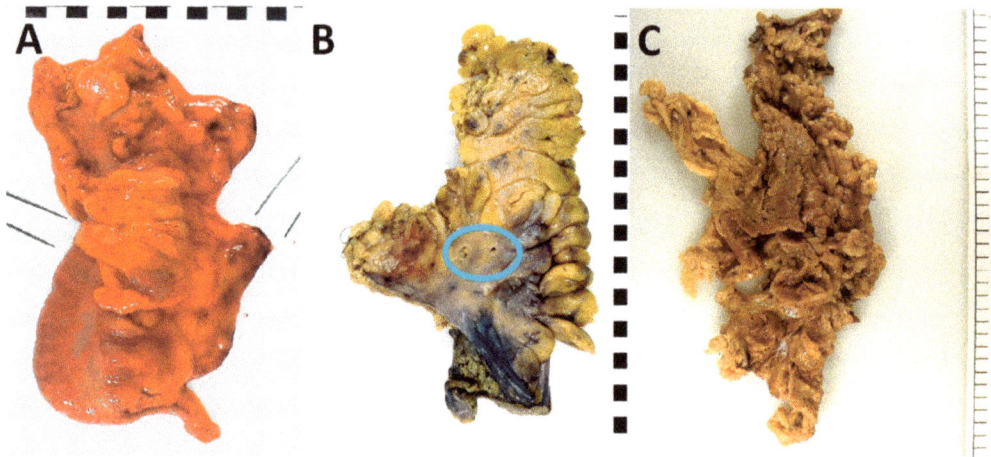

Figure 2. Pathological assessment of the mesocolic plane, showing examples of specimens in the mesocolic plane (**A**), intramesocolic plane (**B**) and muscularis propria plane (**C**). Not the small mesenteric disruptions in B that do not extend down to the muscularis propria (blue circle). The specimen in C shows a ragged mesentery with multiple disruptions down to the muscularis propria.

7. Distance between the Tumour and Point of Central Arterial Ligation

A quality measure of CVL is the distance between the tumour and the arterial ligation point on the pathological specimen. This measure is flawed at the individual level, as the length of the original vessel is not known by the pathologist, and the vessel will contract after removal and even more with formalin fixation [47]. However, from the population perspective, when intermediate-level ligation was compared to central ligation by Hohenberger, the latter was associated with a significantly greater distance between the tumour and ligation point: 81.4 mm vs. 128.7 mm in right-sided tumours; $p < 0.0001$ and 97.0 mm vs. 145.0 mm in left-sided tumours; $p < 0.001$. It was also significantly correlated with a greater lymph node yield [47]. Further studies have corroborated these findings [11,25,50], and associations have been made between optimal-plane specimens and an increased distance between the tumour and high-tie, as well as increased lymph node yield [11,60].

The central ligation height is a key marker for the radicality of CME, but there are challenges. The measure is best conducted on fresh specimens immediately after resection. However, for logistical and clinical reasons, this is often impractical [61]. To optimise this measurement, two solutions have been suggested: in-theatre measuring of the specimen or photography against a metric scale. In addition, there is significant anatomical variation found in the length of the central vessel [25,61], and thus, at the individual level, its measure holds little value. It is, however, useful at the population level because it accurately conveys the radicality of CME and can therefore be used for audit and training.

Assessment of the remaining arterial stump radiologically is another consideration. Despite Swedish and U.K. studies, which cite anatomical variation as reason to suggest the length of the remaining arterial stump does not accurately predict the length of the resected vessel [62,63], stump length is still a strong marker for surgical radicality. A Danish study quantified that the mean stump length measured by CT was 38 mm (95% CI: 33–43 mm), whereas the target within the CME with CVL context is approximately 10 mm [61]. If increased radicality improves outcomes, there is potential to use this post-operatively for immediate feedback, as well as for follow-up, because the arterial stump does not significantly change length over time [64]. However, a CT conducted immediately after surgery is unlikely to be palatable due to increased radiation exposure, so this may need to be done on the routine 12-month post-operative scan.

8. Length of Bowel Resection

A multi-centre study in Japan (where the '10 cm rule' is standard) compared various surgical approaches (CME with CVL, D3 lymph node removal and conventional surgery) in stage III colon cancer and considered bowel resection length [25]. The study found CME bowel length was significantly greater than D3 (median 355 mm vs. 184 mm in right-sided tumours; $p = 0.0003$, 355 mm vs. 146 mm in left-sided tumours; $p < 0.0001$), but the central arterial ligation height was not significantly different (median 115 mm vs. 103 mm in right-sided tumours, 128 mm vs. 120 mm in left-sided tumours). When conventional 'intermediate ligation' surgery is compared to D3, the latter yields significantly shorter bowel resection length and greater arterial ligation height (median central ligation height: 81 mm vs. 103 mm in right-sided tumours; $p = 0.037$, 100 mm vs. 120 mm in left-sided tumours; $p = 0.034$). Unsurprisingly, surgery performed in the conventional way was in the mesocolic plane only 47% of the time versus 72% for D3 surgery [25]. This suggests that, when compared to other CME parameters, the oncological value gained by increasing the length of resection is relatively limited.

Kobayashi et al. found that as the length of bowel resection increases, so does the number of resected lymph nodes [25]. Although this has been corroborated in other studies [24,25,47,48], the number of malignant lymph nodes does not appear to increase, suggesting that there is no benefit to removing large numbers of benign nodes that are well away from the tumour site [24,25]. Longitudinal outcomes from Hohenberger and those in Japan both show comparable results despite significant differences in specimen length. The T-REX study aims to establish a more accurate comparison of optimal resection length and ligation height in centres around the world undertaking both CME and D3 surgery [65].

9. Lymph Node Yield

In general, CME lymph node yield is greater than that of non-CME surgery [66]. Two studies by West et al. quantified CME vs. non-CME: a median of 18 versus 30 nodes [47] and a median of 18 versus 28 nodes [50]. Due to the longer bowel resection in CME, many of the additional nodes are more likely to be of the D1 and D2 types, although the D3 nodes will also be included in CME [47]. There has been international debate as to the optimum number of nodes to harvest and how they should be processed in an effort to stage colorectal cancer accurately. The Royal College of Pathologists advises that every node within the specimen should be examined and that pathologists should regularly audit their practice with the expectation of a minimum average of 12 nodes across 50 cases [67]. However, leading centres regularly harvest 20–40 nodes via careful dissection or the use of ancillary methods such as methylene blue [68]. CME is thought to partially bring benefit from maximised node yield via increased accuracy of staging. Hohenberger found that a yield of 28 was independently associated with 5-year cancer-related survival (96.3% vs. 90.7%, $p = 0.018$) for those patients that were node-negative [7]. Another study found CME to have a significant benefit over non-CME surgery in stage I and II colon cancer for similar reasons [9]. Part of the survival benefit from greater lymph node numbers in early-stage disease arises from stage migration. Much of the benefit is believed to be due to a better immune response, e.g., the relationship between deficient mismatch repair/microsatellite instability, immune response and patient outcomes [69].

A primary reason why staging is of utmost importance is for patient access to adjuvant chemotherapy; low yields reduce the likelihood of a stage III diagnosis, which then precludes access to such therapy [70]. However, node yield as a marker of surgical quality in isolation is not recommended unless the surgical plane is also considered, as even the most radical surgery can occasionally result in low yield, and conversely, specimens that are extensively disrupted may still contain many nodes [71]. Most important is that an exhaustive search be performed that evaluates all paracolic, intermediate and central nodes within 10 cm of the tumour. Morris et al. also investigated whether the practicing pathologist had any influence over the yield; it was found that specialist pathologists (those that regularly undertake this work) were more likely than non-specialists to achieve adequate yield within their specific role (OR, 2.16; 95% CI, 1.93 to 2.41) [70].

10. Photography

The key to recording and documenting specimen quality is standardised specimen photography. This can be utilised by the MDT to facilitate audits of surgical quality, scientific discussion and training. The aforementioned feedback loop is strengthened by this activity; studies show that benefits have been gained in the assessment of specimen quality as well as linked to improved outcomes, especially when used in clinical trial settings [34,72]. More specifically, Munkedal et al. found that by utilising specimen photography within MDT meetings wherein surgeons could derive feedback, mesocolic plane surgery increased (52% to 76%, p = 0.02) [34]. Photography also allows the addition of centralised mesocolic grading across multiple centres, e.g., in a clinical trial, which in turn has been shown to reduce interobserver error [24,25,50]. The recommended standardised approach is outlined below (see Figure 3).

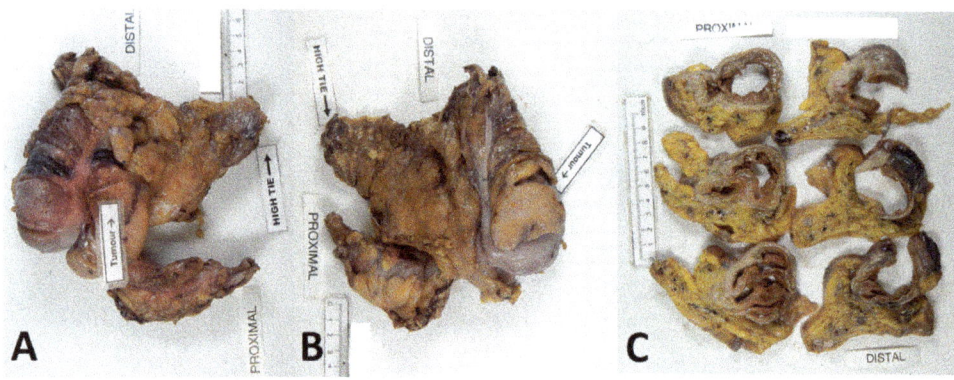

Figure 3. Optimal specimen photography protocol. Three separate images should be captured as a minimum. These include the anterior whole specimen view (**A**), posterior whole specimen view (**B**) and cross-sectional slices (**C**).

Photography should be high-resolution and taken directly above the specimen to reduce distortion artefacts. A fixed stand should ideally be used to mitigate against movement artefacts. Placed next to the specimen should be a metric scale, as this allows for calibration of the software for morphometrical analysis. Ideally, prior to formalin fixing or opening, the anterior and posterior aspects of the whole specimen should be photographed. The mesentery should be laid out flat and without tension, so that the proximal and distal aspects, tumour and vascular ties can be labelled or obviously visualised. Close-ups of any relevant areas should be taken, e.g., mesocolic defects and perforations. Formalin fixation should follow, and the tumour segment should be sliced at 3–4 mm intervals. The slices should be laid out sequentially, with the proximal and distal slices labelled. Finally, clinically important areas should be noted, and close-up photographs taken. This protocol has been used to quality control specimens for a number of studies referenced in this manuscript [24,25,34,47,48,50].

11. Conclusions

TME has improved oncological outcomes and increased overall survival for rectal cancer patients around the world. This has predominantly been achieved by operating within the mesorectal plane, which facilitates intact resection of the cancer. Unsurprisingly, therefore, TME is now internationally standardised and precisely defined. By applying the same principles, CME can provide similar benefits for the resection of colon cancer. Studies to pathologically assess the quality of resection have confirmed that when CME is compared to conventional surgical approaches, the former produces a higher-quality specimen (more likely to be intact and within the mesocolic plane) and facilitates improvements in other quality markers. These include increased lymph node yield and improved radicality of surgery by centrally ligating the supplying vasculature. Operating within the mesocolic plane has been associated with an overall improvement in 5-year survival, especially for patients with stage III colon cancer.

Notwithstanding the suitability of the pathologist for objectively, systematically and promptly reporting an independent assessment of the specimen, it is unfortunate that recent studies comparing CME with non-CME have negated the importance of such an analysis. Lack of standardisation in CME means that inclusion of this analysis in the future is even more important and should be mandatory to interpret trial data. These benefits are only increased further when combined with a well-functioning MDT. Not only can pathological data inform MDT discussions around the individual patient, but it can also be extensively used in training sessions, informing best practices and continually improving the MDT as well as overall patient outcomes. It is therefore essential that any new clinical trials in this area be underpinned by independent pathological quality control.

Author Contributions: R.J. and N.P.W. jointly wrote the review and have approved the submitted version. All authors have read and agreed to the published version of the manuscript.

Funding: R.J. is funded by the Pathological Society of Great Britain and Ireland, London, UK (ref ID 0322 03). N.P.W. is funded by Yorkshire Cancer Research, Harrogate, UK (ref L386).

Institutional Review Board Statement: Not applicable.

Informed Consent Statement: Not applicable.

Data Availability Statement: Not applicable.

Conflicts of Interest: The authors declare no conflict of interest.

References

1. World Cancer Research Fund. Worldwide Cancer Data: Global Cancer Statistics for the Most Common Cancers. 2022. Available online: https://www.wcrf.org/dietandcancer/cancer-trends/worldwide-cancer-data (accessed on 2 January 2022).
2. American Cancer Society. Key Statistics for Colorectal Cancer. 2022. Available online: https://www.cancer.org/cancer/colon-rectal-cancer/about/key-statistics.html (accessed on 2 January 2022).
3. National Cancer Institute. Colon Cancer Treatment. 2022. Available online: https://www.cancer.gov/types/colorectal/patient/colon-treatment-pdq (accessed on 4 January 2022).
4. Heald, R.; Husband, E.; Ryall, R. The mesorectum in rectal cancer surgery—The clue to pelvic recurrence? *Br. J. Surg.* **1982**, *69*, 613–616. [CrossRef] [PubMed]
5. Quirke, P.; Sebag-Montefiore, D.; Steele, R.; Khanna, S.; Monson, J.; Holliday, A.; Thompson, L.; Griffiths, G.; Stephens, R. Local recurrence after rectal cancer resection is strongly related to the plane of surgical dissection and is further reduced by pre-operative short course radiotherapy. Preliminary results of the Medical Research Council (MRC) CR07 trial. *J. Clin. Oncol.* **2006**, *24* (Suppl. S18), 3512. [CrossRef]
6. Quirke, P.; Steele, R.; Monson, J.; Grieve, R.; Khanna, S.; Couture, J.; O'Callaghan, C.; Myint, A.S.; Bessell, E.; Thompson, L.C. Effect of the plane of surgery achieved on local recurrence in patients with operable rectal cancer: A prospective study using data from the MRC CR07 and NCIC-CTG CO16 randomised clinical trial. *Lancet* **2009**, *373*, 821–828. [CrossRef]
7. Hohenberger, W.; Weber, K.; Matzel, K.; Papadopoulos, T.; Merkel, S. Standardized surgery for colonic cancer: Complete mesocolic excision and central ligation--technical notes and outcome. *Color. Dis.* **2009**, *11*, 354–364, discussion 355–364. [CrossRef] [PubMed]
8. Storli, K.; Søndenaa, K.; Furnes, B.; Nesvik, I.; Gudlaugsson, E.; Bukholm, I.; Eide, G. Short term results of complete (D3) vs. standard (D2) mesenteric excision in colon cancer shows improved outcome of complete mesenteric excision in patients with TNM stages I-II. *Tech. Coloproctol.* **2014**, *18*, 557–564. [CrossRef] [PubMed]

9. Bertelsen, C.A.; Neuenschwander, A.U.; Jansen, J.E.; Wilhelmsen, M.; Kirkegaard-Klitbo, A.; Tenma, J.R.; Bols, B.; Ingeholm, P.; Rasmussen, L.A.; Jepsen, L.V. Disease-free survival after complete mesocolic excision compared with conventional colon cancer surgery: A retrospective, population-based study. *Lancet Oncol.* **2015**, *16*, 161–168. [CrossRef] [PubMed]
10. Merkel, S.; Weber, K.; Matzel, K.; Agaimy, A.; Göhl, J.; Hohenberger, W. Prognosis of patients with colonic carcinoma before, during and after implementation of complete mesocolic excision. *Br. J. Surg.* **2016**, *103*, 1220–1229. [CrossRef] [PubMed]
11. Galizia, G.; Lieto, E.; De Vita, F.; Ferraraccio, F.; Zamboli, A.; Mabilia, A.; Auricchio, A.; Castellano, P.; Napolitano, V.; Orditura, M. Is complete mesocolic excision with central vascular ligation safe and effective in the surgical treatment of right-sided colon cancers? A prospective study. *Int. J. Color. Dis.* **2014**, *29*, 89–97. [CrossRef]
12. Culligan, K.; Remzi, F.; Soop, M.; Coffey, J. Review of nomenclature in colonic surgery–proposal of a standardised nomenclature based on mesocolic anatomy. *Surgeon* **2013**, *11*, 1–5. [CrossRef]
13. Abdelkhalek, M.; Setit, A.; Bianco, F.; Belli, A.; Denewer, A.; Youssef, T.F.; Falato, A.; Romano, G.M. Complete Mesocolic Excision with Central Vascular Ligation in Comparison with Conventional Surgery for Patients with Colon Cancer—The Experiences at Two Centers. *Ann. Coloproctol.* **2018**, *34*, 180–186. [CrossRef]
14. Ng, K.-S.; West, N.P.; Scott, N.; Holzgang, M.; Quirke, P.; Jayne, D.G. What factors determine specimen quality in colon cancer surgery? A cohort study. *Int. J. Color. Dis.* **2020**, *35*, 869–880. [CrossRef] [PubMed]
15. Jamieson, J.K.; Dobson, J.F. The Lymphatics of the Colon. *Proc. R. Soc. Med. Surg. Sect.* **1909**, *2*, 149–174. [CrossRef]
16. Byrnes, K.G.; Walsh, D.; Lewton-Brain, P.; McDermott, K.; Coffey, J.C. Anatomy of the mesentery: Historical development and recent advances. *Semin. Cell Dev. Biol.* **2019**, *92*, 4–11. [CrossRef] [PubMed]
17. Coffey, J.C.; Walsh, D.; Byrnes, K.G.; Hohenberger, W.; Heald, R.J. Mesentery—A 'New' organ. *Emerg. Top. Life Sci.* **2020**, *4*, 191–206. [CrossRef] [PubMed]
18. Culligan, K.; Coffey, J.C.; Kiran, R.P.; Kalady, M.; Lavery, I.C.; Remzi, F.H. The mesocolon: A prospective observational study. *Color. Dis.* **2012**, *14*, 421–428, discussion 428–430. [CrossRef]
19. Vandamme, J.-P.; Bonte, J. *Vascular Anatomy in Abdominal Surgery*; Thieme Medical Publishers: New York, NY, USA, 1990.
20. Kijima, S.; Sasaki, T.; Nagata, K.; Utano, K.; Lefor, A.T.; Sugimoto, H. Preoperative evaluation of colorectal cancer using CT colonography, MRI, and PET/CT. *World J. Gastroenterol. WJG* **2014**, *20*, 16964. [CrossRef]
21. Hirai, K.; Yoshinari, D.; Ogawa, H.; Nakazawa, S.; Takase, Y.; Tanaka, K.; Miyamae, Y.; Takahashi, N.; Tsukagoshi, H.; Toya, H. Three-dimensional computed tomography for analyzing the vascular anatomy in laparoscopic surgery for right-sided colon cancer. *Surg. Laparosc. Endosc. Percutaneous Tech.* **2013**, *23*, 536–539. [CrossRef]
22. Hashiguchi, Y.; Muro, K.; Saito, Y.; Ito, Y.; Ajioka, Y.; Hamaguchi, T.; Hasegawa, K.; Hotta, K.; Ishida, H.; Ishiguro, M. Japanese Society for Cancer of the Colon and Rectum (JSCCR) guidelines 2019 for the treatment of colorectal cancer. *Int. J. Clin. Oncol.* **2020**, *25*, 1–42. [CrossRef]
23. West, N.; Hohenberger, W.; Finan, P.; Quirke, P. Mesocolic plane surgery: An old but forgotten technique? *Color. Dis. Off. J. Assoc. Coloproctol. Great Br. Irel.* **2009**, *11*, 988–989. [CrossRef]
24. West, N.P.; Kobayashi, H.; Takahashi, K.; Perrakis, A.; Weber, K.; Hohenberger, W.; Sugihara, K.; Quirke, P. Understanding optimal colonic cancer surgery: Comparison of Japanese D3 resection and European complete mesocolic excision with central vascular ligation. *J. Clin. Oncol.* **2012**, *30*, 1763–1769. [CrossRef]
25. Kobayashi, H.; West, N.P.; Takahashi, K.; Perrakis, A.; Weber, K.; Hohenberger, W.; Quirke, P.; Sugihara, K. Quality of surgery for stage III colon cancer: Comparison between England, Germany, and Japan. *Ann. Surg. Oncol.* **2014**, *21* (Suppl. S3), S398–S404. [CrossRef] [PubMed]
26. Toyota, S.; Ohta, H.; Anazawa, S. Rationale for extent of lymph node dissection for right colon cancer. *Dis. Colon Rectum* **1995**, *38*, 705–711. [CrossRef] [PubMed]
27. Morikawa, E.; Yasutomi, M.; Shindou, K.; Matsuda, T.; Mori, N.; Hida, J.; Kubo, R.; Kitaoka, M.; Nakamura, M.; Fujimoto, K.; et al. Distribution of metastatic lymph nodes in colorectal cancer by the modified clearing method. *Dis. Colon Rectum* **1994**, *37*, 219–223. [CrossRef]
28. Tan, K.Y.; Kawamura, Y.J.; Mizokami, K.; Sasaki, J.; Tsujinaka, S.; Maeda, T.; Nobuki, M.; Konishi, F. Distribution of the first metastatic lymph node in colon cancer and its clinical significance. *Color. Dis.* **2010**, *12*, 44–47. [CrossRef] [PubMed]
29. Cho, M.S.; Baek, S.J.; Hur, H.; Min, B.S.; Baik, S.H.; Kim, N.K. Modified complete mesocolic excision with central vascular ligation for the treatment of right-sided colon cancer: Long-term outcomes and prognostic factors. *Ann. Surg.* **2015**, *261*, 708–715. [CrossRef] [PubMed]
30. Koh, F.H.; Tan, K.-K. Complete mesocolic excision for colon cancer: Is it worth it? *J. Gastrointest. Oncol.* **2019**, *10*, 1215. [CrossRef]
31. Yamamoto, S.; Inomata, M.; Katayama, H.; Mizusawa, J.; Etoh, T.; Konishi, F.; Sugihara, K.; Watanabe, M.; Moriya, Y.; Kitano, S. Short-term surgical outcomes from a randomized controlled trial to evaluate laparoscopic and open D3 dissection for stage II/III colon cancer: Japan Clinical Oncology Group Study JCOG 0404. *Ann. Surg.* **2014**, *260*, 23–30. [CrossRef] [PubMed]
32. Shin, J.K.; Kim, H.C.; Lee, W.Y.; Yun, S.H.; Cho, Y.B.; Huh, J.W.; Park, Y.A.; Chun, H.-K. Laparoscopic modified mesocolic excision with central vascular ligation in right-sided colon cancer shows better short-and long-term outcomes compared with the open approach in propensity score analysis. *Surg. Endosc.* **2018**, *32*, 2721–2731. [CrossRef]
33. Storli, K.E.; Søndenaa, K.; Furnes, B.; Eide, G.E. Outcome after introduction of complete mesocolic excision for colon cancer is similar for open and laparoscopic surgical treatments. *Dig. Surg.* **2013**, *30*, 317–327. [CrossRef]

34. Munkedal, D.; West, N.; Iversen, L.; Hagemann-Madsen, R.; Quirke, P.; Laurberg, S. Implementation of complete mesocolic excision at a university hospital in Denmark: An audit of consecutive, prospectively collected colon cancer specimens. *Eur. J. Surg. Oncol. (EJSO)* **2014**, *40*, 1494–1501. [CrossRef]
35. Bae, S.U.; Saklani, A.P.; Lim, D.R.; Kim, D.W.; Hur, H.; Min, B.S.; Baik, S.H.; Lee, K.Y.; Kim, N.K. Laparoscopic-assisted versus open complete mesocolic excision and central vascular ligation for right-sided colon cancer. *Ann. Surg. Oncol.* **2014**, *21*, 2288–2294. [CrossRef] [PubMed]
36. Kitano, S.; Inomata, M.; Mizusawa, J.; Katayama, H.; Watanabe, M.; Yamamoto, S.; Ito, M.; Saito, S.; Fujii, S.; Konishi, F.; et al. Survival outcomes following laparoscopic versus open D3 dissection for stage II or III colon cancer (JCOG0404): A phase 3, randomised controlled trial. *Lancet Gastroenterol. Hepatol.* **2017**, *2*, 261–268. [CrossRef] [PubMed]
37. Petz, W.; Ribero, D.; Bertani, E.; Borin, S.; Formisano, G.; Esposito, S.; Spinoglio, G.; Bianchi, P. Suprapubic approach for robotic complete mesocolic excision in right colectomy: Oncologic safety and short-term outcomes of an original technique. *Eur. J. Surg. Oncol.* **2017**, *43*, 2060–2066. [CrossRef] [PubMed]
38. Spinoglio, G.; Bianchi, P.P.; Marano, A.; Priora, F.; Lenti, L.M.; Ravazzoni, F.; Petz, W.; Borin, S.; Ribero, D.; Formisano, G. Robotic versus laparoscopic right colectomy with complete mesocolic excision for the treatment of colon cancer: Perioperative outcomes and 5-year survival in a consecutive series of 202 patients. *Ann. Surg. Oncol.* **2018**, *25*, 3580–3586. [CrossRef]
39. Yozgatli, T.K.; Aytac, E.; Ozben, V.; Bayram, O.; Gurbuz, B.; Baca, B.; Balik, E.; Hamzaoglu, I.; Karahasanoglu, T.; Bugra, D. Robotic complete mesocolic excision versus conventional laparoscopic hemicolectomy for right-sided colon cancer. *J. Laparoendosc. Adv. Surg. Tech.* **2019**, *29*, 671–676. [CrossRef]
40. Widmar, M.; Keskin, M.; Strombom, P.; Beltran, P.; Chow, O.S.; Smith, J.J.; Nash, G.M.; Shia, J.; Russell, D.; Garcia-Aguilar, J. Lymph node yield in right colectomy for cancer: A comparison of open, laparoscopic and robotic approaches. *Color. Dis.* **2017**, *19*, 888–894. [CrossRef]
41. Tagliacozzo, S.; Tocchi, A. Extended mesenteric excision in right hemicolectomy for carcinoma of the colon. *Int. J. Color. Dis.* **1997**, *12*, 272–275. [CrossRef]
42. Kotake, K.; Kobayashi, H.; Asano, M.; Ozawa, H.; Sugihara, K. Influence of extent of lymph node dissection on survival for patients with pT2 colon cancer. *Int. J. Color. Dis.* **2015**, *30*, 813–820. [CrossRef]
43. Olofsson, F.; Buchwald, P.; Elmståhl, S.; Syk, I. No benefit of extended mesenteric resection with central vascular ligation in right-sided colon cancer. *Color. Dis.* **2016**, *18*, 773–778. [CrossRef]
44. Mazzarella, G.; Maria Muttillo, E.; Picardi, B.; Rossi, S.; Angelo Muttillo, I. Complete mesocolic excision and D3 lymphadenectomy with central vascular ligation in right-sided colon cancer: A systematic review of postoperative outcomes, tumor recurrence and overall survival. *Surg. Endosc.* **2021**, *35*, 4945–4955. [CrossRef]
45. Karachun, A.; Petrov, A.; Panaiotti, L.; Voschinin, Y.; Ovchinnikova, T. Protocol for a multicentre randomized clinical trial comparing oncological outcomes of D2 versus D3 lymph node dissection in colonic cancer (COLD trial). *BJS Open* **2019**, *3*, 288. [CrossRef] [PubMed]
46. Lu, J.-Y.; Xu, L.; Xue, H.-D.; Zhou, W.-X.; Xu, T.; Qiu, H.-Z.; Wu, B.; Lin, G.-L.; Xiao, Y. The Radical Extent of lymphadenectomy—D2 dissection versus complete mesocolic excision of LAparoscopic Right Colectomy for right-sided colon cancer (RELARC) trial: Study protocol for a randomized controlled trial. *Trials* **2016**, *17*, 582. [CrossRef] [PubMed]
47. West, N.P.; Hohenberger, W.; Weber, K.; Perrakis, A.; Finan, P.J.; Quirke, P. Complete mesocolic excision with central vascular ligation produces an oncologically superior specimen compared with standard surgery for carcinoma of the colon. *J. Clin. Oncol.* **2010**, *28*, 272–278. [CrossRef] [PubMed]
48. West, N.P.; Morris, E.J.; Rotimi, O.; Cairns, A.; Finan, P.J.; Quirke, P. Pathology grading of colon cancer surgical resection and its association with survival: A retrospective observational study. *Lancet Oncol.* **2008**, *9*, 857–865. [CrossRef] [PubMed]
49. Díaz-Vico, T.; Fernández-Hevia, M.; Suárez-Sánchez, A.; García-Gutiérrez, C.; Mihic-Góngora, L.; Fernández-Martínez, D.; Antonio Álvarez-Pérez, J.; Luis Otero-Díez, J.; Electo Granero-Trancón, J.; Joaquín García-Flórez, L. Complete Mesocolic Excision and D3 Lymphadenectomy versus Conventional Colectomy for Colon Cancer: A Systematic Review and Meta-Analysis. *Ann. Surg. Oncol.* **2021**, *28*, 8823–8837. [CrossRef] [PubMed]
50. West, N.P.; Sutton, K.M.; Ingeholm, P.; Hagemann-Madsen, R.H.; Hohenberger, W.; Quirke, P. Improving the quality of colon cancer surgery through a surgical education program. *Dis. Colon Rectum* **2010**, *53*, 1594–1603. [CrossRef]
51. Emmanuel, A.; Haji, A. Complete mesocolic excision and extended (D3) lymphadenectomy for colonic cancer: Is it worth that extra effort? A review of the literature. *Int. J. Color. Dis.* **2016**, *31*, 797–804. [CrossRef]
52. Enker, W.E.; Laffer, U.T.; Block, G.E. Enhanced survival of patients with colon and rectal cancer is based upon wide anatomic resection. *Ann. Surg.* **1979**, *190*, 350. [CrossRef]
53. Bokey, E.; Chapuis, P.; Dent, O.; Mander, B.; Bissett, I.; Newland, R. Surgical technique and survival in patients having a curative resection for colon cancer. *Dis. Colon Rectum* **2003**, *46*, 860–866. [CrossRef]
54. Sheehan-Dare, G.E.; Marks, K.M.; Tinkler-Hundal, E.; Ingeholm, P.; Bertelsen, C.A.; Quirke, P.; West, N.P. The effect of a multidisciplinary regional educational programme on the quality of colon cancer resection. *Color. Dis.* **2018**, *20*, 105–115. [CrossRef]
55. Guo, P.; Ye, Y.; Jiang, K.; Gao, Z.; Wang, T.; Yin, M.; Wang, Y.; Xie, Q.; Yang, X.; Qu, J. Learning curve of complete mesocolic excision for colon cancer. *Zhonghua Wei Chang Wai Ke Za Zhi = Chin. J. Gastrointest. Surg.* **2012**, *15*, 28.

56. Nagtegaal, I.D.; van de Veld, C.; Worp, E.v.d.; Kapiteijn, E.; Quirke, P.; van Krieken, J.H.J. Macroscopic evaluation of rectal cancer resection specimen: Clinical significance of the pathologist in quality control. *J. Clin. Oncol.* **2002**, *20*, 1729–1734. [CrossRef] [PubMed]
57. Guillou, P.J.; Quirke, P.; Thorpe, H.; Walker, J.; Jayne, D.G.; Smith, A.M.; Heath, R.M.; Brown, J.M. Short-term endpoints of conventional versus laparoscopic-assisted surgery in patients with colorectal cancer (MRC CLASICC trial): Multicentre, randomised controlled trial. *Lancet* **2005**, *365*, 1718–1726. [CrossRef]
58. Munkedal, D.L.; Laurberg, S.; Hagemann-Madsen, R.; Stribolt, K.J.; Krag, S.R.; Quirke, P.; West, N.P. Significant Individual Variation between Pathologists in the Evaluation of Colon Cancer Specimens After Complete Mesocolic Excision. *Dis. Colon Rectum* **2016**, *59*, 953–961. [CrossRef]
59. FOxTROT Collaborative Group. Feasibility of preoperative chemotherapy for locally advanced, operable colon cancer: The pilot phase of a randomised controlled trial. *Lancet Oncol.* **2012**, *13*, 1152–1160. [CrossRef]
60. Siani, L.; Pulica, C. Laparoscopic complete mesocolic excision with central vascular ligation in right colon cancer: Long-term oncologic outcome between mesocolic and non-mesocolic planes of surgery. *Scand. J. Surg.* **2015**, *104*, 219–226. [CrossRef] [PubMed]
61. Munkedal, D.; Rosenkilde, M.; Nielsen, D.; Sommer, T.; West, N.; Laurberg, S. Radiological and pathological evaluation of the level of arterial division after colon cancer surgery. *Color. Dis.* **2017**, *19*, O238–O245. [CrossRef] [PubMed]
62. Spasojevic, M.; Stimec, B.V.; Gronvold, L.B.; Nesgaard, J.-M.; Edwin, B.; Ignjatovic, D. The anatomical and surgical consequences of right colectomy for cancer. *Dis. Colon Rectum* **2011**, *54*, 1503–1509. [CrossRef]
63. Kaye, T.L.; West, N.P.; Jayne, D.G.; Tolan, D.J. CT assessment of right colonic arterial anatomy pre and post cancer resection–a potential marker for quality and extent of surgery? *Acta Radiol.* **2016**, *57*, 394–400. [CrossRef]
64. Munkedal, D.L.E.; Rosenkilde, M.; West, N.P.; Laurberg, S. Routine CT scan one year after surgery can be used to estimate the level of central ligation in colon cancer surgery. *Acta Oncol.* **2019**, *58*, 469–471. [CrossRef]
65. Shiozawa, M.; Ueno, H.; Shiomo, A.; Kim, N.; Kim, J.; Tsarkov, P.; Grützmann, R.; Dulskas, A.; Liang, J.; Samalavičius, N. Study protocol for an International Prospective Observational Cohort Study for Optimal Bowel Resection Extent and Central Radicality for Colon Cancer (T-REX Study). *Jpn. J. Clin. Oncol.* **2020**, *51*, 145–155. [CrossRef] [PubMed]
66. Alhassan, N.; Yang, M.; Wong-Chong, N.; Liberman, A.S.; Charlebois, P.; Stein, B.; Fried, G.M.; Lee, L. Comparison between conventional colectomy and complete mesocolic excision for colon cancer: A systematic review and pooled analysis. *Surg. Endosc.* **2019**, *33*, 8–18. [CrossRef] [PubMed]
67. Loughrey, M.B.; Quirke, P.; Shepherd, N.A. Standards and Datasets for Reporting Cancers: Dataset for Histopathological Reporting of Colorectal Cancer (V4, December 2017). The Royal College of Pathologists Website. 2018. Available online: https://www.rcpath.org/profession/publications/cancer-datasets.html (accessed on 2 January 2022).
68. Jepsen, R.K.; Ingeholm, P.; Lund, E.L. Upstaging of early colorectal cancers following improved lymph node yield after methylene blue injection. *Histopathology* **2012**, *61*, 788–794. [CrossRef] [PubMed]
69. Inamori, K.; Togashi, Y.; Fukuoka, S.; Akagi, K.; Ogasawara, K.; Irie, T.; Motooka, D.; Kobayashi, Y.; Sugiyama, D.; Kojima, M.; et al. Importance of lymph node immune responses in MSI-H/dMMR colorectal cancer. *JCI Insight* **2021**, *6*, e137365. [CrossRef] [PubMed]
70. Morris, E.J.A.; Maughan, N.J.; Forman, D.; Quirke, P. Identifying stage III colorectal cancer patients: The influence of the patient, surgeon, and pathologist. *J. Clin. Oncol.* **2007**, *25*, 2573–2579. [CrossRef]
71. Søndenaa, K.; Quirke, P.; Hohenberger, W.; Sugihara, K.; Kobayashi, H.; Kessler, H.; Brown, G.; Tudyka, V.; D'Hoore, A.; Kennedy, R.H.; et al. The rationale behind complete mesocolic excision (CME) and a central vascular ligation for colon cancer in open and laparoscopic surgery: Proceedings of a consensus conference. *Int. J. Color. Dis.* **2014**, *29*, 419–428. [CrossRef]
72. Nakajima, K.; Inomata, M.; Akagi, T.; Etoh, T.; Sugihara, K.; Watanabe, M.; Yamamoto, S.; Katayama, H.; Moriya, Y.; Kitano, S. Quality control by photo documentation for evaluation of laparoscopic and open colectomy with D3 resection for stage II/III colorectal cancer: Japan Clinical Oncology Group Study JCOG 0404. *Jpn. J. Clin. Oncol.* **2014**, *44*, 799–806. [CrossRef]

Disclaimer/Publisher's Note: The statements, opinions and data contained in all publications are solely those of the individual author(s) and contributor(s) and not of MDPI and/or the editor(s). MDPI and/or the editor(s) disclaim responsibility for any injury to people or property resulting from any ideas, methods, instructions or products referred to in the content.

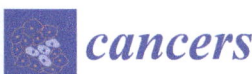

Article

Associations between Response to Commonly Used Neo-Adjuvant Schedules in Rectal Cancer and Routinely Collected Clinical and Imaging Parameters

Masoud Karimi [1,2], Pia Osterlund [1,2,3,*], Klara Hammarström [4], Israa Imam [4], Jan-Erik Frodin [1,2] and Bengt Glimelius [4,*]

1. Department of Gastrointestinal Oncology, Karolinska University Hospital, 171 64 Stockholm, Sweden
2. Department of Oncology and Pathology, Karolinska Institutet, 171 77 Stockholm, Sweden
3. Department of Oncology, Tampere University Hospital, University of Tampere, 33520 Tampere, Finland
4. Department of Immunology, Genetics and Pathology, Uppsala University, 752 36 Uppsala, Sweden
* Correspondence: pia.j.osterlund@regionstockholm.se (P.O.); bengt.glimelius@igp.uu.se (B.G.); Tel.: +46-72-469-4817 (P.O.)

Simple Summary: We studied real-world patients with locally advanced rectal cancer receiving preoperative radiotherapy with or without chemotherapy. The aim was to find factors associated with complete response to therapy, i.e., no remaining tumour, that could be used to identify patients who would not need surgery in the future. Tumour stage and length, intensity of preoperative treatment, and laboratory factors, such as carcinoembryonic antigen (CEA), leucocyte counts, and platelets, were all associated with complete response. Treatment intensity mattered and when radiotherapy was combined with chemotherapy, 21% had a complete response compared to 8% with radiotherapy alone. A model for identifying patients with a better chance of achieving a complete response was developed using tumour stage and length, CEA, and leukocyte levels as factors predicting complete response.

Abstract: Complete pathological response (pCR) is achieved in 10–20% of rectal cancers when treated with short-course radiotherapy (scRT) or long-course chemoradiotherapy (CRT) and in 28% with total neoadjuvant therapy (scRT/CRT + CTX). pCR is associated with better outcomes and a "watch-and-wait" strategy (W&W). The aim of this study was to identify baseline clinical or imaging factors predicting pCR. All patients with preoperative treatment and delays to surgery in Uppsala-Dalarna (n = 359) and Stockholm (n = 635) were included. Comparison of pCR versus non-pCR was performed with binary logistic regression models. Receiver operating characteristics (ROC) models for predicting pCR were built using factors with $p < 0.10$ in multivariate analyses. A pCR was achieved in 12% of the 994 patients (scRT 8% [33/435], CRT 13% [48/358], scRT/CRT + CTX 21% [43/201]). In univariate and multivariate analyses, choice of CRT (OR 2.62; 95%CI 1.34–5.14, scRT reference) or scRT/CRT + CTX (4.70; 2.23–9.93), cT1–2 (3.37; 1.30–8.78; cT4 reference), tumour length ≤ 3.5 cm (2.27; 1.24–4.18), and CEA ≤ 5 µg/L (1.73; 1.04–2.90) demonstrated significant associations with achievement of pCR. Age < 70 years, time from radiotherapy to surgery > 11 weeks, leucocytes ≤ 10^9/L, and thrombocytes ≤ 400^9/L were significant only in univariate analyses. The associations were not fundamentally different between treatments. A model including T-stage, tumour length, CEA, and leucocytes (with scores of 0, 0.5, or 1 for each factor, maximum 4 points) showed an area under the curve (AUC) of 0.66 (95%CI 0.60–0.71) for all patients, and 0.65–0.73 for the three treatments separately. The choice of neoadjuvant treatment in combination with low CEA, short tumour length, low cT-stage, and normal leucocytes provide support in predicting pCR and, thus, could offer guidance for selecting patients for organ preservation.

Keywords: rectal cancer; predictive factors; pre-operative treatment; pathologic complete remission

---

Citation: Karimi, M.; Osterlund, P.; Hammarström, K.; Imam, I.; Frodin, J.-E.; Glimelius, B. Associations between Response to Commonly Used Neo-Adjuvant Schedules in Rectal Cancer and Routinely Collected Clinical and Imaging Parameters. *Cancers* **2022**, *14*, 6238. https://doi.org/10.3390/cancers14246238

Academic Editor: Susanne Merkel

Received: 24 October 2022
Accepted: 13 December 2022
Published: 18 December 2022

Publisher's Note: MDPI stays neutral with regard to jurisdictional claims in published maps and institutional affiliations.

Copyright: © 2022 by the authors. Licensee MDPI, Basel, Switzerland. This article is an open access article distributed under the terms and conditions of the Creative Commons Attribution (CC BY) license (https://creativecommons.org/licenses/by/4.0/).

1. Introduction

Administration of preoperative radiotherapy, either short-course (scRT) or long-course, has been important in decreasing local recurrence rates after rectal cancer surgery [1–5]. In locally advanced rectal cancer (LARC), the addition of chemotherapy to long-course radiotherapy (CRT) further decreases local recurrence rates, whereas the impact on overall survival (OS), except possibly in the most advanced (ugly) cases, is unclear [6–8]. An impact on distant metastasis-free survival rates has only been seen when preoperative chemotherapy (CTX) is added to scRT/CRT, i.e., total neoadjuvant therapy (TNT) [9,10].

The tumour response to neoadjuvant treatment is highly heterogenous, ranging from complete shrinkage of the tumour to lack of effect and, occasionally, to progression. In approximately 10–28% of patients, neoadjuvant treatment results in the disappearance of the rectal tumour with no signs of residual tumour on MRI, proctoscopy, and digital examination (clinical complete response, cCR) or no residual viable cancer cells in the surgical specimen and pathologic complete response (pCR, also denoted ypCR) [9–11]. Patients who achieve pCR exhibit significantly more favourable oncological outcomes with higher 5-year disease-free survival rates (DFS, 83% if pCR versus 66% if non-pCR) and OS rates (88% with pCR versus 76% non-pCR) [12,13]. The achievement of a complete remission provides the possibility for organ-preserving surgery or a non-operative, watch-and-wait (W&W) approach. Research efforts have been directed toward identification of clinical and other parameters that could help predict pCR after preoperative treatment [14–19]. However, several unclear issues, particularly related to the importance of clinical T-stage (cT-stage), tumour length, presence of extramural vascular invasion (cEMVI+), mesorectal fascia (cMRF+) involvement, and clinical laboratory values need to be clarified [14–19].

The primary aim of this study was to identify clinical and imaging factors that can be used to predict pCR (and would thus also be applicable to cCR with the possibility of a W&W strategy), by combining data from two population-based Swedish cohorts, and comparing the three most commonly used schedules, scRT, CRT, or scRT/CRT + CTX; all with a ≥4-week interval to surgery. A secondary aim was to explore if a model based on clinical factors predicting pCR could be built.

2. Materials and Methods

Our study consisted of two independent population-based retrospectively collected cohorts from Uppsala-Dalarna (Cohort A) and Stockholm (Cohort B). All patients living in these regions at the time of diagnosis constituted the study base and were included if they had received preoperative RT with or without chemotherapy with a minimum delay of 4 weeks to surgery. Patients in Cohort A were treated between 1 January 2010 and 31 December 2018; a detailed description of this cohort has been published previously [15]. Cohort B consisted of data for consecutive patients with rectal cancer in the Stockholm region diagnosed between 1 January 2006 and 31 December 2016. Patients were followed for recurrence and survival until 24 March 2022. Several patients in both cohorts were included in randomized trials such as Stockholm III (42 in Cohort A and 54 in Cohort B), EXPERT-C (0/33), or RAPIDO (106/35) [9,20,21].

The results of cohort A have been published [15]; we initially sought to determine whether the two patient datasets demonstrated similar associations between the explored variables and pCR; if so, they could be combined to increase statistical power in the calculations of importance for, above all, the three different treatment schedules most commonly used today.

The study was approved by the local ethical committee at Karolinska Institutet as an extension to the approval by the ethical committee at Uppsala University for the Uppsala/Dalarna study. Through approval, we gained access to the prospectively maintained quality register database including all patients in these regions diagnosed with colorectal cancer. This database is part of the national quality register (Swedish Colorectal Cancer Registry [SCRCR] defined in detail at https://scrcr.se/) (accessed on 7 November 2022).

The same inclusion criteria were applied for both cohorts, except that, patients who achieved cCR (n = 22) and were monitored in a W&W strategy were included in the Uppsala/Dalarna study. However, in this analysis, the cCR patients were excluded to achieve histopathological data from the resected specimen for all patients. The differences in collected data between the cohorts included the presence of metastatic lateral lymph nodes according to MRI and thrombocytes collected only in Cohort B. Of the total 361 cases in cohort A, two patients were inadvertently missed before fusion with Cohort B, leaving 359 patients from cohort A for final analysis. Patients with rectal cancer and M0 disease treated with curative intent who received preoperative neoadjuvant or conversion treatment (hereafter referred to as preoperative) followed by delayed surgery performed $\geq$4 weeks after completion of the RT were eligible. This study excluded patients with concurrent malignant disease and crucial missing information about pathological staging.

Rectal tumours were defined as those located with the caudal limit within 15 cm above the anal verge, the distance being measured by rigid proctoscopy. Low rectal tumours were defined as those 0–5 cm above the anal verge, middle rectum as 6–10 cm, and high tumours as more than 10 cm above the anal verge. The database contains information about clinical, radiological, and histopathological staging, information on all treatments, relapse sites and timepoints, and survival information. This information was retrieved from the SCRCR and the patient's medical files. Cut-off $\leq$ 3.5 cm for tumour length was defined with the ROC/Youden method (area under curve [AUC] 0.55; 95% CI 0.50–0.61, p = 0.050). The other cut-offs were defined as previously published [22–24].

For both cohorts, neoadjuvant treatment was given according to one of three different protocols:

A: scRT: short-course hypo-fractionated 5 Gy $\times$ 5 in one week, and delayed surgery.

B: CRT: Chemoradiation 1.8 Gy $\times$ 28 or 2 $\times$ 25 Gy concomitant with capecitabine 825 mg/m^2 twice daily, days 1–38 or 900 mg/m^2 on RT days, and delayed surgery.

C: scRT/CRT + CTX: neoadjuvant scRT or CRT preceded or followed by chemotherapy as part of the clinical trials EXPERT-C and RAPIDO. The EXPERT-C randomised phase II trial administered four cycles of capecitabine and oxaliplatin (CAPOX) alone or with cetuximab, followed by CRT, TME-surgery, and further four cycles of adjuvant CAPOX [21]. The RAPIDO study compared CRT as standard arm versus an experimental arm starting with 5 Gy $\times$ 5, followed by six courses of CAPOX before surgery [9]. Adjuvant chemotherapy using 8 cycles of CAPOX was provided in the standard arm.

Radiology included pelvic MRI and chest, abdominal, and pelvic CT at baseline used as a basis in these analyses. Restaging 3–6 weeks after completion of the neoadjuvant treatment served as grounds for decision making regarding curative surgery during a multidisciplinary team (MDT) conference, but these results were not included in the analyses.

Statistics

Data were analysed with SPSS (IBM SPSS Statistics for Windows, 2020, Version 27.0.0.1, IBM Corporation, Armonk, NY, USA). Patient demographics are presented as absolute values and percentages, and, for continuous variables, also as median and range. Comparisons of groups were performed by applying the X^2 test for categorical variables. For continuous variables, we applied the non-parametric Mann–Whitney U test or the Wilcoxon signed rank test. Laboratory tests (haemoglobin, leucocytes, thrombocytes, C-reactive protein, and CEA) were analysed as categorical factors. With pCR as a dependent parameter, we used models of binary logistic regression for univariate analyses and calculated odds ratios (OR) and 95% confidence intervals (CI) to predict whether covariates influenced the achievement of pCR. Variables that were associated with pCR in the univariate analyses with $p < 0.05$ for all patients and <0.10 for treatment groups, and with missing values less than 18% were included in the multivariate logistic regression analyses. Receiver operating characteristics (ROC) with Youden optimization and AUC were calculated to discriminate for the model's predictive power. The cut-offs for the factors from the multivariate analysis added to the model were the ones used in the Sorbye consensus [22] and those optimized by the

Youden method as described above. Relapse-free survival (RFS), overall survival (OS), and disease-specific survival (DSS) were calculated with Kaplan–Meier survival estimates and the Cox proportional hazards model. All p-values were two-sided and considered statistically significant when $p < 0.05$.

3. Results

3.1. Patient Characteristics

Patient and tumour characteristics for the 359 patients in Cohort A and the 635 in Cohort B are described in Table S1. Minor differences in age and baseline MRI-derived factors, such as cN-stage, cMRF+, cEMVI+ and mucinous tumour, as well as clinical factors such as elevated carcinoembryonic antigen (CEA) distribution were noted. The proportion of patients treated with the three alternatives, scRT, CRT, or scRT/CRT + CTX, varied between the cohorts because of the differences in inclusion times, with Cohort A formed in 2010–2018, and Cohort B in 2006–2016. Prior to June 2011, when the RAPIDO trial comparing CRT and scRT + CTX was initiated, most LARCs were treated with CRT and after June 2016, and when the trial had closed patient entry, these patients continued to be treated with scRT + CTX within the LARCTC-US study (https://clinicaltrials.gov/ct2/show/NCT03729687) (accessed on 23 November 2022). Different treatment schedules resulted in varying times to surgery. Patient and tumour characteristics in the treatment groups (scRT, CRT, and scRT/CR + CTX) in the two cohorts were also in line.

When the associations between the characteristics and the probability of reaching pCR (12.8% in Cohort A and 12.3% in Cohort B) were compared between the cohorts, similar results were observed (Table S2). Because of this, we concluded that the findings reported from Cohort A [15] were confirmed in an independent cohort (Cohort B) and the two cohorts could be pooled.

The clinical characteristics of the pooled cohort (A + B) by treatment group are described in Table 1. Patients treated with scRT were older and had less advanced tumours (cT1-3, cN0, cMRF-, or cEMVI-) according to treatment indication, and had fewer mucinous tumours and shorter tumour lengths, but higher C-reactive protein (CRP) levels. The most advanced tumours were observed in the scRT/CRT + CTX group.

Table 1. Baseline clinical, imaging, and laboratory characteristics of the pooled cohort of eligible patients (n = 994) according to pre-operative treatment.

Treatment		scRT	CRT	scRT/CRT + CTX	All Patients	p-Value
		n = 435 (44%)	n = 358 (36%)	n = 201 (20%)	n = 994 (100%)	
Age	Median (range)	73 (43–91)	64 (31–81)	64 (23–82)	66 (23–91)	0.003
	≤70 years	183 (42%)	287 (80%)	156 (78%)	626 (63%)	<0.001
	>70 years	252 (58%)	71 (20%)	45 (22%)	368 (37%)	
Sex	Female	173 (40%)	150 (42%)	85 (42%)	408 (41%)	0.768
	Male	262 (60%)	208 (58%)	116 (58%)	586 (59%)	
MRI T-stage	cT1-2	50 (12%)	10 (3%)	2 (1%)	62 (6%)	<0.001
	cT3	260 (60%)	170 (47%)	102 (51%)	532 (54%)	
	cT4	125 (28%)	178 (50%)	96 (48%)	399 (40%)	
	Missing	0 (0%)	0 (0%)	1 (0.5%)	1 (0.1%)	
MRI N-stage	cN0	124 (29%)	37 (10%)	10 (5%)	171 (17%)	<0.001
	cN1-2	309 (71%)	321 (90%)	191 (95%)	821 (83%)	
	Missing	2 (0.5%)	0 (0%)	0 (0%)	2 (0.2%)	
MRI Mesorectal fascia engagement	No	254 (58%)	86 (24%)	61 (30%)	401 (40%)	<0.001
	Yes	175 (40%)	272 (76%)	139 (69%)	586 (59%)	
	Missing	6 (2%)	0 (0%)	1 (0.5%)	7 (0.7%)	
MRI Extramural vascular invasion	No	296 (68%)	201 (56%)	94 (47%)	591 (60%)	<0.001
	Yes	129 (30%)	157 (44%)	105 (52%)	391 (39%)	
	Missing	10 (2%)	0 (0%)	2 (1%)	12 (1%)	

Table 1. Cont.

Treatment		scRT	CRT	scRT/CRT + CTX	All Patients	p-Value
		n = 435 (44%)	n = 358 (36%)	n = 201 (20%)	n = 994 (100%)	
MRI Mucinous tumour	No	369 (85%)	301 (84%)	142 (71%)	812 (82%)	**<0.001**
	Yes	55 (13%)	57 (16%)	56 (28%)	168 (17%)	
	Missing	11 (2%)	0 (0%)	3 (1%)	14 (1%)	
MRI Lateral lymph nodes	No	242 (56%)	202 (56%)	52 (26%)	496 (50%)	**<0.001**
	Yes	44 (10%)	68 (19%)	27 (13%)	139 (14%)	
	Missing	149 (34%)	88 (25%)	122 (61%)	359 (36%)	
MRI Tumour length	≤3.5 cm	87 (20%)	27 (8%)	22 (11%)	136 (14%)	**<0.001**
	>3.5 cm	320 (74%)	319 (89%)	173 (86%)	812 (82%)	
	Missing	27 (6%)	12 (3%)	6 (3%)	45 (4%)	
Distance anal verge	0–5 cm	179 (41%)	144 (40%)	64 (32%)	387 (39%)	0.050
	6–10 cm	164 (38%)	147 (41%)	80 (40%)	391 (39%)	
	11–15 cm	92 (21%)	67 (19%)	57 (28%)	216 (22%)	
Weeks from end of RT to surgery	≤8	244 (56%)	141 (39%)	29 (14%)	414 (42%)	**<0.001**
	8–11	92 (21%)	133 (37%)	18 (9%)	243 (24%)	
	>11	99 (23%)	84 (24%)	154 (77%)	337 (34%)	
Haemoglobin	>110 g/L	291 (67%)	327 (91%)	179 (89%)	797 (80%)	0.100
	≤110 g/L	54 (12%)	30 (8%)	21 (10%)	105 (11%)	
	Missing	90 (21%)	1 (0.2%)	1 (0.5%)	92 (9%)	
Leucocytes	≤10^9/L	257 (59%)	302 (84%)	155 (77%)	714 (72%)	0.122
	>10^9/L	63 (15%)	49 (14%)	28 (14%)	140 (14%)	
	Missing	115 (26%)	7 (2%)	18 (9%)	140 (14%)	
Thrombocytes	≤400^9/L	176 (41%)	239 (67%)	69 (34%)	484 (49%)	0.598
	>400^9/L	19 (4%)	31 (9%)	10 (5%)	60 (6%)	
	Missing	240 (55%)	88 (24%)	122 (61%)	450 (45%)	
C-reactive protein	≤10 mg/L	186 (43%)	251 (70%)	108 (54%)	545 (55%)	**<0.001**
	>10 mg/L	86 (20%)	47 (13%)	45 (22%)	178 (18%)	
	Missing	163 (38%)	60 (17%)	48 (24%)	271 (27%)	
Carcinoembryonic antigen	≤5 µ/L	198 (45%)	187 (52%)	119 (59%)	504 (51%)	0.441
	>5 µ/L	107 (25%)	124 (35%)	76 (38%)	307 (31%)	
	Missing	130 (30%)	47 (13%)	6 (3%)	183 (18%)	
Pathologic complete response	Non-pCR	402 (92%)	310 (87%)	158 (79%)	870 (87%)	**<0.001**
	pCR	33 (8%)	48 (13%)	43 (21%)	124 (13%)	

Abbreviations: CRT: concomitant chemoradiotherapy, MRI: magnetic resonance imaging, pCR: pathologic complete response, RT: radiotherapy, scRT: short course radiotherapy, scRT/CRT + CTX: scRT/CRT combined with systemic chemotherapy, MRI Tumour length: craniocaudal extension of tumour measured by MRI. p-values below 0.05 are marked in bold.

Survival was compared between the pCR and non-pCR groups. The median reverse Kaplan–Meier follow-up was at 64 months (95% CI 63–65). RFS was significantly better in the pCR group (HR 0.22; 95% CI 0.13–0.37), with 5-year RFS rates of 96% in pCR versus 79% in non-pCR groups (Figure S1A). OS was better in the pCR group with a 5-year OS rate of 92% compared with 70% in the non-pCR group (Figure S1B). DSS, considering CRC deaths and censoring deaths from other causes, was also higher in the pCR arm, with a 5-year DSS rate of 96% in the pCR group versus 79% in the non-pCR group (Figure S1C).

3.2. Clinical Factors and pCR

pCR was achieved in 12% of the 994 patients. pCR was noted in 8% (33/435) with scRT, in 13% (48/358) with CRT, and in 21% (43/201) with scRT/CRT + CTX ($p < 0.001$).

Characteristics of the patients who achieved pCR compared to those who did not are presented in Table 2. Tumour characteristics such as cT-stage ($p = 0.027$) and tumour length

(p = 0.010) were statistically significantly associated with pCR. Furthermore, laboratory parameters, including leucocytosis (p = 0.014), thrombocytosis (p = 0.023), elevated CRP (p < 0.001), and CEA (p = 0.001) were statistically significantly different between the pCR and non-pCR groups. The cohort did not show any difference.

Table 2. Differences in baseline clinical, laboratory, and imaging-defined characteristics and treatment groups between the pCR and the non-pCR groups for the pooled cohort (n = 994).

		Non-pCR n = 870 (Row%)	pCR n = 124 (Row%)	p-Value
Age	Median (range) ≤70 years >70 years	68 (23–91) 531 (85%) 339 (92%)	65 (38–84) 95 (15%) 29 (8%)	**0.003** **0.001**
Sex	Female Male	351 (86%) 519 (89%)	57 (14%) 67 (11%)	0.234
MRI T-stage	cT1-2 cT3 cT4 Missing	48 (77%) 464 (87%) 357 (90%) 1	14 (23%) 68 (13%) 42 (10%) 0	**0.027**
MRI N-stage	cN0 cN1-2 Missing	152 (89%) 716 (87%) 2	19 (11%) 105 (13%) 0	0.546
MRI Mesorectal fascia engagement	No Yes Missing	346 (86%) 517 (88%) 7	55 (14%) 69 (12%) 0	0.366
MRI Extramural vascular invasion	No Yes Missing	513 (87%) 348 (89%) 9	78 (13%) 43 (11%) 3	0.190
MRI Mucinous tumour	No Yes Missing	713 (88%) 144 (86%) 13	99 (12%) 24 (14%) 1	0.456
MRI Lateral lymph nodes	No Yes Missing	441 (89%) 116 (84%) 313	55 (11%) 23 (17%) 46	0.083
MRI Tumour length	≤3.5 cm >3.5 cm Missing	109 (80%) 716 (88%) 44	27 (20%) 96 (12%) 1	**0.010**
Distance anal verge	0–5 cm 6–10 cm 11–15 cm	332 (86%) 347 (89%) 191 (88%)	55 (14%) 44 (11%) 25 (12%)	0.414
Weeks from end of RT to surgery	≤8 8–11 >11	371 (90%) 214 (88%) 285 (85%)	43 (10%) 29 (12%) 52 (15%)	0.110
Haemoglobin	>110 g/L ≤110 g/L Missing	689 (86%) 97 (92%) 84	108 (14%) 8 (8%) 8	0.088
Leucocytes	≤10^9/L >10^9/L Missing	614 (86%) 131 (94%) 125	100 (14%) 9 (6%) 15	**0.014**
Thrombocytes	≤400^9/L >400^9/L Missing	418 (86%) 58 (97%) 394	66 (14%) 2 (2%) 56	**0.023**
C-reactive protein	≤10 mg/L >10 mg/L Missing	468 (86%) 160 (90%) 242	77 (14%) 18 (10%) 29	**<0.001**
Carcinoembryonic antigen	≤5 μ/L >5 μ/L Missing	424 (84%) 281 (92%) 165	80 (16%) 26 (8%) 18	**0.001**
Treatment group	scRT CRT scRT/CRT + CTX	402 (92%) 310 (87%) 158 (79%)	33 (8%) 48 (13%) 43 (21%)	**<0.001**
Cohort	A Uppsala/Dalarna B Stockholm	313 (87%) 557 (88%)	46 (13%) 78 (12%)	0.808

Abbreviations: CRT: concomitant chemoradiotherapy, MRI: magnetic resonance imaging, pCR: pathologic complete response, RT: radiotherapy, scRT: short course radiotherapy, scRT/CRT + CTX: scRT/CRT combined with systemic chemotherapy, MRI Tumour length: craniocaudal extension of tumour measured by MRI. p-values below 0.05 are marked in bold.

Data regarding the probability of reaching pCR according to treatment are shown in Table 3. Significant differences for all patients were noted for age, cT-stage, cN-stage, cMRF, cEMVI, mucinous tumour, and weeks from RT to surgery for treatment (exact *p*-values not shown). Differences in pCR rates for the scRT group were noted for cT-stage, cMRF, cEMVI, and CEA. For the CRT group, differences in pCR versus non-pCR were noted for cT-stage, tumour length, and elevated CEA. For the scRT/CRT + CTX arm, only sex was statistically significant in the pCR versus non-pCR comparison.

Table 3. Observed frequencies of pCR according to major clinical parameters in the treatment groups.

		scRT			CRT			scRT/CRT + Chemo			Total		
		Total 435	pCR 33	Row %	Total 358	pCR 48	Row %	Total 201	pCR 43	Row %	Total 994	pCR 124	Row %
Sex	Female	173	10	6%	150	23	15%	85	24	28%	408	57	14%
	Male	262	23	9%	208	25	12%	116	19	16%	586	67	11%
Age	≤70 years	183	19	10%	287	42	15%	156	34	22%	626	95	15%
	>70 years	252	14	6%	71	6	8%	45	9	20%	368	29	8%
MRI T-stage	cT1-2	50	9	18%	10	5	50%	2	0	0%	62	14	23%
	cT3	260	19	7%	170	23	14%	102	26	25%	532	68	13%
	cT4	125	5	4%	178	20	11%	96	17	18%	399	42	11%
	Missing	0	0		0	0		1	0	0%	1	0	0%
MRI N-stage	cN0	124	12	10%	37	5	14%	10	2	20%	171	19	11%
	cN1-2	309	21	7%	321	43	13%	191	41	21%	821	105	13%
	Missing	2	0	0%	0	0		0	0		2	0	0%
MRI Mesorectal fascia	MRF-	254	26	10%	86	14	16%	61	15	25%	401	55	14%
	MRF+	175	7	4%	272	34	13%	139	28	20%	586	69	12%
	Missing	6	0	0%	0	0		1	0	0%	7	0	0%
MRI Extramural vascular invasion	EMVI-	296	28	9%	201	30	15%	94	20	21%	591	78	13%
	EMVI+	129	4	3%	157	18	11%	105	21	20%	391	43	11%
	Missing	10	1	10%	0	0		2	2	100%	12	3	25%
MRI Mucinous tumour	Non-mucinous	369	30	8%	301	40	13%	142	29	20%	812	99	12%
	Mucinous	55	2	4%	57	8	14%	56	14	25%	168	24	14%
	Missing	11	1	9%	0	0		3	0	0%	14	1	7%
MRI Lateral lymph nodes	No lat. nodes	242	18	7%	202	26	13%	52	11	21%	496	55	11%
	Lateral nodes	44	5	11%	68	11	16%	27	7	26%	139	23	17%
	Missing	149	10	7%	88	11	13%	122	25	20%	359	46	13%
MRI Tumour length	≤3.5 cm	87	10	11%	27	9	33%	22	8	36%	136	27	20%
	>3.5 cm	320	23	7%	319	38	12%	173	35	20%	812	96	12%
	Missing	27	0	0%	12	1	8%	6	0	0%	45	1	2%
Distance anal verge	0–5 cm	179	16	9%	144	22	15%	64	17	27%	387	55	14%
	6–10 cm	164	10	6%	147	17	12%	80	17	21%	391	44	11%
	11–15 cm	92	7	8%	67	9	13%	57	9	16%	216	25	12%
Weeks from RT to surgery	≤8	244	22	9%	141	17	12%	29	4	14%	414	43	10%
	8–11	92	7	8%	133	20	15%	18	2	11%	243	29	12%
	>11	99	4	4%	84	11	13%	154	37	24%	337	52	15%
Haemoglobin	>110 g/L	291	22	8%	327	47	14%	179	39	22%	797	108	14%
	≤110 g/L	54	3	6%	30	1	3%	21	4	19%	105	8	8%
	Missing	90	8	9%	1	0	0%	1	0	0%	92	8	9%
Leucocytes	≤10^9/L	257	19	7%	302	44	15%	155	37	24%	714	100	14%
	>10^9/L	63	3	5%	49	3	6%	28	3	11%	140	9	6%
	Missing	115	11	10%	7	1	14%	18	3	17%	140	15	11%
Thrombocytes	≤400^9/L	176	13	7%	239	35	15%	69	18	26%	484	66	14%
	>400^9/L	19	0	0%	31	2	6%	10	0	0%	60	2	3%
	Missing	240	20	8%	88	11	13%	122	25	20%	450	56	12%
C-reactive protein	≤10 mg/L	186	14	8%	251	36	14%	108	27	25%	545	77	14%
	>10 mg/L	86	4	5%	47	5	11%	45	9	20%	178	18	10%
	Missing	163	15	9%	60	7	12%	48	7	15%	271	29	11%
Carcinoembryonic antigen	≤5 μ/L	198	18	9%	187	32	17%	119	30	25%	504	80	16%
	>5 μ/L	107	3	3%	124	11	9%	76	12	16%	307	26	8%
	Missing	130	12	9%	47	5	11%	6	1	17%	183	18	10%

Abbreviations: CRT: concomitant chemoradiotherapy, MRI: magnetic resonance imaging, pCR: pathologic complete response, RT: radiotherapy, scRT: short course radiotherapy, scRT/CRT + CTX: scRT/CRT combined with systemic chemotherapy, MRI Tumour length: craniocaudal extension of tumour measured by MRI. Differences that are statistically significant (X^2-test) in the different treatments are marked in bold.

3.3. Univariate and Multivariate Analyses for pCR

Patients achieving pCR were compared to non-pCR patients for clinical and tumour-related factors (Table 4). In the univariate binary logistic regression analyses for pCR, statistical significance was noted for age $\leq$ 70 years (OR 2.09, 95% CIs in Table 4), cT1-2 (OR 2.47, with T4 as reference), tumour length $\leq$ 3.5 cm (OR 1.84), time from RT to surgery (OR 1.57), normal leucocytes (OR 2.37), normal thrombocytes (OR 4.57), normal CEA (OR 2.03), or CRT (OR 1.89, with scRT as reference), and scRT/CRT + CTX (OR 3.32 with scRT as reference).

Table 4. Univariate and multivariate logistic regression analyses of the pooled cohort (n = 994 and 735, respectively) for clinical, laboratory, and imaging-defined factors predicting pCR status.

		Univariate Analyses n = 994		Multivariable Model n = 735	
		OR (95% CI)	p-Value	OR (95% CI)	p-Value
Age	Continuous	0.97 (0.95–0.99)	**0.002**		
	>70 years	1.00		1.00	
	$\leq$70 years	2.09 (1.35–3.23)	**0.001**	1.35 (0.77–2.37)	0.291
Sex	Male	1.00			
	Female	1.25 (0.86–1.83)	0.234		
MRI T-stage	cT4	1.00		1.00	
	cT3	1.24 (0.82–1.87)	0.292	1.38 (0.85–2.28)	0.193
	cT1-2	2.47 (1.26–4.87)	**0.008**	3.37 (1.30–8.78)	**0.013**
MRI N-stage	cN1-2	1.00			
	cN0	1.173 (0.70–1.97)	0.546		
MRI Mesorectal fascia engagement	MRF+	1.00			
	MRF-	1.19 (0.81–1.74)	0.367		
MRI Extramural vascular invasion	EMVI+	1.00			
	EMVI-	1.23 (0.82–1.82)	0.305		
MRI Mucinous tumour	Mucinous	1.00			
	Non-mucinous	1.20 (0.72–1.94)	0.456		
MRI Lateral lymph nodes	Lateral lymph nodes	1.00			
	No lateral lymph nodes	0.62 (0.37–1.06)	0.085		
MRI Tumour length	>3.5 cm	1.00		1.00	
	$\leq$3.5 cm	1.84 (1.15–2.96)	**0.011**	2.27 (1.24–4.18)	**0.008**
Distance anal verge	0–5 cm	1.00			
	6–10 cm	0.76 (0.50–1.17)	0.217		
	11–15 cm	0.79 (0.47–1.30)	0.154		
Weeks from RT to Surg.	$\leq$8	1.00		1.00	
	8–11	1.16 (0.70–1.92)	0.540	1.61 (0.87–2.98)	0.131
	>11	1.57 (1.02–2.42)	**0.040**	1.45 (0.79–2.67)	0.227
Haemoglobin	$\leq$110 g/L	1.00			
	>110 g/L	1.90 (0.89–4.01)	0.093		
Leucocytes	>10^9/L	1.00		1.00	
	$\leq$10^9/L	2.37 (1.16–4.81)	**0.017**	2.02 (0.93–4.37)	0.075
Thrombocytes	>400^9/L	1.00			
	$\leq$400^9/L	4.57 (1.09–19.2)	**0.037**		
C-reactive protein	$\leq$10 mg/L	1.00			
	>10 mg/L	1.46 (0.85–2.52)	0.171		
Carcinoembryonic antigen	>5 µ/L	1.00		1.00	
	$\leq$5 µ/L	2.03 (1.27–3.25)	**0.003**	1.73 (1.04–2.90)	**0.034**
Treatment group	scRT	1.00		1.00	
	CRT	1.89 (1.18–3.01)	**0.008**	2.621 (1.34–5.14)	**0.005**
	scRT/CRT + CTX	3.32 (2.03–5.41)	**<0.001**	4.70 (2.23–9.93)	**<0.001**

Abbreviations: CRT: concomitant chemoradiotherapy, MRI: magnetic resonance imaging, pCR: pathologic complete response, RT: radiotherapy, scRT: short course radiotherapy, scRT/CRT + CTX: scRT/CRT combined with systemic chemotherapy, MRI Tumour length: craniocaudal extension of tumour measured by MRI. p-values below 0.05 are marked in bold.

In multivariate analysis (n = 735 with 98 events), seven covariates with p-value < 0.05 in the univariate analyses were included, excluding thrombocytes not collected in Cohort A. Factors that were statistically significant for pCR in the multivariate model included cT1-2 (OR 3.37 with cT4 as reference), tumour length $\leq$ 3.5 cm (OR 2.27), non-elevated CEA

(OR 1.73), and CRT (OR 2.61 with scRT as reference) or scRT/CRT + CTX (OR 4.70 with scRT as reference). Interaction terms for the significant factors were not significant and thus not included in the multivariate model (p-value for cT-stage + tumour length was 0.963, cT-stage + CEA was 0.957, and cT-stage + treatment group was 0.850).

We examined predictive factors associated with pCR for the three treatments separately. In the scRT group (n = 435), univariate analyses demonstrated that age ≤ 70 years, cT1-2, cMRF-, cEMVI-, and normal thrombocytes were associated with higher pCR rates (Table S3), with none of the factors remaining statistically significant in the multivariate analysis (n = 294). In the CRT population (n = 358), cT1-2, tumour length ≤ 3.5 cm, and normal CEA were associated with a higher pCR rate in the univariate analyses, and cT1-2 (OR 5.94) remained statistically significant in the multivariate analysis (n = 301, Table S4). In the scRT/CRT + CTX group (n = 201), female sex with OR 2.00 was the only statistically significant factor in the univariate analyses (Table S5).

3.4. Predictive Model for pCR

A predictive model for pCR was developed based on factors identified in the multivariable analysis (Table S6, Figure S2). Cut-offs were based on TNM classification, the literature, and the ROC defined.

The scoring points for cT-stage (cT1-2 = 0, cT3 = 0.5, and cT4 = 1), tumour length (≤3.5 cm = 0, 4–7 cm = 0.5, and >7 cm = 1), CEA (≤3 μg/L = 0, 3–5 μg/L = 0.5, and >5 μg/L = 1), and leucocytes (≤8.2-10^9/L = 0, 8.3-10^9/L = 0.5, and >10^9/L = 1) were combined, thus resulting in a maximum score of 4. ORs and 95% CIs are presented in Table S6.

The performance of the combined pCR effects model obtained an AUC of 0.65 (95% CI 0.60–0.71), with cut-off < 1.75 points for the whole cohort ($p < 0.001$), of which 25% had pCR. In the subgroup treated with scRT, AUC was 0.73 (0.62–0.83) and cut-off < 1.25 points and 16% had pCR; in the CRT group, AUC was 0.67 (0.58–0.76) with cut-off < 1.75 points and 31% had pCR; and for scRT/CRT + CTX, AUC was 0.65 (0.55–0.75) with cut-off < 1.75 points and 50% had pCR (all statistically significant).

4. Discussion

The highest pCR rates of 21% were achieved with scRT/CRT + CTX compared with 13% with CRT and 8% with scRT in this pooled analysis of rectal cancer patients who underwent surgery after a delay following pre-treatment. Independent factors associated with pCR were cT1-2, tumour length ≤ 3.5 cm, normal CEA, and treatment modality. Leucocytosis also adds to the model. This may have practical importance when discussing whether a non-surgical W&W approach could be recommended prior to treatment initiation.

Our population-based results indicate that treatment with RT, either preceded or followed by systemic chemotherapy, i.e., TNT, is the most effective treatment modality for achieving pCR. In recent years, the focus has been directed towards more extensive administration of chemotherapy in the neoadjuvant setting and several clinical trials have been performed or are ongoing [9,10,25,26]. Results from the RAPIDO study demonstrated the superiority of scRT + CTX versus CRT in preventing disease-related events, predominantly systemic recurrences, and support our findings regarding the hierarchy of preoperative treatments in achieving pCR [9]. Despite a two-fold higher chance of pCR in the experimental group (28% versus 14%) [9], a 5-year update of the trial has revealed more locoregional failures in the experimental group (12% vs. 8%, $p = 0.07$) [27]. Results from the US OPRA study with CRT and chemotherapy either as induction or consolidation showed better organ preservation rates (3-year TME-free survival rate 41% vs. 53%), when the chemotherapy was given as consolidation after CRT [11].

Several studies have reported cT-stage as an independent variable to predict pCR [28,29], in line with our findings. Our cohort of patients with cT1-2 tumours was limited (n = 62, as most patients with cT1-2 tumours underwent surgery directly or were treated with scRT without a delay to surgery and were thus excluded from analysis), but achieved a pCR rate of 23%, and this was as high as 50% in the CRT group. With a corresponding rate for cT3 tumours of 13% we can conclude that, not surprisingly, cT1-2-stage can be used as predictive factor for pCR when using scRT or CRT. Most cT2-stage patients are regularly not candidates for pre-surgical treatment, and too few patients with cT1-2 tumours were treated with scRT/CRT + CTX to draw any conclusions. In Cohort A, a subdivision of cT3-stage into the substages a-d was explored [15]; however, this was not recorded in cohort B. It is possible that the best discriminator is not between cT2 and cT3 but rather within cT3. Separation of cT2 from cT3a is also difficult using MRI [30].

Length of tumour persistently demonstrated statistically significant associations with pCR in our examination for the entire cohort. We found a cut-off of ≤3.5 cm to be a break point for tumours responding with pCR. The calculated AUC 0.55 indicates, however, a limited discriminative strength and necessitates incorporation of other parameters when predicting pCR. A study by Jankowski et al. [31] showed that a tumour length > 7 cm and circumferent extension of the tumour meant that only 1.6% could achieve a sustained cCR with a sensitivity as low as 23% [31]. In our study, we did not retrieve data for the extent of circumferential tumour engagement of the rectal wall; thus, our results are not comparable with the Polish study. It is fully plausible that cT-stage and tumour length overlap as larger tumours are more often associated, but not necessarily always (reflected in non-significant interaction term), with higher cT-stage with deeper invasion into the rectal wall. In this way, their significance as predictive factors may intertwine.

The serum marker CEA has been used to predict prognosis both pre- and post-operatively, and it is an important tool for surveillance of colorectal patients to detect recurrence post-operatively [24]. CEA has also been the subject of interest as a predictor for response to neo-adjuvant therapy in rectal cancer, most studies of which have found associations with pCR rates [14,15,28,32–34]. In a report from Joye et al., a CEA cut-off of 4.6 µg/L was applied and an association between pre-treatment CEA and probability for pCR was found in a multivariable analysis [14]. Furthermore, in our study, a pre-treatment CEA value below reference (≤5 µg/L) had a positive association with an OR of 1.28 for reaching pCR (whereas the ROC-defined subgroup with ≤3 µg/L had an OR of 2.39). CEA was the only laboratory parameter in the full cohort that demonstrated statistically significant associations with pCR in both univariate and multivariable analyses; however, the number of patients with missing values for the other laboratory tests was quite high (9–45%).

The significance of age in univariate analyses is probably related to the active selection of younger fit patients for more intense treatment. Older patients, often with comorbidities, may not always tolerate these treatments and are left with scRT alone, which has less cell killing effect and, thus, fewer pCRs, as seen in a systematic review [35].

Our findings of both leucocytosis and thrombocytosis being significant covariate factors in univariate analyses are in accordance with previous reports in LARC [17,36–39]. These associations were most pronounced in the scRT/CRT + CTX-group. Thrombocytosis could not be added to the multivariate model as this information was available only in Cohort B. Pre-treatment haemoglobin value and its relation to oncologic treatment response (particularly RT) and prognosis in solid tumours, including rectal cancer, have been the focus of several studies [14,28,40]. A higher pre-treatment haemoglobin value is associated with pCR likelihood [14,28], in line with a trend in our study. Clinically, haemoglobin values are probably of limited relevance.

MRI-defined cMRF+ and cEMVI+ were significantly associated with pCR in the scRT group but not in the CRT or scRT/CRT + CTX groups. Both involved MRF and positive EMVI indicate a more advanced tumour and the reference treatment is either CRT or scRT/CRT + CTX. Thus, scRT was provided only to fragile patients not tolerating the reference treatment. Therefore, if a suboptimal treatment must be given, with scRT for an advanced tumour, both MRF+ and EMVI+ mean a lower chance of pCR. If the reference treatment is applied, neither of these factors are important for predicting pCR (or potentially for a cCR if a W&W policy is applied).

In summary, besides treatment protocol, early tumour stage (cT1-2), tumour length ≤ 3.5 cm, normal routine blood counts, and CEA can assist in predicting pCR and, ultimately, cCR state in a setting before neoadjuvant treatment initiation. The decision to aim for organ preservation by giving more active neoadjuvant treatment than indicated can thus be supported by our model, with the caveat of its limitation as AUCs were in the range of 0.65–0.73, sensitivity and specificity 59–70%, and pCR carried rates of 16–50%. The predictive factors and the model also need to be validated in other large patient series, preferably prospective, and we will start with the RAPIDO [9] dataset. In this regard, other markers, serial examinations with MRI, PET-CT, and functional radiology measuring the tumour's metabolic activity before and early during the treatment could improve the baseline model in the future [41].

Better survival has also been observed in patients achieving pCR [12,13] in line with our findings for OS, DSS, and RFS (with 5-year rates of 92%, 96%, and 92%, respectively). pCR status thus helps in decisions to omit adjuvant therapy [42]. A third decision our prognostic factors may support is to sustain from surgery in cCR and offer a W&W strategy. Today, this is normally based on tumour-free proctoscopy, digital examination, and MRI. Still, in this situation, there is a clear risk that tumour cells persist [43]. It has been reported that a near-pCR situation is not associated with the same favourable prognosis as pCR [44,45]. This adds to the dilemma and necessitates incorporation of further tools to judge durable tumour control probability with better certainty.

Our study has limitations associated with retrospective studies. The exclusion of cCR patients also reduced the number of favourable outcome patients in cohort A. Undeniably, there has been a selection bias as many patients were selected for different treatment protocols based on age and comorbidities. In terms of strengths, this was a comprehensive study that included a large number of patients treated with the three most widely utilized neoadjuvant protocols after up-to-date staging, including an MRI for all patients.

5. Conclusions

The choice of neoadjuvant treatment in combination with low CEA, short tumour length, low cT-stage, and normal leucocytes provide support in predicting pCR and, thus, could offer guidance for selection of patients for organ preservation strategies at baseline, i.e., to provide neoadjuvant rather than adjuvant treatments and W&W strategies.

Supplementary Materials: The following supporting information can be downloaded at: https://www.mdpi.com/article/10.3390/cancers14246238/s1, Table S1: Comparison of major clinical and imaging characteristics of cohort A and cohort B; Table S2: Comparison of clinical, laboratory, and imaging-defined characteristics between pCR vs. non-pCR groups for cohort A (n = 359) and cohort B (n = 635); Table S3: Univariate and multivariate analyses of the scRT cohort (n = 435) for clinical, laboratory, and imaging-defined factors predicting pCR status; Table S4: Univariate and multivariate analyses of the CRT cohort (n = 358) for clinical, laboratory, and imaging-defined factors predicting pCR status; Table S5: Univariate and multivariate analyses of the scRT/CRT + CTX cohort (n = 201) for clinical, laboratory, and imaging-defined factors predicting pCR status; Table S6: Score board for the predictive pCR model; Figure S1: Relapse-free survival (RFS; panel A), overall survival (OS; panel B), and disease-specific survival (DSS) of patients with tumours achieving a pathologic complete response (pCR) compared to non-pCR; Figure S2: Receiver operator characteristics (ROC) and area under the curve (AUC) with cut-offs optimized by Youden for the model including MRI cT-stage, tumour length, elevated CEA, and leucocytosis for all patients (ALL; panel A), short-course radiotherapy (scRT; panel B), chemoradiation (CRT, panel C), and scRT/CRT aS2: and chemotherapy (scRT/CRT + CTX, panel D) groups.

Author Contributions: Conceptualization, M.K., K.H., I.I., J.-E.F. and B.G.; Data curation, M.K., P.O., K.H., I.I. and B.G.; Formal analysis, P.O., J.-E.F. and B.G.; Funding acquisition, J.-E.F. and B.G.; Investigation, B.G.; Methodology, M.K., P.O., J.-E.F. and B.G.; Project administration, J.-E.F. and B.G.; Resources, P.O., J.-E.F. and B.G.; Supervision, P.O., J.-E.F. and B.G.; Validation, M.K., P.O., J.-E.F. and B.G.; Visualization, M.K., P.O. and B.G.; Writing—original draft, M.K., P.O., J.-E.F. and B.G.;

Writing—review and editing, M.K., P.O., K.H., I.I, J.-E.F. and B.G. All authors have read and agreed to the published version of the manuscript.

Funding: This research was funded by Swedish Cancer Society, grant number 180306, and Stockholm Cancer Society, grant number 211111.

Institutional Review Board Statement: The study was conducted in accordance with the Declaration of Helsinki and approved by the Institutional Review Boards/Ethics committee of Karolinska Institutet and Uppsala University (U-a 2011/092, 2012/224, 2015/419; 2018/490; U-a 2017/235).

Informed Consent Statement: Patient consent was waived due to the retrospective registry design (according to Swedish law, informed consent is not needed in this setting).

Data Availability Statement: Data can be made available by written request to the corresponding author.

Acknowledgments: The authors want to thank Celina Österlund for visualization of the results, and statistician Tuija Poussa for the valuable statistical advice.

Conflicts of Interest: The authors declare no conflict of interest. The funders had no role in the design of the study; in the collection, analyses, or interpretation of data; in the writing of the manuscript; or in the decision to publish the results.

References

1. Swedish_Rectal_Cancer_Trial; Cedermark, B.; Dahlberg, M.; Glimelius, B.; Påhlman, L.; Rutqvist, L.E.; Wilking, N. Improved survival with preoperative radiotherapy in resectable rectal cancer. *N. Engl. J. Med.* **1997**, *336*, 980–987. [CrossRef] [PubMed]
2. Glimelius, B.; Isacsson, U.; Jung, B.; Påhlman, L. Radiotherapy in addition to radical surgery in rectal cancer: Evidence for a dose-response effect favoring preoperative treatment. *Int. J. Radiat. Oncol. Biol. Phys.* **1997**, *37*, 281–287. [CrossRef] [PubMed]
3. Colorectal Cancer Collaborative Group. Adjuvant radiotherapy for rectal cancer: A systematic overview of 8507 patients from 22 randomised trials. *Lancet* **2001**, *358*, 1291–1304. [CrossRef] [PubMed]
4. Kapiteijn, E.; Marijnen, C.A.; Nagtegaal, I.D.; Putter, H.; Steup, W.H.; Wiggers, T.; Rutten, H.J.; Pahlman, L.; Glimelius, B.; van Krieken, J.H.; et al. Preoperative radiotherapy combined with total mesorectal excision for resectable rectal cancer. *N. Engl. J. Med.* **2001**, *345*, 638–646. [CrossRef]
5. Sebag-Montefiore, D.; Stephens, R.J.; Steele, R.; Monson, J.; Grieve, R.; Khanna, S.; Quirke, P.; Couture, J.; de Metz, C.; Myint, A.S.; et al. Preoperative radiotherapy versus selective postoperative chemoradiotherapy in patients with rectal cancer (MRC CR07 and NCIC-CTG C016): A multicentre, randomised trial. *Lancet* **2009**, *373*, 811–820. [CrossRef]
6. Bosset, J.F.; Collette, L.; Calais, G.; Mineur, L.; Maingon, P.; Radosevic-Jelic, L.; Daban, A.; Bardet, E.; Beny, A.; Ollier, J.C. Chemotherapy with preoperative radiotherapy in rectal cancer. *N. Engl. J. Med.* **2006**, *355*, 1114–1123. [CrossRef]
7. Gérard, J.P.; Conroy, T.; Bonnetain, F.; Bouché, O.; Chapet, O.; Closon-Dejardin, M.T.; Untereiner, M.; Leduc, B.; Francois, E.; Maurel, J.; et al. Preoperative radiotherapy with or without concurrent fluorouracil and leucovorin in T3-4 rectal cancers: Results of FFCD 9203. *J. Clin. Oncol.* **2006**, *24*, 4620–4625. [CrossRef]
8. Braendengen, M.; Tveit, K.M.; Berglund, A.; Birkemeyer, E.; Frykholm, G.; Påhlman, L.; Wiig, J.N.; Byström, P.; Bujko, K.; Glimelius, B. Randomized phase III study comparing preoperative radiotherapy with chemoradiotherapy in nonresectable rectal cancer. *J. Clin. Oncol.* **2008**, *26*, 3687–3694. [CrossRef]
9. Bahadoer, R.R.; Dijkstra, E.A.; van Etten, B.; Marijnen, C.A.M.; Putter, H.; Kranenbarg, E.M.; Roodvoets, A.G.H.; Nagtegaal, I.D.; Beets-Tan, R.G.H.; Blomqvist, L.K.; et al. Short-course radiotherapy followed by chemotherapy before total mesorectal excision (TME) versus preoperative chemoradiotherapy, TME, and optional adjuvant chemotherapy in locally advanced rectal cancer (RAPIDO): A randomised, open-label, phase 3 trial. *Lancet Oncol.* **2021**, *22*, 29–42. [CrossRef]
10. Conroy, T.; Bosset, J.F.; Etienne, P.L.; Rio, E.; François, É.; Mesgouez-Nebout, N.; Vendrely, V.; Artignan, X.; Bouché, O.; Gargot, D.; et al. Neoadjuvant chemotherapy with FOLFIRINOX and preoperative chemoradiotherapy for patients with locally advanced rectal cancer (UNICANCER-PRODIGE 23): A multicentre, randomised, open-label, phase 3 trial. *Lancet Oncol.* **2021**, *22*, 702–715. [CrossRef]
11. Garcia-Aguilar, J.; Patil, S.; Gollub, M.J.; Kim, J.K.; Yuval, J.B.; Thompson, H.M.; Verheij, F.S.; Omer, D.M.; Lee, M.; Dunne, R.F.; et al. Organ Preservation in Patients with Rectal Adenocarcinoma Treated with Total Neoadjuvant Therapy. *J. Clin. Oncol.* **2022**, *40*, 23. [CrossRef] [PubMed]
12. Martin, S.T.; Heneghan, H.M.; Winter, D.C. Systematic review and meta-analysis of outcomes following pathological complete response to neoadjuvant chemoradiotherapy for rectal cancer. *Br. J. Surg.* **2012**, *99*, 918–928. [CrossRef] [PubMed]
13. Li, J.Y.; Huang, X.Z.; Gao, P.; Song, Y.X.; Chen, X.W.; Lv, X.E.; Fu, Y.; Xiao, Q.; Ye, S.Y.; Wang, Z.N. Survival landscape of different tumor regression grades and pathologic complete response in rectal cancer after neoadjuvant therapy based on reconstructed individual patient data. *BMC Cancer* **2021**, *21*, 1214. [CrossRef] [PubMed]
14. Joye, I.; Debucquoy, A.; Fieuws, S.; Wolthuis, A.; Sagaert, X.; D'Hoore, A.; Haustermans, K. Can clinical factors be used as a selection tool for an organ-preserving strategy in rectal cancer? *Acta Oncol.* **2016**, *55*, 1047–1052. [CrossRef] [PubMed]

15. Hammarström, K.; Imam, I.; Mezheyeuski, A.; Ekström, J.; Sjöblom, T.; Glimelius, B. A Comprehensive Evaluation of Associations between Routinely Collected Staging Information and the Response to (Chemo)Radiotherapy in Rectal Cancer. *Cancers* **2020**, *13*, 16. [CrossRef] [PubMed]
16. McDermott, D.M.; Singh, S.A.; Renz, P.B.; Hasan, S.; Weir, J. Predictors of Pathologic Response after Total Neoadjuvant Therapy in Patients with Rectal Adenocarcinoma: A National Cancer Database Analysis. *Cureus* **2021**, *13*, e17233. [CrossRef]
17. Kang, B.H.; Song, C.; Kang, S.B.; Lee, K.W.; Lee, H.S.; Kim, J.S. Nomogram for Predicting the Pathological Tumor Response from Pre-treatment Clinical Characteristics in Rectal Cancer. *Anticancer Res.* **2020**, *40*, 2171–2177. [CrossRef]
18. Mahadevan, L.S.; Zhong, J.; Venkatesulu, B.; Kaur, H.; Bhide, S.; Minsky, B.; Chu, W.; Intven, M.; van der Heide, U.A.; van Triest, B.; et al. Imaging predictors of treatment outcomes in rectal cancer: An overview. *Crit. Rev. Oncol. Hematol.* **2018**, *129*, 153–162. [CrossRef]
19. Shao, K.; Zheng, R.; Li, A.; Li, X.; Xu, B. Clinical predictors of pathological good response in locally advanced rectal cancer. *Radiat. Oncol.* **2021**, *16*, 10. [CrossRef]
20. Erlandsson, J.; Holm, T.; Pettersson, D.; Berglund, A.; Cedermark, B.; Radu, C.; Johansson, H.; Machado, M.; Hjern, F.; Hallbook, O.; et al. Optimal fractionation of preoperative radiotherapy and timing to surgery for rectal cancer (Stockholm III): A multicentre, randomised, non-blinded, phase 3, non-inferiority trial. *Lancet Oncol.* **2017**, *18*, 336–346. [CrossRef]
21. Dewdney, A.; Cunningham, D.; Tabernero, J.; Capdevila, J.; Glimelius, B.; Cervantes, A.; Tait, D.; Brown, G.; Wotherspoon, A.; Gonzalez de Castro, D.; et al. Multicenter randomized phase II clinical trial comparing neoadjuvant oxaliplatin, capecitabine, and preoperative radiotherapy with or without cetuximab followed by total mesorectal excision in patients with high-risk rectal cancer (EXPERT-C). *J. Clin. Oncol.* **2012**, *30*, 1620–1627. [CrossRef] [PubMed]
22. Sorbye, H.; Köhne, C.H.; Sargent, D.J.; Glimelius, B. Patient characteristics and stratification in medical treatment studies for metastatic colorectal cancer: A proposal for standardization of patient characteristic reporting and stratification. *Ann. Oncol.* **2007**, *18*, 1666–1672. [CrossRef] [PubMed]
23. Salerno, G.; Sinnatamby, C.; Branagan, G.; Daniels, I.R.; Heald, R.J.; Moran, B.J. Defining the rectum: Surgically, radiologically and anatomically. *Colorectal. Dis.* **2006**, *8* (Suppl. S3), 5–9. [CrossRef] [PubMed]
24. Nicholson, B.D.; Shinkins, B.; Pathiraja, I.; Roberts, N.W.; James, T.J.; Mallett, S.; Perera, R.; Primrose, J.N.; Mant, D. Blood CEA levels for detecting recurrent colorectal cancer. *Cochrane Database Syst. Rev.* **2015**, *2015*, Cd011134. [CrossRef] [PubMed]
25. Kasi, A.; Abbasi, S.; Handa, S.; Al-Rajabi, R.; Saeed, A.; Baranda, J.; Sun, W. Total Neoadjuvant Therapy vs Standard Therapy in Locally Advanced Rectal Cancer: A Systematic Review and Meta-analysis. *JAMA Netw. Open* **2020**, *3*, e2030097. [CrossRef]
26. Jin, J.; Tang, Y.; Hu, C.; Jiang, L.M.; Jiang, J.; Li, N.; Liu, W.Y.; Chen, S.L.; Li, S.; Lu, N.N.; et al. Multicenter, Randomized, Phase III Trial of Short-Term Radiotherapy Plus Chemotherapy Versus Long-Term Chemoradiotherapy in Locally Advanced Rectal Cancer (STELLAR). *J. Clin. Oncol.* **2022**, *40*, 1681–1692. [CrossRef]
27. Bahadoer, R.; Dijkstra, E. Patterns of locoregional failure and distant metastases in patients treated for locally advanced rectal cancer in the RAPIDO trial. *Eur. J. Surg. Oncol.* **2022**, *48*, e34. [CrossRef]
28. Armstrong, D.; Raissouni, S.; Price Hiller, J.; Mercer, J.; Powell, E.; MacLean, A.; Jiang, M.; Doll, C.; Goodwin, R.; Batuyong, E.; et al. Predictors of Pathologic Complete Response after Neoadjuvant Treatment for Rectal Cancer: A Multicenter Study. *Clin. Colorectal. Cancer* **2015**, *14*, 291–295. [CrossRef]
29. Al-Sukhni, E.; Attwood, K.; Mattson, D.M.; Gabriel, E.; Nurkin, S.J. Predictors of Pathologic Complete Response Following Neoadjuvant Chemoradiotherapy for Rectal Cancer. *Ann. Surg. Oncol.* **2016**, *23*, 1177–1186. [CrossRef]
30. Beets-Tan, R.G.; Beets, G.L.; Vliegen, R.F.; Kessels, A.G.; Van Boven, H.; De Bruine, A.; von Meyenfeldt, M.F.; Baeten, C.G.; van Engelshoven, J.M. Accuracy of magnetic resonance imaging in prediction of tumour-free resection margin in rectal cancer surgery. *Lancet* **2001**, *357*, 497–504. [CrossRef]
31. Jankowski, M.; Pietrzak, L.; Rupiński, M.; Michalski, W.; Hołdakowska, A.; Paciorek, K.; Rutkowski, A.; Olesiński, T.; Cencelewicz, A.; Szczepkowski, M.; et al. Watch-and-wait strategy in rectal cancer: Is there a tumour size limit? Results from two pooled prospective studies. *Radiother. Oncol.* **2021**, *160*, 229–235. [CrossRef] [PubMed]
32. Das, P.; Skibber, J.M.; Rodriguez-Bigas, M.A.; Feig, B.W.; Chang, G.J.; Wolff, R.A.; Eng, C.; Krishnan, S.; Janjan, N.A.; Crane, C.H. Predictors of tumor response and downstaging in patients who receive preoperative chemoradiation for rectal cancer. *Cancer* **2007**, *109*, 1750–1755. [CrossRef] [PubMed]
33. Wallin, U.; Rothenberger, D.; Lowry, A.; Luepker, R.; Mellgren, A. CEA—A predictor for pathologic complete response after neoadjuvant therapy for rectal cancer. *Dis. Colon. Rectum.* **2013**, *56*, 859–868. [CrossRef] [PubMed]
34. Moreno García, V.; Cejas, P.; Blanco Codesido, M.; Feliu Batlle, J.; de Castro Carpeño, J.; Belda-Iniesta, C.; Barriuso, J.; Sánchez, J.J.; Larrauri, J.; González-Barón, M.; et al. Prognostic value of carcinoembryonic antigen level in rectal cancer treated with neoadjuvant chemoradiotherapy. *Int. J. Colorectal. Dis.* **2009**, *24*, 741–748. [CrossRef] [PubMed]
35. Hoendervangers, S.; Burbach, J.P.M.; Lacle, M.M.; Koopman, M.; van Grevenstein, W.M.U.; Intven, M.P.W.; Verkooijen, H.M. Pathological Complete Response Following Different Neoadjuvant Treatment Strategies for Locally Advanced Rectal Cancer: A Systematic Review and Meta-analysis. *Ann. Surg. Oncol.* **2020**, *27*, 4319–4336. [CrossRef]
36. Diefenhardt, M.; Hofheinz, R.D.; Martin, D.; Beißbarth, T.; Arnold, D.; Hartmann, A.; von der Grün, J.; Grützmann, R.; Liersch, T.; Ströbel, P.; et al. Leukocytosis and neutrophilia as independent prognostic immunological biomarkers for clinical outcome in the CAO/ARO/AIO-04 randomized phase 3 rectal cancer trial. *Int. J. Cancer* **2019**, *145*, 2282–2291. [CrossRef]

37. Kim, H.J.; Choi, G.S.; Park, J.S.; Park, S.; Kawai, K.; Watanabe, T. Clinical significance of thrombocytosis before preoperative chemoradiotherapy in rectal cancer: Predicting pathologic tumor response and oncologic outcome. *Ann. Surg. Oncol.* **2015**, *22*, 513–519. [CrossRef]
38. Belluco, C.; Forlin, M.; Delrio, P.; Rega, D.; Degiuli, M.; Sofia, S.; Olivieri, M.; Pucciarelli, S.; Zuin, M.; De Manzoni, G.; et al. Elevated platelet count is a negative predictive and prognostic marker in locally advanced rectal cancer undergoing neoadjuvant chemoradiation: A retrospective multi-institutional study on 965 patients. *BMC Cancer* **2018**, *18*, 1094. [CrossRef]
39. Ramsay, G.; Ritchie, D.T.; MacKay, C.; Parnaby, C.; Murray, G.; Samuel, L. Can Haematology Blood Tests at Time of Diagnosis Predict Response to Neoadjuvant Treatment in Locally Advanced Rectal Cancer? *Dig. Surg.* **2019**, *36*, 495–501. [CrossRef]
40. Khan, A.A.; Klonizakis, M.; Shabaan, A.; Glynne-Jones, R. Association between pretreatment haemoglobin levels and morphometric characteristics of the tumour, response to neoadjuvant treatment and long-term outcomes in patients with locally advanced rectal cancers. *Colorectal. Dis.* **2013**, *15*, 1232–1237. [CrossRef]
41. Pyo, D.H.; Choi, J.Y.; Lee, W.Y.; Yun, S.H.; Kim, H.C.; Huh, J.W.; Park, Y.A.; Shin, J.K.; Cho, Y.B. A Nomogram for Predicting Pathological Complete Response to Neoadjuvant Chemoradiotherapy Using Semiquantitative Parameters Derived from Sequential PET/CT in Locally Advanced Rectal Cancer. *Front. Oncol.* **2021**, *11*, 742728. [CrossRef] [PubMed]
42. Glynne-Jones, R.; Wyrwicz, L.; Tiret, E.; Brown, G.; Rödel, C.; Cervantes, A.; Arnold, D. Rectal cancer: ESMO Clinical Practice Guidelines for diagnosis, treatment and follow-up. *Ann. Oncol.* **2017**, *28*, iv22–iv40. [CrossRef] [PubMed]
43. Hughes, R.; Glynne-Jones, R.; Grainger, J.; Richman, P.; Makris, A.; Harrison, M.; Ashford, R.; Harrison, R.A.; Livingstone, J.I.; McDonald, P.J.; et al. Can pathological complete response in the primary tumour following pre-operative pelvic chemoradiotherapy for T3-T4 rectal cancer predict for sterilisation of pelvic lymph nodes, a low risk of local recurrence and the appropriateness of local excision? *Int. J. Colorectal. Dis.* **2006**, *21*, 11–17. [CrossRef] [PubMed]
44. Swellengrebel, H.A.; Bosch, S.L.; Cats, A.; Vincent, A.D.; Dewit, L.G.; Verwaal, V.J.; Nagtegaal, I.D.; Marijnen, C.A. Tumour regression grading after chemoradiotherapy for locally advanced rectal cancer: A near pathologic complete response does not translate into good clinical outcome. *Radiother. Oncol.* **2014**, *112*, 44–51. [CrossRef]
45. Erlandsson, J.; Lorinc, E.; Ahlberg, M.; Pettersson, D.; Holm, T.; Glimelius, B.; Martling, A. Tumour regression after radiotherapy for rectal cancer—Results from the randomised Stockholm III trial. *Radiother. Oncol.* **2019**, *135*, 178–186. [CrossRef]

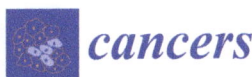

Article

Beyond Total Mesorectal Excision (TME)—Results of MRI-Guided Multivisceral Resections in T4 Rectal Carcinoma and Local Recurrence

Sigmar Stelzner [1,2,*], Thomas Kittner [3], Michael Schneider [4], Fred Schuster [4], Markus Grebe [5], Erik Puffer [6], Anja Sims [1] and Soeren Torge Mees [1]

1. Department of General and Visceral Surgery, Dresden-Friedrichstadt General Hospital, Teaching Hospital of the Technical University of Dresden, D-01067 Dresden, Germany; anja.sims@klinikum-dresden.de (A.S.); soeren-torge.mees@klinikum-dresden.de (S.T.M.)
2. Department of Visceral, Transplant, Thoracic, and Vascular Surgery, University Hospital of Leipzig, D-04103 Leipzig, Germany
3. Department of Radiology, Dresden-Friedrichstadt General Hospital, Teaching Hospital of the Technical University of Dresden, D-01067 Dresden, Germany; thomas.kittner@klinikum-dresden.de
4. Department of Urology, Dresden-Friedrichstadt General Hospital, Teaching Hospital of the Technical University of Dresden, D-01067 Dresden, Germany; michael.schneider@klinikum-dresden.de (M.S.); fred.schuster@klinikum-dresden.de (F.S.)
5. Department of Gynaecology, Dresden-Friedrichstadt General Hospital, Teaching Hospital of the Technical University of Dresden, D-01067 Dresden, Germany; markus.grebe@klinikum-dresden.de
6. Institut of Pathology, Dresden-Friedrichstadt General Hospital, Teaching Hospital of the Technical University of Dresden, D-01067 Dresden, Germany; erik.puffer@klinikum-dresden.de
* Correspondence: sigmar.stelzner@medizin.uni-leipzig.de; Tel.: +49-341-9719153; Fax: +49-341-9717209

Citation: Stelzner, S.; Kittner, T.; Schneider, M.; Schuster, F.; Grebe, M.; Puffer, E.; Sims, A.; Mees, S.T. Beyond Total Mesorectal Excision (TME)—Results of MRI-Guided Multivisceral Resections in T4 Rectal Carcinoma and Local Recurrence. *Cancers* **2023**, *15*, 5328. https://doi.org/10.3390/cancers15225328

Academic Editor: Arnaud Alves

Received: 18 September 2023
Revised: 31 October 2023
Accepted: 2 November 2023
Published: 8 November 2023

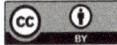

Copyright: © 2023 by the authors. Licensee MDPI, Basel, Switzerland. This article is an open access article distributed under the terms and conditions of the Creative Commons Attribution (CC BY) license (https:// creativecommons.org/licenses/by/ 4.0/).

Simple Summary: Surgery for rectal cancer involving adjacent organs (T4 primary tumors) or for locally recurrent rectal cancer requires dissection planes beyond the well-defined perimesorectal space. It is, therefore, of paramount importance to define the extent of surgery preoperatively. Magnetic resonance imaging (MRI) provides adequate guidance for the surgeon to achieve a clear resection margin. In this study, the diagnostic performance of MRI against histopathology and oncological outcomes that can be achieved with MRI-guided surgery are studied using an MRI-based division of the pelvis into seven compartments. Overall, the accuracy of MRI is good, yielding excellent results for T4 tumors and good results for locally recurrent tumors. Complete histopathologic (R0) resection is the most important determinant of outcome.

Abstract: Rectal cancer invading adjacent organs (T4) and locally recurrent rectal cancer (LRRC) pose a special challenge for surgical resection. We investigate the diagnostic performance of MRI and the results that can be achieved with MRI-guided surgery. All consecutive patients who underwent MRI-based multivisceral resection for T4 rectal adenocarcinoma or LRRC between 2005 and 2019 were included. Pelvic MRI findings were reviewed according to a seven-compartment staging system and correlated with histopathology. Outcomes were investigated by comparing T4 tumors and LRRC with respect to cause-specific survival in uni- and multivariate analysis. We identified 48 patients with T4 tumors and 28 patients with LRRC. Overall, 529 compartments were assessed with an accuracy of 81.7%, a sensitivity of 88.6%, and a specificity of 79.2%. Understaging was as low as 3.0%, whereas overstaging was 15.3%. The median number of resected compartments was 3 (interquartile range 3–4) for T4 tumors and 4 (interquartile range 3–5) for LRRC ($p = 0.017$). In 93.8% of patients with T4 tumors, a histopathologically complete R0(local)- resection could be achieved compared to 57.1% in LRRC ($p < 0.001$). Five-year overall survival for patients with T4 tumors was 53.3% vs. 32.1% for LRRC ($p = 0.085$). R0-resection and M0-category emerged as independent prognostic factors, whereas the number of resected compartments was not associated with prognosis in multivariate analysis. MRI predicts compartment involvement with high accuracy and especially avoids understaging. Surgery based on MRI yields excellent loco-regional results for T4 tumors and good results for LRRC. The number of resected compartments is not independently associated with prognosis, but R0-resection remains the crucial surgical factor.

Keywords: pelvic compartments; locally advanced rectal cancer; locally recurrent rectal cancer; MRI assessment; MRI-guided surgery; prognosis

1. Introduction

The standard of surgical care for patients with rectal cancer is total mesorectal excision (TME)-based surgery with five-year local recurrence rates of approximately 5% and even lower in contemporary surgical series [1,2]. Nevertheless, locally recurrent rectal cancer (LRRC) remains an issue in rectal cancer treatment, and if detected, salvage surgery should be considered as a potentially curative option [3]. In addition, about 10% of patients with rectal cancer present with infiltration of adjacent organs (T4-tumors) [4]. Both LRRC and T4-primary tumors require complex surgical management with en bloc removal of involved organs and structures beyond the well-defined planes of TME surgery [5]. These often exenterative operations may result in considerable morbidity and functional sequelae [6,7]. It is, therefore, of paramount importance to carefully select patients for surgery. MRI has emerged as the gold standard for assessment of the tumor spread in the small pelvis [8–10]. However, beyond-TME surgery is rather a surgical strategy than a clearly defined procedure. Therefore, it is common clinical practice to divide the pelvis into compartments and remove those parts that are involved. Surgery is guided by the findings of MRI and depends on its accuracy. This approach enables the surgeon, on the one hand, to achieve a clear surgical margin and, on the other hand, to spare uninvolved compartments and, hence, function. Georgiou et al. established an MRI staging system based on seven pelvic compartments and reported excellent results with respect to diagnostic performance [11]. Meanwhile, the usefulness of the proposed pelvic compartmentation was confirmed on an anatomical base [12].

The aim of this study is to investigate the performance of this MRI compartment assessment with respect to histopathology and report the results achieved by MRI-guided beyond-TME surgery. Our hypothesis is that the number of resected compartments is not associated with prognosis if the MRI assessment is accurate.

2. Materials and Methods

The database of the colorectal unit of Dresden-Friedrichstadt General Hospital was queried for all consecutive patients with resection of rectal cancer infiltrating adjacent organs or exhibiting positive lateral lymph nodes (Figure 1B) that required en bloc resection of the lateral pelvic compartment (primary tumor group). Additionally, all patients operated on for a local recurrence of rectal cancer were retrieved (local recurrence group). The chosen time interval ranged from 2005 to 2019. Inclusion criteria were histologically confirmed adenocarcinoma, resection of either an adjacent organ or en bloc resection of one or both lateral compartments and attempt of complete tumor removal. Patients with histology other than adenocarcinoma or without an MRI of the pelvis were excluded. The extracted data were supplemented by an extensive chart review. We documented patient, treatment, and tumor characteristics. Additionally, initial MRI scans and reports were reviewed with respect to the extent of infiltration according to the seven compartments described by Georgiou et al. (Figure 1) [11]. If tumor infiltration was detected within the confines of one compartment, the compartment was judged infiltrated irrespective of the extent of infiltration. Investigators of the MRI scans were blinded against the pathology reports. Likewise, all histopathology reports were screened for the description of adjacent organ infiltration, and the declaration of compartment involvement followed the definitions of Georgiou et al. [11]. If a compartment was described as positive in MRI and negative in histopathology, the combination was judged as overstaging; likewise, if a compartment was negative in MRI and positive in histopathology, it was declared as understaging.

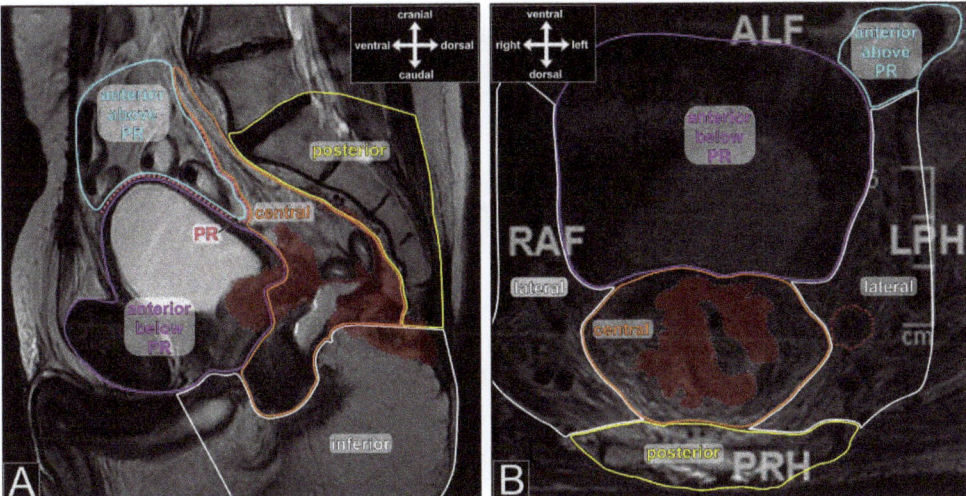

Figure 1. Pelvic MRI with delineation of the pelvic compartments (different colors, T2-weighted fast spin echo sequence). (**A**) sagittal image with a locally recurrent rectal cancer (anastomotic recurrence in a 68-year-old male) after anterior resection. The recurrent tumor is delineated with a grey dotted line and colored burgundy. PR—peritoneal reflection; (**B**) axial image with a cT3 primary tumor (marked as in A) and a positive lymph node in the left lateral compartment (red dotted line) in a 70-year-old male. The lymph node proved to be infiltrated by adenocarcinoma on histopathology after RCT and en bloc resection of the central and left lateral compartments.

All patients were discussed in a multidisciplinary team (MDT) and offered radiochemotherapy for downsizing whenever possible. As a rule, a second pelvic MRI was performed after preoperative therapy in order to document tumor response. It was, however, not considered for the assessment of this study.

MRI examinations were performed with a 1.5-Tesla General Electrics scanner (General Electrics Company, Boston, MA, USA). According to protocol, two phased-array surface coils equipped with four receiving channels were employed for signal detection. The positioning of the coils was on the pelvis and underneath the patient. For gross orientation, a sagittal T2-weighted turbo spin-echo was used in order to detect the tumor location. In primary rectal cancer, the protocol followed the recommendations of the MERCURY study, including high-resolution T2 fast relaxation fast spin echo images perpendicular to the longitudinal axis of the rectum [13,14]. For these images, a small field of view (20 cm) and a slice thickness of 3 mm (gap 0.3 mm) were chosen. Scan acquisition parameters were: echo time (TE) 110.0 ms, repetition time (TR) 3357.0 ms, Echo Train Length (ETL) 15, and Receiver Bandwidth 31.25 kHz. Neither contrast agents nor diffusion-weighted imaging (DWI) were systematically employed in the considered time period. In local recurrence, image acquisition was tailored to the tumor location in the turbo spin-echo images.

All patients were treated by laparotomy. The extent of the operation was guided by the pretherapeutic MRI imaging and intraoperative assessment. If performed, pelvic side wall dissection was done en bloc, usually with resection of the internal iliac vessels of the involved side [15]. Further details of anatomical landmarks and surgical strategies have only recently been described elsewhere [12,16].

Follow-up was realized in our outpatient clinic with at least annual visits and appropriate investigations as recommended by the German guidelines [17]. A detailed description has formerly been given [18].

All parameters were compared for the two groups. MRI findings were analyzed with regard to the pathology findings as the gold standard. We evaluated accuracy, specificity, sensitivity, negative predictive value, and positive predictive value for all compartments and repeated the analysis for every single compartment. As appropriate, patient, treatment, and tumor characteristics were compared with the χ2-test, Fisher exact test, and Mann–Whitney-U test. Survival was calculated as overall survival (OS) according to Kaplan–Meier and potential prognostic factors were tested with the log-rank test. These potential prognosticators were included in a multivariate Cox proportional model to elicit independent associations. The starting point for survival analysis was the date of multivisceral resection. Death of any cause was counted as an event. Patients who were lost to follow-up or had less than 60 months of observation time at the closing date of the study (31 March 2023) were censored. A p-value of <0.05 was considered significant. Statistical analysis was performed with SPSS® version 29 (IBM Corp., Armonk, NY, USA).

3. Results

We identified 75 consecutive patients with a multivisceral resection in the predefined time period. Four patients were excluded because of a missing MRI ($n = 3$) and a sacral resection for an abscess ($n = 1$), leaving 71 to be considered. Five patients recurred after initial multivisceral resection and underwent further exenterative surgery for their recurrence. They were analyzed in both groups; thus, 76 cases (25 (32.9%) females) were included in the analysis. Forty-eight patients (63.2%) were operated for their primary tumor (including two cT3 tumors with positive lateral lymph nodes) and 28 (36.8%)) for a LRRC (Figure 2). Median age was 66.5 (interquartile range (IQR) 58–73) years, with patients in the LRRC group slightly older than in the primary tumor group (68 vs. 65 years). Median follow-up for surviving patients was 72.6 months, with only one patient lost. Further patients and tumor characteristics are given in Table 1.

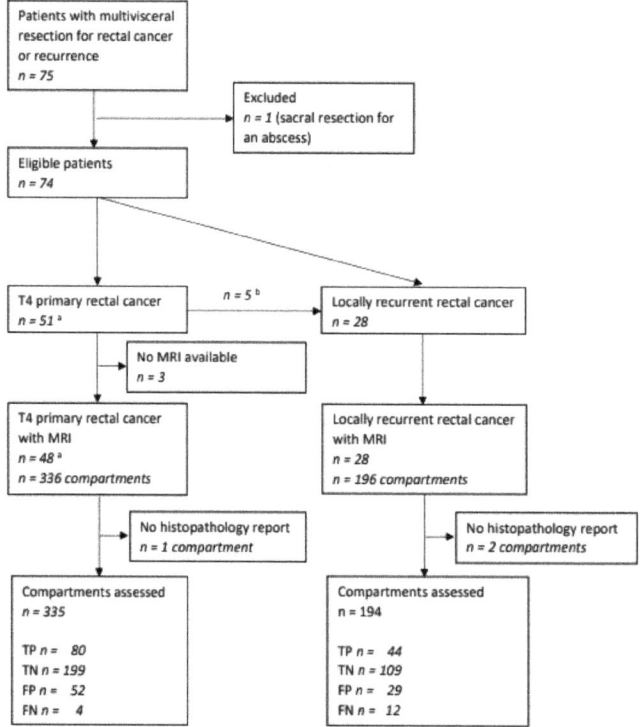

Figure 2. Flow chart of the study population/MRI assessment. TP—true positive, TN—true negative, FP—false positive, FN—false negative. [a]—including two cT3 tumors with positive lateral lymph nodes; [b]—five patients were operated on for a local recurrence after multivisceral resection for a T4 primary tumor and were investigated in both groups.

Table 1. Patient and tumor characteristics.

Parameter	Primary Tumor Group (n = 48)	Local Recurrence Group (n = 28)	Total (n = 76)	p
Age (median (IQR) in years)	65 (58–73)	68 (58–74)	66.5 (58–73)	0.477 [a]
Sex				0.618 [b]
Male	31 (64.6)	20 (71.4)	51 (67.1)	
Female	17 (35.4)	8 (28.6)	25 (32.9)	
Follow-up (median (IQR) in months)	72.6 (63.2–111.2)	74.3 (47.5–112.4)	72.6 (61.6–111.2)	0.674 [a]
Pretherapeutic CEA				0.816 [b]
Normal	22 (45.8)	12 (42.9)	34 (44.7)	
Elevated	25 (54.2)	16 (57.1)	42 (55.3)	
Values in ng/L (median (IQR) in months)	7.0 (3.0–41.8)	8.6 (2.1–24.8)	7.9 (3.0–32.0)	
Tumor extent				1.000 [b]
(r)cT0–3 [c]	2 (4.2)	1 (3.6)	3 (3.9)	
(r)cT4	46 (95.8)	27 (100)	73 (97.3)	
Lateral lymph nodes				0.142 [b]
No	40 (83.3)	27 (96.4)	67 (88.2)	
Yes	8 (16.7)	1 (3.6)	9 (11.8)	
Distant metastases				1.000 [b]
No	32 (66.7)	19 (67.9)	51 (67.1)	
Yes	16 (33.3)	9 (32.1)	25 (32.9)	
Preoperative irradiation of the small pelvis				0.001 [b]
No	7 (14.6)	14 (50.0)	21 (27.6)	
Yes	41 (85.4)	14 (50.0)	55 (72.4)	

Values in parentheses are percentages if not otherwise specified. IQR—interquartile range; CEA—carcinoembryonic antigen. [a]—Mann–Whitney-U test, [b]—Fisher exact test, [c]—patients with lateral lymph nodes.

A median of 3 compartments were involved in both groups on MRI. However, significantly more compartments were resected in patients with recurrent disease (median 4 (IQR 3–5) vs. 3 (IQR 3–4), $p = 0.017$). Cystectomy was performed in half of the patients with LRRC compared to one-third in those with T4 primary tumor. Vascular resections and sacral resections were performed significantly more often in LRRC, whereas significantly more hysterectomies were performed in women with T4 tumors. A pelvic floor reconstruction with a VRAM flap was significantly more often necessary in exenterative surgery for LRRC. In histopathologic work-up, a local R0-resection was achieved in 45 (93.8%) patients with primary tumors and 16 (57.1%) with recurrent tumors ($p < 0.001$). However, the median of involved compartments on histopathology was equal in both groups (2 (IQR 1–2) in primary tumor, 2 (IQR 1–3) in LRRC, $p = 0.480$) (Table 2).

Overall, 529 compartments were assessed, with three missing statements in the pathology report (Figure 2). Overall, accuracy was 81.7%, with a sensitivity of 88.6%, a specificity of 79.2%, a positive predictive value of 60.5% and a negative predictive value of 95.1%. Accuracy was somewhat higher for patients with T4 tumors compared to those with LRRC (83.3% vs. 78.9%). Likewise, sensitivity was better for patients with T4 tumors than for patients with LRRC (95.2% vs. 78.6%). Accuracy was highest for the anterior above peritoneal reflection (AAPR) compartment (90.8) and lowest for the lateral compartment (70.7). Overstaging summed up to 15.3%, whereas understaging was as low as 3.0%. Detailed figures for diagnostic performance are given in Table 3.

Table 2. Operative, histopathologic, and MRI characteristics.

Parameter	Primary Tumor Group (n = 48)	Local Recurrence Group (n = 28)	Total (n = 76)	p
Resected organs				
Cystectomy	15 (31.3)	14 (50.0)	29 (38.2)	0.143 [a]
partial resection of the bladder	2 (4.2)	0	2 (2.6)	0.528 [a]
Hysterectomy [b]	14 (82.4)	1 (12.5)	15 (60.0)	0.002 [a]
Vaginal resection [b]	9 (52.9)	6 (75.0)	15 (60.0)	0.402 [a]
Vascular resection	8 (16.7)	12 (42.9)	20 (26.3)	0.016 [a]
Sacral resection	2 (4.2)	7 (25.0)	9 (11.8)	0.010 [a]
en bloc resection lateral compartment	25 (52.1)	19 (67.9)	44 (57.9)	0.231 [a]
Flap reconstruction				
none	38 (79.2)	11 (39.3)	49 (64.5)	<0.001 [c]
V-Y	5 (10.4)	3 (10.7)	8 (10.5)	
VRAM	5 (10.4)	14 (50.0)	19 (25.0)	
(r)pT-category [d]				
0	1 (2.1)	2 (7.1)	3 (3.9)	
1	1 (2.1)	0	1 (1.3)	
2	3 (6.3)	1 (3.6)	4 (5.3)	
3	21 (43.8)	2 (7.1)	23 (30.3)	
4	22 (45.8)	23 (82.1)	45 (59.2)	0.003 [a,e]
(r)pN-category [d]				
0	27 (56.3)	22 (78.6)	49 (64.5)	0.044 [c]
1	13 (27.1)	6 (21.4)	19 (25.0)	
2	8 (16.7)	0	8 (10.5)	
R-classification (local)				
0	45 (93.8)	16 (57.1)	61 (80.3)	<0.001 [a]
1/2	3 (6.3)	12 [f] (42.9)	15 (19.7)	
Involved compartments on MRI, median (IQR)	3 (2–3)	3 (2–3)	3 (2–3)	0.717 [g]
Resected compartments, median (IQR)	3 (3–4)	4 (3–5)	3 (3–4)	0.017 [g]
Involved compartments on histopathology, median (IQR)	2 (1–2)	2 (1–3)	2 (1–2)	0.480 [g]

Values in parentheses are percentages if not otherwise specified. V-Y—VY advancement flap; VRAM—vertical rectus abdominis myocutaneous flap; IQR—interquartile range. [a]—Fisher-exact test; [b]—female patients only; [c]—χ^2-test; [d]—including yp and p categories; [e]—(r)pT4 vs. all other categories, [f]—two patients R2; [g]—Mann-Withney-U test.

Table 3. Diagnostic performance MRI vs. histopathology.

Parameter	All-Comp.	T4-Comp.	LR-Comp.	PR	AAPR	ABPR	Central	Lateral	Posterior	Inferior
Accuracy—TP+TN/all	81.7	83.3	78.9	78.7	90.8	76.3	89.5	70.7	86.8	78.7
Sensitivity—TP/TP+FN	88.6	95.2	78.6	-	71.4	100	93.5	77.8	71.4	87.5
Specificity—TN/TN+FP	79.2	79.3	79.0	81.9	92.8	56.1	71.4	67.2	88.4	77.6
PPV—TP/TP+FP	60.5	60.0	60.3	-	50.0	66.0	93.5	43.8	38.5	31.8
NPV—TN/TN+FN	95.1	98.0	90.1	95.2	97.0	100	71.4	90.7	96.8	98.1
Overstaging FP/all	15.3	15.5	14.9	17.3	6.6	23.7	5.3	24.0	10.5	20.0
Unterstaging FN/all	3.0	1.2	6.2	4.0	2.6	0	5.3	5.3	2.6	1.3

All values are percentages. Comp.—all compartments; LR—local recurrence; PR—peritoneal reflection compartment; AAPR—anterior above peritoneal reflection compartment; ABPR—anterior below peritoneal reflection compartment; TP—true positive; TN—true negative; FP—false positive; FN—false negative; PPV—positive predictive value; NPV—negative predictive value.

The 5-year OS rate was 45.2 [33.8; 56.6 (95% CI)]% for all patients, with a difference between patients with T4-tumors (53.3%) and LRRC (32.1%, $p = 0.085$, Figure 3). In patients with a complete local pathohistological (R0) resection, the 5-year OS rate was 54.9% compared to 6.7% in patients with an R1/2 resection ($p < 0.001$, Figure 4). There was also a difference of 53.2% vs. 34.0% for patients with 1–3 vs. 4–6 resected compartments ($p = 0.144$, Figure 5). Patients without distant metastases had a clear survival advantage (Figure 6), whereas pretherapeutic CEA level was only non-significantly associated with prognosis (Table 4). In multivariate analysis, R0-resections and M0 category emerged as independent prognosticators, whereas the number of resected compartments showed no independent association with prognosis (Table 5).

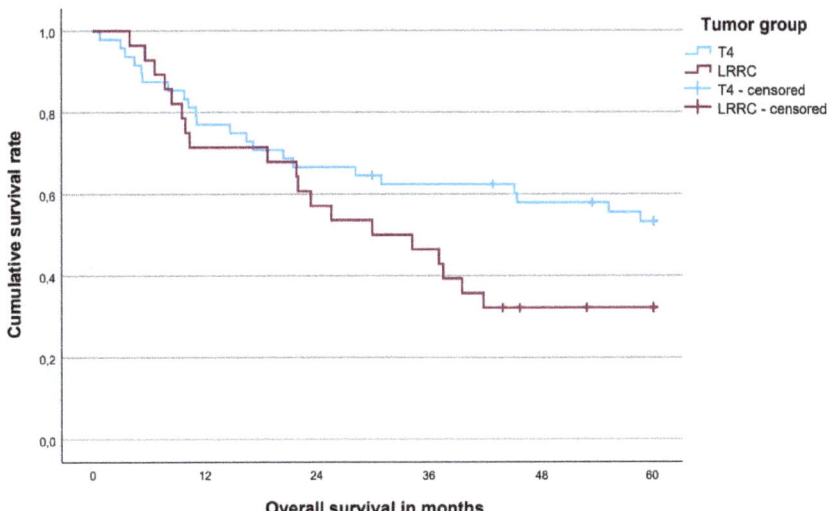

Figure 3. Five-year overall survival for primary tumors vs. locally recurrent rectal cancer. Five-year overall survival rates: T4 primary tumors ($n = 48$) 53.3%, locally recurrent rectal cancer ($n = 28$) 32.1% ($p = 0.085$). LRRC—locally recurrent rectal cancer.

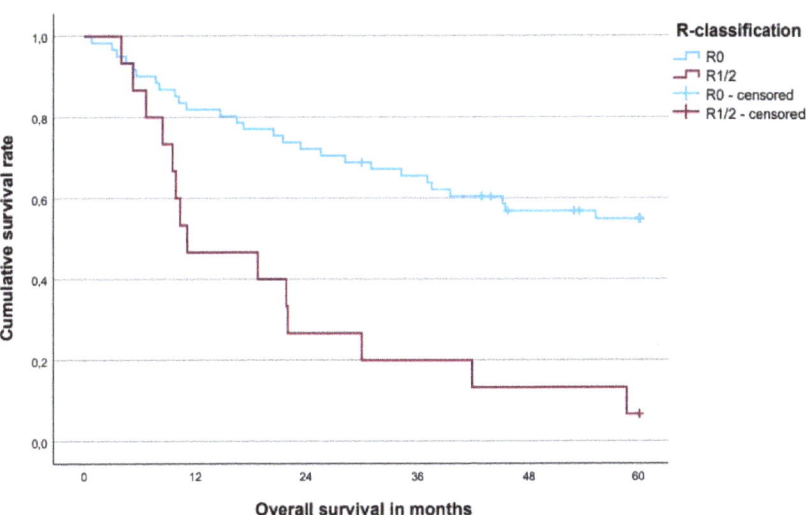

Figure 4. Five-year overall survival for locally R0- vs. R1/2-resected tumors. Five-year overall survival rates: R0 ($n = 61$) 54.9%, R1/2 ($n = 15$) 6.7% ($p < 0.001$).

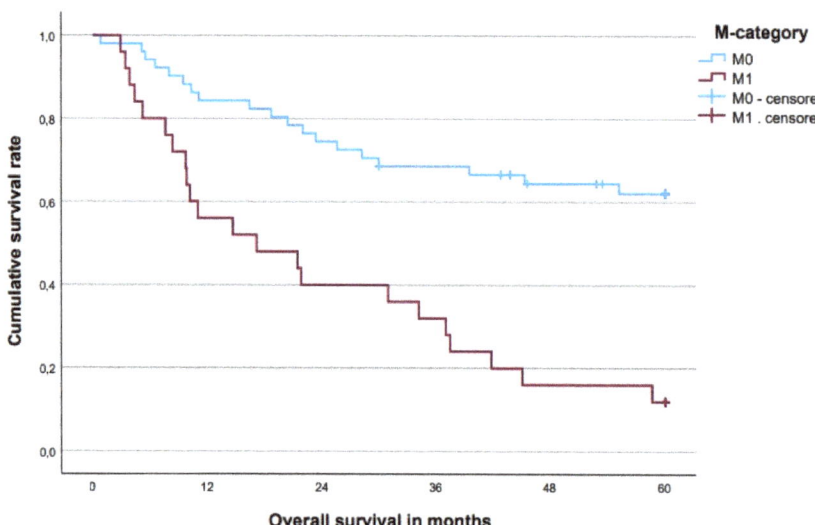

Figure 5. Five-year overall survival for M0 vs. M1 tumors. Five-year overall survival rates: M0 (*n* = 51) 62.1%, M1 (*n* = 25) 12.0% (*p* < 0.001).

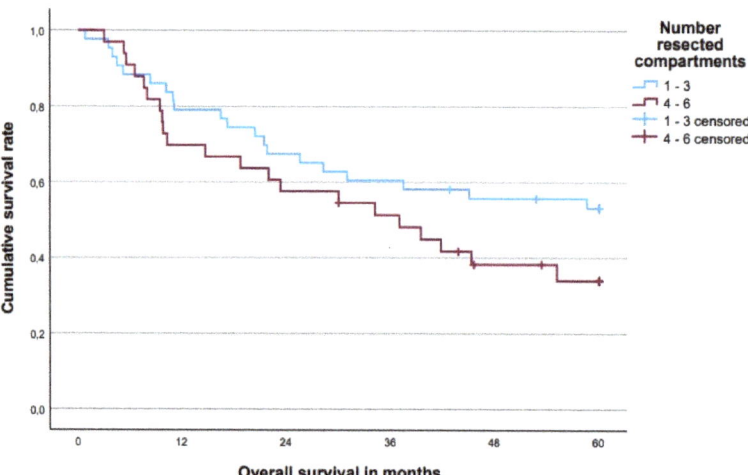

Figure 6. Five-year overall survival for a number of resected compartments. Five-year overall survival rates: one to three compartments (*n* = 43) 53.2%, four to six compartments (*n* = 33) 34.0% (*p* = 0.144).

Table 4. Five-year overall survival rates.

Parameter	n	5-Year Overall Survival in % [95% CI (%)]	Events	p
Total	76	45.2 [33.8; 56.6]	41	
Group				0.085
Primary tumor	48	53.3 [39.0; 67.6]	22	
Local recurrence	28	32.1 [14.8; 49.3]	19	
R-classification				<0.001
0	61	54.9 [42.2; 67.6]	27	
1/2	15	6.7 [0; 19.2]	14	
Number resected compartments				0.144
1–3	43	53.2 [38.1; 68.3]	20	
4–6	33	34.0 [16.9; 51.1]	21	
M-category				<0.001
0	51	62.1 [48.6; 75.6]	19	
1	25	12.0 [0; 24.7]	22	
Pretherapeutic CEA				0.112
Normal	34	54.9 [37.8; 72.0]	15	
Elevated	42	37.5 [22.6; 52.4]	26	

CI—confidence interval; CEA—carcinoembryonic antigen.

Table 5. Cox regression analysis for 5-year overall survival.

Parameter	Univariate			Multivariate		
	Hazard Ratio	95% CI	p	Hazard Ratio	95% CI	p
Group						
Primary tumor	Ref.			Ref.		
Local recurrence	1.712	0.923; 3.177	0.088	0.988	0.455; 2.147	0.975
R-classification						
0	Ref.			Ref.		
1/2	3.617	1.868; 7.004	<0.001	2.509	1.168; 5.391	0.018
No. resected compartments						
1–3	Ref.			Ref.		
4–6	1.575	0.852; 2.912	0.147	1.633	0.795; 3.355	0.182
Distant metastases						
M0	Ref.			Ref.		
M1	3.820	2.049; 7.123	<0.001	3.479	1.810; 6.688	<0.001
Pretherapeutic CEA						
Normal	Ref.			Ref.		
Elevated	1.667	0.882; 3.151	0.116	1.378	0.692; 2.745	0.362

CI—confidence interval; CEA—carcinoembryonic antigen.

4. Discussion

Our study demonstrates that MRI is able to predict the status of the pelvic compartments correctly in 81.7%. The proportion of understaging, including the risk of leaving an involved compartment behind, was only 3.0%. This translates into a favorable local R0 resection rate for patients with T4 primary rectal cancer and a good R0 resection rate for patients with local recurrence. The number of resected compartments was not independently associated with prognosis in multivariate testing. This is an indicator that the attempt at resection of a tumor, which has extended beyond surgical TME planes, is warranted as long as an R0 resection seems possible. The high precision of MRI to identify involved compartments (sensitivity of 88.6%) makes this diagnostic tool the first choice in planning extended procedures.

4.1. Diagnostic Accuracy

Overall, the possibility of detecting an LRRC by MRI correctly was given with a sensitivity of 77–100% and a specificity of 29–86% in a recent review [19]. Data on diagnostic performance with regard to different pelvic compartments are scarce. Georgiou et al. achieved an overall accuracy of 93.1% [11]. These excellent results are attributable to their strive to keep the interval between MRI acquisition and surgery as short as possible, including post-neoadjuvant therapy imaging for assessment. Our study examines the initial MRI, which in many cases was then followed by neoadjuvant radio(chemo)therapy. Neoadjuvant therapy has the potential to downsize the tumor with the possibility of tumor withdrawal from involved tissues. However, it may be difficult to differentiate remaining fibrosis from a tumor on MRI; therefore, we planned surgery according to the pretherapeutic images [3]. If, on histopathology, no tumor was detectable, the compartment in question was counted as a false positive. This resulted in a rather high sensitivity (88.6%) but a somewhat lower specificity (79.2%). For comparison, Georgiou et al. achieved 96.0% and 90.7%, respectively [11]. The high diagnostic reliability of MRI for the absence of tumor invasion into adjacent structures was also confirmed by a Dutch group with negative predictive values between 93% and 100% [20]. The problem of fibrosis and scarring was especially evident in LRRC. Accordingly, Brown et al. examining exclusively LRRC achieved an accuracy of 82.8% with a sensitivity of 77.4% and a specificity of 85.0% [21]. Another pitfall of compartment assessment is the common recognition that posterior compartment involvement is described only on histopathology if bony infiltration can be demonstrated [22]. While tumors can often be found to have breached the posterior mesorectal fascia, an infiltration into or beyond the periost rarely occurs. Furthermore, the assessment of the lateral compartment was repeatedly reported to be problematic [11,20,21,23]. The multitude of anatomical structures and possible pathways of tumor spread along lymphatic and vascular structures may be the reason for difficulties in correct assessment [24].

4.2. R0-Rates

The strategy of beyond-TME surgery is to resect the adjacent compartment or at least parts of it if the tumor extends the boundaries of the mesorectal fascia and infiltrates into the compartment in question. The rationale behind it is twofold: first, to obtain a clear margin and not to risk inadvertent exposure of the tumor surface to the operation field; second, to address the possible potential pathways of further tumor spread of the adjacent compartment. The latter has hitherto not yet been fully elucidated. Whereas involvement of the lateral compartment often results from a lateral route of lymphatic spread prone to continue to more central lymphatic stations, e.g., the common iliacal or paraaortal nodes, the spread along the lymphatic or vascular routes of an involved urogenital organ or the bony pelvis remains unclear. Furthermore, the anatomical boundaries of the pelvic compartments do, in part, overlap and are not delineated as clearly as the mesorectal compartment [12]. It is, therefore, of paramount importance to surgically interpret the radiological MRI findings within multidisciplinary sessions in order to define an individual MRI-guided surgical strategy on a patient basis [10,25]. However, for comparisons of results and the determination of the case mix, a description of involved well-defined compartments remains indispensable.

Tumor biology of primary T4 tumors and locally recurrent tumors is obviously different [26]. Primary T4 tumors represent a continuous tumor mass with compact cell formations. Clearance rates are excellent, and the prognosis is very good if no distant metastases are present. The R0 resection rates are reported to range between 72% and 91% [27–29]. Our rate of 93.8% compares favorably with these figures and translates into a 5-year OS rate of 53.3%. On the contrary, LRRC is disadvantaged by the fact that in the majority of cases, tumor cells have already escaped the confines of the mesorectal compartment and have inadvertently been left behind after TME surgery. Moreover, primary surgery disrupts tissue planes, restricts local blood supply, and results in scarring, all of which pave the way for diffuse and maybe discontinuous tumor spread in local recurrence. Correspondingly, an R0 resection is much more difficult to achieve with R0 rates given in the literature between 55% and 76% [26,27,30–32]. Our results (57.1%) are within the range of these figures, although we surgically removed significantly more compartments than in T4 tumors. Again, the lateral and the posterior compartments are repeatedly reported to set limitations to radical resection [33–36].

4.3. Prognosis

Given meticulous staging, multimodal treatment, and dedicated surgery, the survival rates of cT4 rectal cancer approach that of cT3 tumors. Determinants of prognosis after R0 resection are metastatic disease, pathological lymph node status, and status of the circumferential resection margin [37]. A multicenter observational study from the PelvEx Group reported a 3-year OS of R0-resected patients of 56.4% ($n = 1030$) [29]. In a large single-center study from Wales ($n = 174$), the 5-year OS was 56.4% [37]. If we restricted our analysis to overall R0 patients, the respective 3- and 5-year OS data were 64.4% and 57.1% (data not shown). These figures, however, have to be interpreted with caution because T4 tumors include tumors from stages II to IV, and survival data depend on the proportion of the different stages.

The prognosis for LRRC from the time point of recurrence detection is much worse. The aforementioned PelvEx Group analyzed 656 patients after R0 resection for local recurrence and estimated a 3-year OS of 48.1% [30]. In a meta-analysis, Banghu et al. reported 5y OS rates to range from 28 to 92% [38]. The 3- and 5-year rates of R0-resected patients with LRRC from our study population were 68.8% and 50.0% (data not shown). Again, the prognosis depends on tumor load and patient selection and has to be interpreted with caution.

The strengths of our study are the high rate of pretherapeutic MRI and an almost complete follow-up. There are some limitations which should be discussed. First, although based on a prospective database, the study is retrospective in nature, with all limitations inherent in this kind of study. However, direct comparison of MRI and histopathological data by a compartment-for-compartment base permits insights into the robustness of MRI staging in daily clinical practice. Second, more sophisticated imaging techniques like DWI were not systematically used. The MRI protocol followed the suggestions of the MERCURY group, and involved radiologists were trained as participants of the Low Rectal Cancer study [39]. Third, only resected compartments could be investigated on histopathology. There was no systematic attempt to investigate the remaining compartments after surgery. Thus, compartments judged by the surgeon to be free of tumor and left behind were counted as not involved. Fourth, the proportion of false positive compartments was rather high, in part owing to the use of pretherapeutic images for assessment. Albeit results, especially for primary T4 tumors, are favorable, a change of strategy with careful assessment of post-neoadjuvant treatment MRI and preservation of non-involved compartments deserves further evaluation.

5. Conclusions

MRI is able to predict pelvic compartment involvement by T4 or LRRC tumors with high accuracy and an especially low percentage of understaging. This translates into excellent results of surgery for T4 tumors and good results for the more challenging LRRC. The number of resected compartments is not independently associated with outcomes as long as an R0 resection can be achieved.

Author Contributions: Conceptualization, S.S., T.K., M.S., F.S., M.G., E.P., A.S. and S.T.M.; Data curation, S.S., T.K. and E.P.; Formal analysis, S.S., T.K. and A.S.; Investigation, S.S., T.K., M.S., F.S., M.G. and E.P.; Methodology, S.S. and T.K.; Project administration, S.S., T.K. and S.T.M.; Resources, S.S., T.K., M.S., F.S., M.G. and E.P.; Software, S.S.; Supervision, S.S., T.K. and S.T.M.; Validation, S.S., T.K., M.S., F.S., M.G., E.P., A.S. and S.T.M.; Visualization, S.S. and T.K.; Writing—original draft, S.S. and A.S.; Writing—review and editing, S.S., T.K., M.S., F.S., M.G., E.P., A.S. and S.T.M.; Funding acquisition, S.S. All authors have read and agreed to the published version of the manuscript.

Funding: The maintenance of the database at the Coloproctologic Unit of Dresden-Friedrichstadt General Hospital was supported by a grant from the Tumor Center Dresden.

Institutional Review Board Statement: Ethical review and approval were waived for this study. The responsible review board is the "Ethikkommission der Sächsischen Landesärztekammer". Regulations regarding studies that need ethics approval are recorded under: https://www.slaek.de/de/arzt/ethikkommission.php. Our study does not fulfill any criterion that is listed here (AMG (§ 40 Abs. 1 Satz 2); Good Clinical Practice (GCP)-Rechtsverordnung (§ 7 Absatz 1); § 17 Abs. 1 Nr. 16 Sächsisches Heilberufekammergesetz (SächsHKaG) in Verbindung mit § 15 Abs. 1 der Berufsordnung der Sächsischen Landesärztekammer (BO).

Informed Consent Statement: Not applicable.

Data Availability Statement: The data presented in this study are available upon reasonable request from the corresponding author.

Acknowledgments: The authors are indebted to Lisa Domichowski and Anja Willing, Medical Data Managers, for their support in data acquisition, and Tillmann Heinze, Center of Clinical Anatomy, Kiel, for editing Figure 1.

Conflicts of Interest: The authors state that there is no conflict of interest.

References

1. Ruppert, R.; Junginger, T.; Kube, R.; Strassburg, J.; Lewin, A.; Baral, J.; Maurer, C.A.; Sauer, J.; Lauscher, J.; Winde, G.; et al. Risk-adapted neoadjuvant chemoradiotherapy in rectal cancer: Final report of the OCUM study. *J. Clin. Oncol.* **2023**, *41*, 4025–4034. [CrossRef] [PubMed]
2. Jacob, A.; Albert, W.; Jackisch, T.; Jakob, C.; Sims, A.; Witzigmann, H.; Mees, S.T.; Stelzner, S. Association of certification, improved quality and better oncological outcomes for rectal cancer in a specialized colorectal unit. *Int. J. Colorectal Dis.* **2021**, *36*, 517–533. [CrossRef] [PubMed]
3. PelvEx Collaborative. Contemporary management of locally advanced and recurrent rectal cancer: Views from the PelvEx Collaborative. *Cancers* **2022**, *14*, 1161. [CrossRef] [PubMed]
4. Detering, R.; Saraste, D.; de Neree Tot Babberich, M.P.M.; Dekker, J.W.T.; Wouters, M.W.J.M.; van Geloven, A.A.W.; Bemelman, W.A.; Tanis, P.J.; Martling, A.; Westerterp, M.; et al. International evaluation of circumferential resection margins after rectal cancer resection: Insights from the Swedish and Dutch audits. *Colorectal Dis.* **2020**, *22*, 416–429. [CrossRef] [PubMed]
5. The Beyond TME Collaborative. Consensus statement on the multidisciplinary management of patients with recurrent and primary rectal cancer beyond total mesorectal excision planes. *Br. J. Surg.* **2013**, *100*, 1009–1014. [CrossRef] [PubMed]
6. Peacock, O.; Waters, P.S.; Kong, J.C.; Warrier, S.K.; Wakeman, C.; Eglinton, T.; Heriot, A.G.; Frizelle, F.A.; McCormick, J.J. Complications after extended radical resections for locally advanced and recurrent pelvic malignancies: A 25-year experience. *Ann. Surg. Oncol.* **2020**, *27*, 409–414. [CrossRef]
7. Harji, D.P.; Griffiths, B.; Velikova, G.; Sagar, P.M.; Brown, J. Systematic review of health-related quality of life in patients undergoing pelvic exenteration. *Eur. J. Surg. Oncol.* **2016**, *42*, 1132–1145. [CrossRef]
8. Inoue, A.; Sheedy, S.P.; Wells, M.L.; Mileto, A.; Goenka, A.H.; Ehman, E.C.; Yalon, M.; Murthy, N.S.; Mathis, K.L.; Behm, K.T.; et al. Rectal cancer pelvic recurrence: Imaging patterns and key concepts to guide treatment planning. *Abdom. Radiol.* **2023**, *48*, 1867–1879. [CrossRef]
9. Ng, K.S.; Lee, P.J.M. Pelvic exenteration: Pre-, intra-, and post-operative considerations. *Surg. Oncol.* **2021**, *37*, 101546. [CrossRef]
10. PelvEx Collaborative. Minimum standards of pelvic exenterative practice: PelvEx Collaborative guideline. *Br. J. Surg.* **2022**, *109*, 1251–1263. [CrossRef]
11. Georgiou, P.A.; Tekkis, P.P.; Constantinides, V.A.; Patel, U.; Goldin, R.D.; Darzi, A.W.; Nicholls, J.R.; Brown, G. Diagnostic accuracy and value of magnetic resonance imaging (MRI) in planning exenterative pelvic surgery for advanced colorectal cancer. *Eur. J. Cancer* **2013**, *49*, 72–81. [CrossRef] [PubMed]
12. Stelzner, S.; Heinze, T.; Heimke, M.; Gockel, I.; Kittner, T.; Brown, G.; Mees, S.T.; Wedel, T. Beyond total mesorectal excision—Compartment-based anatomy of the pelvis revisited for exenterative pelvic surgery. *Ann. Surg.* **2023**, *278*, e58–e67. [CrossRef]
13. Mercury Study Group. Diagnostic accuracy of preoperative magnetic resonance imaging in predicting curative resection of rectal adenocarcinoma: Prospective observational study. *BMJ* **2006**, *333*, 749–782.

14. Brown, G.; Daniels, I.R.; Richardson, C.; Revell, P.; Peppercorn, D.; Bourne, M. Techniques and trouble-shooting in high spatial resolution thin slice MRI for rectal cancer. *Br. J. Radiol.* 2005, *78*, 245–251. [CrossRef]
15. Austin, K.K.; Solomon, M.J. Pelvic exenteration with en bloc iliac vessel resection for lateral pelvic wall involvement. *Dis. Colon. Rectum.* 2009, *52*, 1223–1233. [CrossRef] [PubMed]
16. Jackisch, J.; Jackisch, T.; Roessler, J.; Sims, A.; Nitzsche, H.; Mann, P.; Mees, S.T.; Stelzner, S. Tailored concept for the plastic closure of pelvic defects resulting from extralevator abdominoperineal excision (ELAPE) or pelvic exenteration. *Int. J. Colorectal Dis.* 2022, *37*, 1669–1679. [CrossRef]
17. Guideline Programme Oncology (German Cancer Society, German Cancer Aid, AWMF): Level3-Guideline Colorectal Carcinoma, Long Version 2.1, 2019, AWMF Registry No. 021/007OL. (In German). Available online: https://www.leitlinienprogramm-onkologie.de/leitlinen/kolorektales-karzinom/ (accessed on 17 July 2023).
18. Fischer, J.; Hellmich, G.; Jackisch, T.; Puffer, E.; Zimmer, J.; Bleyl, D.; Kittner, T.; Witzigmann, H.; Stelzner, S. Outcome for stage II and III rectal and colon cancer equally good after treatment improvement over three decades. *Int. J. Colorectal Dis.* 2015, *30*, 797–806. [CrossRef]
19. Colosio, A.; Fornès, P.; Soyer, P.; Lewin, M.; Loock, M.; Hoeffel, C. Local colorectal cancer recurrence: Pelvic MRI evaluation. *Abdom. Imaging* 2013, *38*, 72–81. [CrossRef]
20. Dresen, R.C.; Kusters, M.; Daniels-Gooszen, A.W.; Cappendijk, V.C.; Nieuwenhuijzen, G.A.; Kessels, A.G.; de Bruïne, A.P.; Beets, G.L.; Rutten, H.J.; Beets-Tan, R.G. Absence of tumor invasion into pelvic structures in locally recurrent rectal cancer: Prediction with preoperative MR imaging. *Radiology* 2010, *256*, 143–150. [CrossRef]
21. Brown, W.E.; Koh, C.E.; Badgery-Parker, T.; Solomon, M.J. Validation of MRI and surgical decision making to predict a complete resection in pelvic exenteration for recurrent rectal cancer. *Dis. Colon. Rectum* 2017, *60*, 144–151. [CrossRef]
22. Yamada, K.; Ishizawa, T.; Niwa, K.; Chuman, Y.; Akiba, S.; Aikou, T. Patterns of pelvic invasion are prognostic in the treatment of locally recurrent rectal cancer. *Br. J. Surg.* 2001, *88*, 988–993. [CrossRef]
23. Messiou, C.; Chalmers, A.G.; Boyle, K.; Wilson, D.; Sagar, P. Pre-operative MR assessment of recurrent rectal cancer. *Br. J. Radiol.* 2008, *81*, 468–473. [CrossRef]
24. Heinze, T.; Fletcher, J.; Miskovic, D.; Stelzner, S.; Bayer, A.; Wedel, T. The middle rectal artery: Revisited anatomy and surgical implications of a neglected blood vessel. *Dis. Colon. Rectum* 2023, *66*, 477–485. [CrossRef]
25. Akash, M.; Mehta, D.B.; Jenkins, J.T. Preoperative assessment of tumor anatomy and surgical resectability. *Surg. Manag. Adv. Pelvic Cancer* 2021, 17–31.
26. van Kessel, C.S.; Solomon, M.J. Understanding the philosophy, anatomy, and surgery of the extra-TME plane of locally advanced and locally recurrent rectal cancer; single institution experience with international benchmarking. *Cancers* 2022, *14*, 5058. [CrossRef] [PubMed]
27. Lau, Y.C.; Jongerius, K.; Wakeman, C.; Heriot, A.G.; Solomon, M.J.; Sagar, P.M.; Tekkis, P.P.; Frizelle, F.A. Influence of the level of sacrectomy on survival in patients with locally advanced and recurrent rectal cancer. *Br. J. Surg.* 2019, *106*, 484–490. [CrossRef] [PubMed]
28. Bhangu, A.; Ali, S.M.; Brown, G.; Nicholls, R.J.; Tekkis, P. Indications and outcome of pelvic exenteration for locally advanced primary and recurrent rectal cancer. *Ann. Surg.* 2014, *259*, 315–322. [CrossRef] [PubMed]
29. PelvEx Collaborative. Surgical and survival outcomes following pelvic exenteration for locally advanced primary rectal cancer: Results from an international collaboration. *Ann. Surg.* 2019, *269*, 315–321. [CrossRef]
30. PelvEx Collaborative. Factors affecting outcomes following pelvic exenteration for locally recurrent rectal cancer. *Br. J. Surg.* 2018, *105*, 650–657. [CrossRef]
31. Bird, T.G.; Ngan, S.Y.; Chu, J.; Kroon, R.; Lynch, A.C.; Heriot, A.G. Outcomes and prognostic factors of multimodality treatment for locally recurrent rectal cancer with curative intent. *Int. J. Colorectal Dis.* 2018, *33*, 393–401. [CrossRef]
32. Nordkamp, S.; Voogt, E.L.K.; van Zoggel, D.M.G.I.; Martling, A.; Holm, T.; Jansson Palmer, G.; Suzuki, C.; Nederend, J.; Kusters, M.; Burger, J.W.A.; et al. Locally recurrent rectal cancer: Oncological outcomes with different treatment strategies in two tertiary referral units. *Br. J. Surg.* 2022, *109*, 623–631. [CrossRef] [PubMed]
33. Belli, F.; Sorrentino, L.; Gallino, G.; Gronchi, A.; Scaramuzza, D.; Valvo, F.; Cattaneo, L.; Cosimelli, M. A proposal of an updated classification for pelvic relapses of rectal cancer to guide surgical decision-making. *J. Surg. Oncol.* 2020, *122*, 350–359. [CrossRef] [PubMed]
34. Iversen, H.; Martling, A.; Johansson, H.; Nilsson, P.J.; Holm, T. Pelvic local recurrence from colorectal cancer: Surgical challenge with changing preconditions. *Colorectal Dis.* 2018, *20*, 399–406. [CrossRef] [PubMed]
35. Rahbari, N.N.; Ulrich, A.B.; Bruckner, T.; Münter, M.; Nickles, A.; Contin, P.; Löffler, T.; Reissfelder, C.; Koch, M.; Büchler, M.W.; et al. Surgery for locally recurrent rectal cancer in the era of total mesorectal excision: Is there still a chance for cure? *Ann. Surg.* 2011, *253*, 522–533. [CrossRef]
36. van Ramshorst, G.H.; O'Shannassy, S.; Brown, W.E.; Kench, J.G.; Solomon, M.J. A qualitative study of the development of a multidisciplinary case conference review methodology to reduce involved margins in pelvic exenteration surgery for recurrent rectal cancer. *Colorectal Dis.* 2018, *20*, 1004–1013. [CrossRef]
37. Radwan, R.W.; Jones, H.G.; Rawat, N.; Davies, M.; Evans, M.D.; Harris, D.A.; Beynon, J.; Swansea Pelvic Oncology Group. Determinants of survival following pelvic exenteration for primary rectal cancer. *Br. J. Surg.* 2015, *102*, 1278–1284. [CrossRef]

38. Bhangu, A.; Ali, S.M.; Darzi, A.; Brown, G.; Tekkis, P. Meta-analysis of survival based on resection margin status following surgery for recurrent rectal cancer. *Colorectal Dis.* **2012**, *14*, 1457–1466. [CrossRef]
39. Battersby, N.J.; How, P.; Moran, B.; Stelzner, S.; West, N.P.; Branagan, G.; Strassburg, J.; Quirke, P.; Tekkis, P.; Pedersen, B.G.; et al. Prospective Validation of a Low Rectal Cancer Magnetic Resonance Imaging Staging System and Development of a Local Recurrence Risk Stratification Model: The MERCURY II Study. *Ann. Surg.* **2016**, *263*, 751–760. [CrossRef]

Disclaimer/Publisher's Note: The statements, opinions and data contained in all publications are solely those of the individual author(s) and contributor(s) and not of MDPI and/or the editor(s). MDPI and/or the editor(s) disclaim responsibility for any injury to people or property resulting from any ideas, methods, instructions or products referred to in the content.

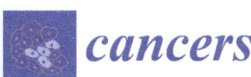

Article

Proposal of a T3 Subclassification for Colon Carcinoma

Susanne Merkel [1,2,*], Maximilian Brunner [1,2], Carol-Immanuel Geppert [2,3], Robert Grützmann [1,2], Klaus Weber [1,2] and Abbas Agaimy [2,3]

1. Department of Surgery, Friedrich-Alexander-Universität Erlangen-Nürnberg, 91054 Erlangen, Germany
2. Comprehensive Cancer Center Erlangen-European Metropolitan Area of Nürnberg (CCC ER-EMN), 91054 Erlangen, Germany
3. Institute of Pathology, Friedrich-Alexander-Universität Erlangen-Nürnberg, 91054 Erlangen, Germany
* Correspondence: susanne.merkel@uk-erlangen.de

Simple Summary: One of the most important prognostic factors for patients with colon cancer is the anatomical extent at the time of surgery. It is described by the TNM classification, which is the basis for treatment planning. T refers to the extent of the primary tumor. Usually, four T categories are distinguished. T3 describes invasion into the pericolic tissue and is the most frequent category found in colon carcinomas. A subclassification of T3, as we present here in this retrospective study, helps to better predict prognosis and further optimize treatment and therapeutic standards.

Abstract: The TNM classification system is one of the most important factors determining prognosis for cancer patients. In colorectal cancer, the T category reflects the depth of tumor invasion. T3 is defined by a tumor that invades through the muscularis propria into pericolorectal tissues. The data of 1047 patients with complete mesocolic excision were analyzed. The depth of invasion beyond the outer border of the muscularis propria into the subserosa or into nonperitonealized pericolic tissue was measured and categorized in 655 pT3 patients: pT3a ($\leq$1 mm), pT3b,c (>1–15 mm) and pT3d (>15 mm). The prognosis of these categories was compared. Five-year distant metastasis increased significantly from pT3a (5.7%) over pT3b,c (17.7%) to pT3d (37.2%; $p = 0.001$). There was no difference between pT2 (5.3%) and pT3a or between pT3d and pT4a (42.1%) or pT4b (33.7%). The 5-year disease-free survival decreased significantly from pT3a (77.4%) over pT3b,c (65.4%) to pT3d (50.1%; $p = 0.015$). No significant difference was found between pT2 (80.5%) and pT3a or between pT3d and pT4a (43.9%; $p = 0.296$) or pT4b (53.4%). The prognostic inhomogeneity in pT3 colon carcinoma has been demonstrated. A three-level subdivision of T3 for colon carcinoma in the TNM system into T3a ($\leq$1 mm), T3b (>1–15 mm), and T3c (>15 mm) is recommended.

Keywords: colon carcinoma; pT3; T3 subdivision; distant metastasis; survival; prognosis; prognostic factor; TNM classification

1. Introduction

The TNM classification system [1,2] is one of the most important factors determining treatment and prognosis for patients diagnosed with solid cancer. Advances in diagnostics and treatment require regular optimization of the staging system. The T-category reflects the primary tumor, either defined by tumor size (largest diameter) as in many organs, by the depth of the tumor invasion as in colorectal cancer (CRC), or by combined sets of criteria. In CRC, T3 is defined by a tumor that invades through the muscularis propria into pericolorectal tissues. T4a and T4b tumors penetrate through the visceral peritoneum (T4a) or invade directly or adhere to adjacent organs or structures (T4b).

Prognostic inhomogeneity of the pT3 category has already been shown for rectal carcinoma after primary surgical treatment [3] and after preoperative neoadjuvant chemoradiation followed by surgery [4]. A proposal for a subdivision of the pT3 category was

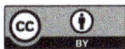

presented for both rectal and colon carcinomas in the various editions of the TNM supplements [5–8]. However, thus far, it has not been included in the official TNM classification. Here, we present a subclassification of pT3 in colon carcinoma to demonstrate the wide range of prognoses of these tumors. Furthermore, we wanted to show the overlap of pT3 with pT2 at a low invasion depth and the overlap of pT3 with pT4 at an advanced invasion depth.

2. Materials and Methods

2.1. Inclusion and Exclusion Criteria of the Study

Data from patients with the following inclusion criteria were analyzed: invasive colon carcinoma, no appendix carcinoma; pT-category > pT1; more than 16 cm from the anal verge; treatment by complete mesocolic excision (CME) at the Department of Surgery of the University Hospital Erlangen, Germany, between 1998 and 2015; curative resection (R0 by macroscopic and microscopic examination); no neoadjuvant treatment; no distant metastases at diagnosis; carcinoma not arising in the setting of familial adenomatous polyposis, ulcerative colitis or Crohn's disease. Thirty-four of 1081 patients (3.1%) had to be excluded: 22 patients because of missing data on the depth of invasion into subserosa or into nonperitonealized pericolic tissue and 12 patients because of missing follow-up information. In summary, data from 1047 consecutive patients were analyzed.

2.2. Description of the pT3 Subdivision

In pT3 carcinomas, the depth of invasion beyond the outer border of the muscularis propria into the subserosa or into nonperitonealized pericolic tissue was measured and categorized by the pathologist into four groups: pT3a, ≤ 1 mm; pT3b, >1–5 mm; pT3c, >5–15 mm; pT3d, >15 mm (Figure 1); then, the two intermediate subgroups pT3b and pT3c were combined into a single subgroup for statistical analysis. Here, we distinguish between the three categories: pT3a (invasion up to 1 mm), pT3b,c (invasion more than 1 mm up to 15 mm), and pT3d (invasion more than 15 mm).

2.3. Tumor Documentation

Epidemiological data, treatment, histopathological findings, and follow-up data were collected prospectively at the Erlangen Registry for Colorectal Carcinomas (ERCRC). The detailed documentation of the histopathological examinations allowed the classification of all carcinomas in accordance with the 8th edition of the UICC TNM classification [2].

According to its embryologic origin, the right colon was defined from the cecum to the proximal two-thirds of the transverse colon; the left colon extended from the distal third of the transverse colon to the sigmoid colon.

2.4. Surgical Procedure, Adjuvant Treatment, and Follow-Up

Complete mesocolic excision (CME) [9] was introduced and developed in 1985 and has consequently been implemented since 1995 [10]. With the exception of 11 patients who underwent laparoscopic surgery, all patients were operated on by an open approach. The median number of regional lymph nodes that were examined in the specimens was 29 (range 8–145). In 1041 of 1047 patients (99.4%), twelve or more lymph nodes were examined.

Adjuvant treatment was administered in 244 of 373 patients (65.4%) with stage III disease and in 13 of 472 patients (2.8%) with high-risk stage II disease, mostly using 5-fluorouracil and folinic acid with or without oxaliplatin according to the evidence-based German guideline for colorectal cancer that was valid at the time of treatment [11].

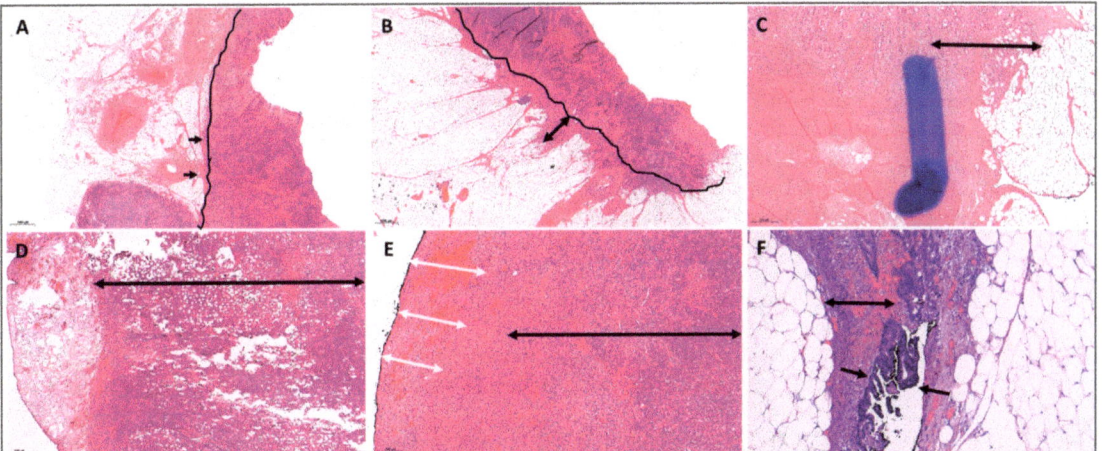

Figure 1. Histological presentation of the categories pT3a-d and pT4 in colorectal carcinoma. Double-headed black arrows highlight the depth of the subserosal invasion; arrows highlight neoplastic cells. (**A**): CRC completely obliterating the lamina muscularis propria (black line) and showing early involvement of the subserosa (arrows), indicating pT3a. (**B**): Similar illustration as in (**A**), but with 4 mm subserosal extension indicated by the double-head arrow (pT3b). (**C**): This case showed subserosal invasion >5 but <15 mm, corresponding to pT3c. (**D**): Example of pT3d showing extensive (>15 mm) subserosal invasion covered by edematous but tumor-free subserosa on the left. (**E**): This case formally qualifies as pT3d. However, the residual subserosa was replaced by a hemorrhagic granulating inflammatory reaction (double-headed white arrows), so sealed serosal penetration cannot be reliably ruled out in such cases. (**F**): Classic pT4 status showing neoplastic tissue on top of the serosa (arrows). However, a hemorrhagic granulating inflammatory reaction is seen (double head arrow), resulting in partially sealed serosal penetration (such cases might later seal completely and hence mimic the case shown in (**E**)).

Patients were followed up for at least 5 years with physical examination, estimation of carcinoembryonic antigen (CEA) levels, abdominoperineal ultrasonography, chest X-ray, and colonoscopy. Thereafter, vital status was checked annually.

2.5. Statistical Analysis

The chi-square test and Fisher's exact test were used to compare categorical data, and the Mann–Whitney U test was used to compare continuous data. The Kaplan–Meier method was applied to analyze the rates of distant metastases, disease-free survival, overall survival, and cancer-related survival. For the analysis of disease-free survival, the first occurrence of locoregional or distant recurrence or death from any cause was defined as an event. For estimation of overall survival, we defined death from any cause as an event. For the analysis of cancer-related survival, an event was defined as death from colon cancer, either because of recurrence (locoregional or distant) or because of postoperative death following reoperation. The 95% confidence intervals (CIs) were calculated according to the method described by Greenwood [12]. The survival curves were compared using a log-rank test. Cox regression analysis was used for multivariate analyses and was adjusted for age in survival analyses. For the identification of independent prognostic factors, all variables with $p < 0.05$ in univariate analysis were included in the multivariate model. A p-value < 0.05 was considered significant. All analyses were performed using the statistical software package SPSS® version 24.0 (IBM, Armonk, New York, NY, USA).

3. Results

3.1. Patient Characteristics

The demographic and clinicopathological characteristics of the 1047 patients are shown in Table 1. A total of 655 patients were classified as pT3 and divided into subgroups pT3a, n = 155 (23.7%); pT3b,c, n = 433 (66.1%); and pT3d, n = 67 (10.2%). Table 2 presents the distribution of typical prognostic factors. We found significant differences in the distribution of prognostic factors between pT3a, pT3b,c, and pT3d carcinomas. High-grade carcinomas and those with lymphatic invasion were found to be significantly less frequent in pT3a than in pT3b,c ($p = 0.016$ and $p < 0.001$). Lymph node-positive carcinomas and those with lymphatic and/or venous invasion were found significantly more frequently in pT3d than in pT3b,c carcinomas ($p < 0.001$, $p = 0.001$, and $p = 0.006$). At the same time, pT3a carcinomas showed a similar distribution of these prognostic factors as pT2 carcinomas, and pT3d carcinomas had a similar distribution as pT4a and pT4b carcinomas. No differences were identified with respect to the location of the tumors within the right or left colon.

Table 1. Patient and tumor characteristics for 1047 patients.

		n	(%)
Age median (range) (years)		69 (21–99)	
Sex	Male	602	57.5
	Female	445	42.5
ASA *	ASA I–II	730	70.9
	ASA III–IV	300	28.7
Tumor site	Right colon	511	48.8
	Left colon	536	51.2
Emergencies	Elective surgery	931	88.9
	Emergency presentation	116	11.1
Surgical procedure	Colon standard resection	787	75.2
	Colon extended resection	260	24.8
Multivisceral resection	No	928	88.6
	Yes	119	11.4
Adjuvant treatment	No	790	75.5
	Yes	257	24.5
pT category	pT2 (muscularis propria)	265	25.3
	pT3a ($\leq$1 mm)	155	14.8
	pT3b,c (>1–15 mm)	433	41.4
	pT3d (>15 mm)	67	6.4
	pT4a (serosa)	75	7.2
	pT4b (other organs)	52	5.0
pN category	pN0	674	64.4
	pN1	261	24.9
	pN2	112	10.7
Grading	G1,2	699	66.8
	G3,4	348	33.2
Lymphatic invasion	L0	737	70.5
	L1	309	29.5
Venous invasion	V0	1012	96.7
	V1	34	3.3

ASA American Society of Anesthesiologists Classification; * ASA missing in 17 patients.

Table 2. Distribution of prognostic factors (n = 1047).

	pT2	p	pT3a (≤1 mm)	p	pT3b,c (>1–15 mm)	p	pT3d (>15 mm)	p	pT4a	p	pT4b	p overall
n	265		155		433		67		75		52	
	n (%)		n (%)		n (%)		n (%)		n (%)		n (%)	
Right colon	131 (49.4)		79 (51.0)		211 (48.7)		28 (42)		38 (51)		24 (46)	
Left colon	134 (50.6)	0.564	76 (49.0)	0.632	222 (51.3)	0.290	39 (58)	0.290	37 (49)	0.617	28 (54)	0.862
pN0	202 (76.2)		106 (68.4)		273 (63.0)		29 (43)		34 (45)		30 (58)	
pN1	54 (20.4)		38 (24.5)		110 (25.4)		19 (28)		21 (28)		19 (37)	
pN2	9 (3.4)	0.175	11 (7.1)	0.257	50 (11.5)	<0.001	19 (28)	0.965	20 (27)	0.011	3 (6)	<0.001
G1,2	204 (77.0)		115 (74.2)		275 (63.5)		40 (60)		39 (52)		26 (50)	
G3,4	61 (23.0)	0.592	40 (25.8)	0.016	158 (36.5)	0.548	27 (40)	0.356	36 (48)	0.825	26 (50)	<0.001
L0	225 (85.2)		129 (83.2)		285 (65.8)		30 (45)		35 (47)		33 (64)	
L1	39 (14.8)	0.653	26 (16.8)	<0.001	148 (34.2)	0.001	37 (55)	0.821	40 (53)	0.062	19 (37)	<0.001
V0	262 (99.2)		153 (98.7)		419 (96.8)		60 (90)		69 (92)		49 (94)	
V1	2 (0.8)	0.587	2 (1.3)	0.202	14 (3.2)	0.006	7 (10)	0.614	6 (8)	0.630	3 (6)	<0.001

The median follow-up of all patients was 8 years (range 0–22 years). During follow-up, locoregional recurrences were observed in 27 patients (2.6%), and distant metastases were observed in 173 patients (16.5%). At the time of analysis, 512 patients (48.9%) had died: 39 (3.7%) postoperatively, 139 (13.3%) related to recurrent disease, 62 (5.9%) from other malignancies, and 272 (26.0%) due to other nonmalignant diseases.

3.2. Locoregional Recurrences

The 5-year rate of locoregional recurrence for all patients was 2.9% (95% CI 1.7–4.1%; Table S1).

3.3. Distant Metastases

The 5-year rate of distant metastases for all patients was 16.4% (95% CI 14.0–18.8%). Distant metastases increased significantly from pT3a over pT3b,c to pT3d, i.e., from 5.7% via 17.7% to 37.2% ($p = 0.002$ and 0.001; Table 3a, Figure 2a) within 5 years. At the same time, there was no difference between pT2 and pT3a with 5.3% and 5.7% ($p = 0.993$) or between pT3d and pT4a and pT4b with 37.2%, 42.1% and 33.7% ($p = 0.579$ and $p = 0.403$). In patients without regional lymph node metastases (pN0), a significant difference in the frequency of distant metastasis was identified between pT3a and pT3b,c (4.1% vs. 13.0%; $p = 0.011$), which could be confirmed in multivariate analysis (Table S2). In contrast, in lymph node-positive patients (pN1,2), a significant difference was found between pT3b,c and pT3d (26.1% vs. 56.2%; $p = 0.001$).

Thirty patients developed peritoneal metastases, 20 of whom had distant metastases in other locations. This was observed extremely rarely in pT2 and pT3a patients (1/265 and 1/155) and was rare in pT3b,c and pT3d patients (12/433 and 1/67). pT4a patients were diagnosed with peritoneal metastases much more frequently (12/75; 16%), followed by pT4b patients (3/52; 6%).

3.4. Disease-Free Survival

A 5-year disease-free survival rate of 67.9% (65.2–70.6%) was observed for all patients. The differences between the pT categories were similar to those for distant metastasis. The 5-year disease-free survival decreased significantly from pT3a (77.4%) over pT3b,c (65.4%) to pT3d (50.1%; $p = 0.015$ and 0.033; Table 3b, Figure 2b). No significant difference was found between pT2 (80.5%) and pT3a (77.4%; $p = 0.844$) or between pT3d (50.1%) and pT4a (43.9%; $p = 0.296$) and pT4b (53.4%; $p = 0.177$). In pN0 patients, a significantly better 5-year disease-free survival was found in pT3a (80.2%) compared to pT3b,c (68.7%; $p = 0.012$), while in pN1,2 patients, it was significantly better in pT3b,c (59.9%) compared to pT3d (34.2%; $p = 0.007$).

Table 3. Distant metastases and disease-free survival (n = 1047).

	pT2	p	pT3a (≤1 mm)	p	pT3b,c (>1–15 mm)	p	pT3d (>15 mm)	p	pT4a (Serosa)	p	pT4b (Other Organs)
(a) Distant metastases											
Any pN 5-year rate (95% CI)	n = 265 5.3% (2.6–8.0)	0.993	n = 155 5.7% (1.8–9.6)	0.002	n = 433 17.7% (14.0–21.4)	0.001	n = 67 37.2% (24.7–49.7)	0.579	n = 75 42.1% (30.3–53.9)	0.403	n = 52 33.7% (20.2–47.2)
pN0 5-year rate (95% CI)	n = 202 3.8% (1.1–6.5)	0.936	n = 106 4.1% (0.2–8.0)	0.011	n = 273 13.0% (8.9–17.1)	0.951	n = 29 12.1% (0–25.0)	0.263	n = 34 25.3% (10.0–40.6)	0.212	n = 30 14.7% (1.4–28.0)
pN1,2 5-year rate (95% CI)	n = 63 10.1% (2.5–17.7)	0.803	49 9.2% (0.6–17.8)	0.069	160 26.1% (18.8–33.4)	0.001	n = 38 56.2% (39.1–73.3)	0.855	n = 41 53.2% (37.1–69.3)	0.623	n = 22 59.9% (38.3–81.5)
(b) Disease-free survival											
Any pN 5-year rate (95% CI)	n = 265 80.5% (75.6–85.4)	0.844	n = 155 77.4% (70.7–84.1)	0.015	n = 433 65.4% (60.9–69.9)	0.033	n = 67 50.1% (37.9–62.3)	0.296	n = 75 43.9% (32.7–55.1)	0.177	n = 52 53.4% (39.7–67.1)
pN0 5-year rate (95% CI)	n = 202 79.9% (74.4–85.4)	0.161	n = 106 80.2% (72.6–87.8)	0.012	n = 273 68.7% (63.2–74.2)	0.619	n = 29 71.7% (55.0–88.4)	0.226	n = 34 58.8% (42.3–75.3)	0.157	n = 30 73.3% (57.4–89.2)
pN1,2 5-year rate (95% CI)	n = 63 82.3% (72.9–91.7)	0.054	49 71.4% (58.7–84.1)	0.508	160 59.9% (52.3–67.5)	0.007	n = 38 34.2% (19.1–49.3)	0.667	n = 41 31.7% (17.4–46.0)	0.805	n = 22 26.0% (7.2–44.8)

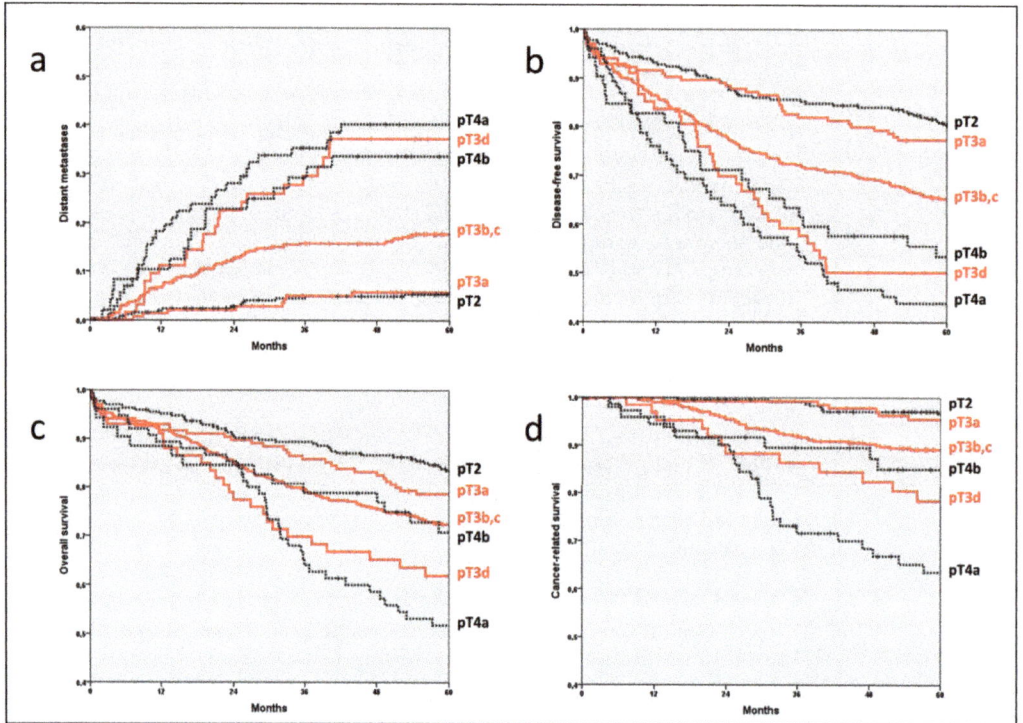

Figure 2. Comparison of the prognosis between patients with pT2 (n = 265), pT3a (n = 155) and pT3b,c (n = 433) and pT3d (n = 67), pT4a (n = 75) and pT4b (n = 52) colon carcinomas: (**a**) distant metastases, (**b**) disease-free survival, (**c**) overall survival, (**d**) cancer-related survival.

3.5. Overall Survival

The 5-year overall survival rate was 73.9% (71.2–76.6%) for all patients. The overall survival rates decreased from pT3a (78.6%) over pT3b,c (72.4%) to pT3d (61.9%; Table 4a, Figure 2c). However, the significance level was not reached. Only in pN1,2 patients was there a significant decrease in the 5-year rate from 68.6% in pT3b,c to 48.9% in pT3d carcinomas ($p = 0.011$).

Table 4. Overall survival and cancer-related survival (n = 1047).

	pT2	p	pT3a (≤1 mm)	p	pT3b,c (>1–15 mm)	p	pT3d (>15 mm)	p	pT4a (Serosa)	p	pT4b (Other Organs)
(a) Overall survival											
Any pN 5-year rate (95% CI)	n = 265 83.5% (79.0–88.0)	0.634	n = 155 78.6% (72.1–85.1)	0.119	n = 433 72.4% (68.1–76.7)	0.249	n = 67 61.9% (50.1–73.7)	0.108	n = 75 51.8% (40.4–63.2)	0.068	n = 52 70.7% (58.2–83.2)
pN0 5-year rate (95% CI)	n = 202 82.4% (77.1–87.7)	0.300	n = 106 81.1% (73.7–88.5)	0.058	n = 273 74.6% (69.5–79.7)	0.162	n = 29 78.8% (63.7–93.9)	0.058	n = 34 70.5% (55.2–85.8)	0.182	n = 30 83.3% (70.0–96.6)
pN1,2 5-year rate (95% CI)	n = 63 87.1% (79.0–95.3)	0.006	49 73.5% (61.2–85.8)	0.988	160 68.6% (61.3–75.9)	0.011	n = 38 48.9% (32.6–65.2)	0.480	n = 41 36.6% (21.9–51.3)	0.459	n = 22 53.6% (32.4–74.8)
(b) Cancer-related survival											
Any pN 5-year rate (95% CI)	n = 265 96.6% (94.2–99.0)	0.300	n = 155 95.5% (92.0–99.0)	0.025	n = 433 89.2% (86.1–92.3)	0.039	n = 67 78.3% (67.3–89.3)	0.049	n = 75 63.5% (51.9–75.1)	0.042	n = 52 85.1% (74.9–95.3)
pN0 5-year rate (95% CI)	n = 202 97.7% (95.5–99.9)	0.541	n = 106 96.7% (93.0–100)	0.071	n = 273 92,9 (89.6–96.2)	0.087	n = 29 100%	0.006	n = 34 84.0% (71.1–96.9)	0.071	n = 30 96.2% (88.8–100)
pN1,2 5-year rate (95% CI)	n = 63 93.2% (86.7–99.7)	0.565	49 92.8% (85.0–100)	0.217	160 82.8 (76.5–89.1)	0.004	n = 38 61.8% (44.4–79.2)	0.287	n = 41 46.5% (28.5–64.5)	0.428	n = 22 69.6% (49.2–90.0)

3.6. Cancer-Related Survival

Finally, the 5-year rate of cancer-related survival of all patients was 89.3% (87.3–91.3%). It decreased significantly from 95.5% in pT3a patients over 89.2% in pT3b,c ($p = 0.025$) to 78.3% in pT3d ($p = 0.039$; Table 4b, Figure 2d). Again, a significant difference in pN1,2 patients was found between pT3c,d and pT3d (82.8% vs. 61.8%; $p = 0.004$).

In nearly all the analyses, a nonsignificant rather worse prognosis was observed in pT4a patients than in pT4b patients, possibly due to the higher rate of metachronous peritoneal metastases in pT4a carcinomas.

3.7. Cox Regression Analysis

In univariate and multivariate Cox regression analyses (Tables 5 and 6), pT3b,c was defined as the reference group and set as 1.0. This enabled us to investigate whether the prognosis of pT3a is significantly better and the prognosis of pT3d patients is significantly worse compared to pT3b,c. In the multivariate analysis of distant metastasis, we found that metastases were diagnosed significantly less frequently in pT3a carcinomas than in pT3b,c, while they occurred almost significantly more frequently in pT3d carcinomas. In multivariate analysis of disease-free survival, the prognosis of pT3a patients was found to be significantly better, and the prognosis of pT3d patients was nonsignificantly worse when compared to pT3b,c.

Table 5. Distant metastases, multivariate Cox regression analysis (n = 1047).

			Univariate Analysis			Multivariate Analysis		
		n	Hazard Ratio	95% CI	p	Hazard Ratio	95% CI	p
Sex	Male	602	1.0					
	Female	445	0.8	0.6–1.1	0.126			
ASA*	ASA I-II	730	1.0					
	ASA III-IV	300	1.3	0.9–1.8	0.148			
Tumor site	Right colon	511	1.0					
	Left colon	536	1.3	1.0–1.8	0.082			
Emergencies	Elective surgery	931	1.0			1.0		
	Emergency presentation	116	2.5	1.7–3.6	<0.001	1.8	1.2–2.7	0.003
Surgical procedure	Colon standard resection	787	1.0					
	Colon extended resection	260	1.2	0.9–1.7	0.308			
pT category	pT2 (muscularis propria)	265	0.4	0.2–0.6	<0.001	0.5	0.3–0.8	0.004
	pT3a (≤1 mm)	155	0.4	0.2–0.7	0.002	0.4	0.2–0.8	0.007
	pT3b,c (>1–15 mm)	433	1.0			1.0		
	pT3d (>15 mm)	67	2.2	1.4–3.6	0.001	1.6	1.0–2.5	0.074
	pT4a (serosa)	75	2.6	1.7–3.9	<0.001	2.1	1.4–3.2	0.001
	pT4b (other organs)	52	2.0	1.1–3.4	0.015	2.0	1.1–3.4	0.017
pN category	pN0	674	1.0			1.0		
	pN1	261	2.3	1.6–3.3	<0.001	2.0	1.4–2.9	<0.001
	pN2	112	5.2	3.6–7.6	<0.001	3.4	2.2–5.3	<0.001
Grading	G1,2	699	1.0			1.0		
	G3,4	348	1.4	1.0–1.9	0.031	1.0	0.7–1.3	0.831
Lymphatic invasion	No	737	1.0			1.0		
	Yes	309	2.7	2.0–3.7	<0.001	1.3	0.9–1.8	0.197
Venous invasion	No	1012	1.0			1.0		
	Yes	34	2.3	1.3–4.3	0.007	1.2	0.7–2.3	0.513

Table 6. Disease-free survival, multivariate Cox regression analysis (n = 1047).

			Univariate Analysis			Multivariate Analysis Adjusted for Age		
		n	Hazard Ratio	95% CI	p	Hazard Ratio	95% CI	p
Sex	Male	602	1.0					
	Female	445	0.9	0.7–1.0	0.072			
ASA*	ASA I-II	730	1.0			1.0		
	ASA III-IV	300	2.4	2.0–2.9	<0.001	1.7	1.4–2.0	<0.001
Tumor site	Right colon	511	1.0					
	Left colon	536	0.9	0.8–1.1	0.265			
Emergencies	Elective surgery	931	1.0			1.0		
	Emergency presentation	116	2.2	1.7–2.7	<0.001	1.5	1.2–1.9	0.002
Surgical procedure	Colon standard resection	787	1.0					
	Colon extended resection	260	1.0	0.9–1.3	0.649			
pT category	pT2 (muscularis propria)	265	0.7	0.6–0.9	0.007	0.8	0.7–1.0	0.096
	pT3a (≤1 mm)	155	0.7	0.5–0.9	0.015	0.7	0.5–1.0	0.024
	pT3b,c (>1–15 mm)	433	1.0			1.0		
	pT3d (>15 mm)	67	1.5	1.1–2.1	0.020	1.2	0.9–1.7	0.281
	pT4a (serosa)	75	1.8	1.4–2.4	<0.001	1.4	1.1–2.0	0.018
	pT4b (other organs)	52	1.4	0.9–1.9	0.095	1.2	0.8–1.7	0.365

Table 6. Cont.

			Univariate Analysis			Multivariate Analysis Adjusted for Age		
		n	Hazard Ratio	95% CI	p	Hazard Ratio	95% CI	p
pN category	pN0	674	1.0			1.0		
	pN1	261	1.1	0.9–1.4	0.175	1.1	0.9–1.4	0.255
	pN2	112	2.1	1.6–2.7	<0.001	1.6	1.2–2.2	0.001
Grading	G1,2	699	1.0					
	G3,4	348	1.1	0.9–1.3	0.208			
Lymphatic invasion	No	737	1.0			1.0		
	Yes	309	1.5	1.3–1.8	<0.001	1.2	1.0–1.5	0.051
Venous invasion	No	1012	1.0			1.0		
	Yes	34	1.7	1.2–2.6	0.008	1.3	0.8–2.0	0.251

3.8. Adjuvant Chemotherapy

In Stage II, 7 of 408 patients (1.7%) received adjuvant chemotherapy (pT3a: n = 1/106, pT3b,c: n = 5/273, pT3d: n = 1/28). None of these patients with adjuvant chemotherapy developed distant metastases. One patient died within five years from distant metastases of an unknown primary.

In stage III, 161 of 247 patients (65.2%) received adjuvant chemotherapy (pT3a: n = 30/49, pT3b,c: n = 108/160, pT3d: n = 23/38). The 5-year rates of distant metastases were 39.7% (95% CI 27.4–52.0) in stage III patients who did not receive chemotherapy and 22.4% (15.9–28.9) in patients who underwent adjuvant chemotherapy ($p = 0.003$). In the 86 patients with stage III who did not receive adjuvant chemotherapy, the 5-year rates of distant metastases were as follows: pT3a (n = 19) 7.1%; pT3b,c (n = 52) 10.2%; pT3d (n = 15) 87.2%; pT3a vs. pT3b,c: $p = 0.151$; pT3b,c vs. pT3d: $p = 0.051$; pT3a vs. pT3d: $p < 0.001$. In patients with stage III disease who underwent adjuvant chemotherapy, the 5-year rates of distant metastases also increased with the depth of invasion: pT3a (n = 30) 10.2%; pT3b,c (n = 108) 21.2%; pT3d (n = 23) 44.1%; pT3a vs. pT3b,c: $p = 0.171$; pT3b,c vs. pT3d; $p = 0.024$; pT3a vs. pT3d: $p = 0.003$. Further details on the prognosis for pT3 subclassification in stage III patients with and without adjuvant chemotherapy are presented in Table S3.

4. Discussion

The depth of the invasion beyond the muscularis propria is an important prognostic factor in colon carcinoma. The TNM classification system classifies carcinomas that invade the pericolic fat tissue as pT3. In contrast, carcinomas that already have involved the serosa or adjacent organs or structures are classified as pT4, more precisely, pT4a and pT4b, respectively. The TNM system does not provide a subclassification for pT3. The prognostic inhomogeneity of pT3 and ypT3 has been discussed in previous studies for rectal carcinomas [3,4]. Our analyses also show that there is a wide range of prognoses in colon carcinomas depending on the depth of infiltration into the pericolic fat.

In all resected pT3 specimens, tumor invasion beyond the muscularis propria into the pericolic fat was measured in mm and transformed to an ordinal scale. Initially, during data collection, we used a four-level scale of pT3a, b, c, and d. Different from the analysis of rectal carcinoma, where we proposed a subdivision of up to 5 mm and more than 5 mm, we found in colon carcinomas that pT3b (invasion of >1–5 mm) and pT3c (>5–15 mm) had a very similar prognosis. Therefore, we suggest a three-level subdivision of pT3 for colon carcinomas into pT3a ($\leq$1 mm), pT3b,c (>1–15 mm), and pT3d (>15 mm).

The majority of patients, approximately two-thirds, belong to the intermediate risk group (pT3b,c) with a depth of invasion of more than 1 mm but not more than 15 mm. However, patients with a minimal invasion of up to 1 mm (pT3a) have a favorable prognosis that is comparable to patients with pT2 carcinomas. This is the case for 26% of pT3 patients without lymph node metastases and for almost 21% of pT3 patients with lymph node metastases. In contrast, patients with tumor invasion into the pericolic fat tissue of more than 15 mm (pT3d) have a significantly worse prognosis, comparable to patients with pT4 carcinomas. This concerns 7% of pT3 pN0 patients and 12% of pT3 pN1,2 patients.

The inhomogeneity of pT3 could be confirmed for stage III patients without and with adjuvant chemotherapy. The 5-year rate of distant metastases increased with the depth of invasion in the group of patients without adjuvant chemotherapy and in the patients with adjuvant treatment. Patients with pT3d pN1,2 carcinomas without adjuvant chemotherapy had the worst prognosis, with a 5-year rate of distant metastasis of 87.2% and a 5-year rate of disease-free survival of only 6.7%. Between 1998 and 2015, adjuvant chemotherapy regimens evolved from 5-FU/FS to combinations with oxaliplatin, such as FOLFOX or XELOX. The different chemotherapy regimens were not included in the analyses. Currently, the chemotherapy regimen is selected primarily with regard to the age and comorbidities of the patients. Whether different regimens can be recommended for the different pT3 subcategories will be an important future question.

Recently, Panarelli et al. [13] highlighted the lack of consistent reproducibility of the AJCC/UICC criteria for classifying deeply invasive colon cancers, in particular, the distinction between deep pT3 (comparable to pT3d) and pT4a (invasion of the serosa). In general, moderate agreement ($\kappa = 0.52$) was achieved by gastrointestinal pathologists when the tumor had a well-delineated pushing deep border. Still, it was only slight ($\kappa = 0.16$) when an inflammatory reaction was present at the advancing tumor edge. The problems with assigning deep T3 versus T4a status reflect the ambiguous definition of serosal penetration as a defining feature of pT4a. In our own experience and as highlighted in the aforementioned Panarelli et al.'s study, this issue is complicated by several factors, including limited reliability on gross findings that are considered suspicious for serosal penetration and the degree of sampling for its verification. On occasion, grossly suspected serosal penetration turns out to be just a deep T3 with an associated inflammatory reaction at the advancing deep tumor edge. Diffusely infiltrating carcinomas are frequently associated with fibroinflammatory and fibrovascular granulating tissues that may result in complete obliteration of the residual subserosal tissue at the advancing tumor edge. This issue has been highlighted in the study by Panarelli et al. as one of the major confusing factors in assigning a pT3 versus pT4a category. Another confounding factor is the tendency of inured or preached serosal tissue to undergo a process of healing, which ultimately results in an apparently intact fibroinflammatory layer between the advancing tumor edge and the serosal surface. This finding might justify assigning a T3 instead of T4a category by general surgical pathologists. Adherence of adjacent omental, mesenteric, or other peritoneal fatty tissue may seal such foci of serosal penetration, suggesting pT3. In their study, Panarelli et al. concluded that the histologic criteria for recognizing serosal penetration represent a persistent source of diagnostic ambiguity for both gastrointestinal and general surgical pathologists in assigning the pT category for colon carcinomas. This significant overlap and confusion regarding deep pT3 versus pT4 could explain the very similar prognosis of the two categories observed in our current study.

The most important difference in the treatment between pN0 and pN+ colon cancer patients is that adjuvant chemotherapy is generally recommended for stage III (pN+) patients. In stage II (pN0), adjuvant chemotherapy is limited to high-risk groups. Therefore, identifying high-risk and low-risk groups is particularly important in stage II. pT3d cancers mainly behave like pT4 cancers. Therefore, these patients belong to a high-risk group for whom adjuvant therapy should also be discussed in stage II [14].

Another risk factor that plays an important role in prognosis, especially in node-negative colon cancer, is the number of regional lymph nodes examined [15,16]. However, in the cohort that we analyzed, only six of 1047 patients had fewer than 12 lymph nodes examined. Swanson et al. also found the left colon to be a risk factor in stage II colon cancer [16]. This could not be confirmed by our data. However, in a previous analysis, including patients treated between 1981 and 1997 at our department, we identified left-sided carcinomas of the sigmoid or descending colon, emergency presentation, a depth of invasion of >15 mm beyond the outer border of the muscularis propria and pT4 lesions as the major risk factors for stage II colon carcinoma [14]. The current German S3 guideline for colorectal carcinoma recommends considering adjuvant chemotherapy in stage II patients with selected risk situations (pT4, tumor perforation, emergency presentation, <12 regional lymph nodes examined). In cases of proven microsatellite instability (MSI-H), adjuvant chemotherapy should not be applied in stage II. This is based on the better long-term prognosis of patients with MSI-H colon carcinoma [17].

The distribution of prognostic factors in the different subcategories of pT3 colon carcinomas showed an increasing rate of lymph node metastases, high-grade carcinomas, lymphatic invasion, and venous invasion with increasing depth of invasion. The attempt to present the subcategories of pT3 as an independent prognostic factor in multivariate Cox regression analysis has been successful only with limitations, most likely for distant metastasis. However, multivariate Cox regression analyses may represent a certain over-adjustment in this case. Nevertheless, we can prove for distant metastasis that if we set pT3b,c to 1.0, distant metastasis in pT3a and pT2 is similarly less frequent, and distant metastasis in pT3d and pT4a,b is similarly more frequent. The hazard ratios and their confidence intervals are similar in both cases. For disease-free survival, this could be shown less clearly.

To our knowledge, this is the only published study that examines a subdivision of pT3 in colon carcinoma patients. Further studies are therefore encouraged to confirm our results. In addition to the different treatment methods for colon and rectal carcinomas, the differences in the optimized subclassifications for colon (pT3a $\leq$ 1 mm; pT3b,c > 1–15 mm; pT3d > 15 mm) and rectal (pT3a,b $\leq$ 5 mm; pT3c,d > 5 mm) [3,4] carcinomas are one more reason to separate the TNM classification for colon and rectal carcinomas.

Our study has some limitations regarding the thickness of pericolic fat tissue. Usually, the pericolic fat is thinner in slim people than in overweight patients. Consequently, there could be subgroups of patients for whom the subclassification may be less meaningful. To the best of our knowledge, there is no study on the distribution patterns of pericolic fatty tissue, e.g., depending on age, sex, or body mass index. For low rectal cancer, Wong et al. [18] examined the thickness of mesorectal fat in 25 Chinese patients with T3 rectal carcinoma. They found the lateral mesorectal fat on the left and right sides to be thicker than the anterior or posterior. The mean thickness at 10 cm from the anal verge was <5 mm in 71% and <15 mm in 95% of the Chinese patients. Allen et al. [19] found a strong correlation between the volume of the visceral compartment area and the mesorectal area in both sexes but not for body mass index. Further limitations of this study are the long study duration with changes in adjuvant treatment over time, the retrospective character, and the single-center analysis.

5. Conclusions

The depth of the invasion beyond the muscularis propria is an important independent prognostic factor in pT3 colon carcinoma. A three-level subdivision of T3 in the TNM system into T3a ($\leq$1 mm), T3b (>1–15 mm), and T3c (>15 mm) is recommended (Figure 3).

T3 subclassification	Depth of invasion	Proposal for a new subclassification for T3 rectal carcinoma	Proposal for a new subclassification for T3 colon carcinoma
T3a	≤1 mm	T3a	T3a
T3b	>1-5 mm	T3a	T3b
T3c	>5-15 mm	T3b	T3b
T3d	>15 mm	T3b	T3c

Figure 3. Proposal for a new subclassification for T3 rectal and colon carcinoma.

Supplementary Materials: The following supporting information can be downloaded at: https://www.mdpi.com/article/10.3390/cancers14246186/s1, Table S1: Locoregional recurrences (n = 1047); 5-year rate all patients 2.9% (1.7–4.1%); Table S2: Overall survival, multivariate Cox regression analysis; Table S3: Prognosis in patients with stage III with and without adjuvant chemotherapy (n = 247).

Author Contributions: Conceptualization, S.M. and A.A.; methodology, S.M.; software, S.M.; validation, S.M. and A.A.; formal analysis, S.M.; investigation, S.M.; resources, S.M., M.B., C.-I.G., R.G., K.W. and A.A.; data curation, S.M.; writing—original draft preparation, S.M. and A.A.; writing—review and editing, S.M., M.B., C.-I.G., R.G., K.W. and A.A.; visualization, S.M.; supervision, A.A.; project administration, S.M. All authors have read and agreed to the published version of the manuscript.

Funding: This research received no external funding.

Institutional Review Board Statement: The study was conducted in accordance with the Declaration of Helsinki and approved by the Institutional Research Ethics Committee of Friedrich-Alexander Universität Erlangen-Nürnberg, Germany (protocol code 132_20 Bc, date of approval 30-04-2020).

Informed Consent Statement: Not required in this registry study.

Data Availability Statement: The data presented in the study are available on request from the corresponding author with the permission of the Institutional Research Ethics Committee of Friedrich-Alexander Universität Erlangen-Nürnberg, Germany.

Conflicts of Interest: The authors declare no conflict of interest.

References

1. AJCC (American Joint Commitee of Cancer). *Cancer Staging Manual*, 8th ed.; Amin, M.B., Edge, S.B., Greene, F.L., Compton, C.C., Gershenwald, J.E., Brookland, R.K., Meyer, L., Gress, D.M., Byrd, D.R., Winchester, D.P., Eds.; Springer: New York, NY, USA, 2017.
2. UICC (International Union of Cancer). *TNM Classification of Malignant Tumours*, 8th ed.; Brierley, J.D., Gospodarowicz, M.K., Wittekind, C., Eds.; Wiley Blackwell: Oxford, UK, 2017.
3. Merkel, S.; Mansmann, U.; Siassi, M.; Papadopoulos, T.; Hohenberger, W.; Hermanek, P. The prognostic inhomogeneity in pT3 rectal carcinomas. *Int. J. Colorectal. Dis.* **2001**, *16*, 298–304. [CrossRef] [PubMed]
4. Merkel, S.; Weber, K.; Schellerer, V.; Gohl, J.; Fietkau, R.; Agaimy, A.; Hohenberger, W.; Hermanek, P. Prognostic subdivision of ypT3 rectal tumours according to extension beyond the muscularis propria. *Br. J. Surg.* **2014**, *101*, 566–572. [CrossRef] [PubMed]
5. UICC (International Union of Cancer). *TNM Supplement. A Commentary on Uniform Use*, 2nd ed.; Wittekind, C., Henson, D.E., Hutter, R.V.P., Sobin, L.H., Eds.; Wiley & Sons: New York, NY, USA, 2001.
6. UICC (International Union of Cancer). *TNM Supplement. A Commentary on Uniform Use*, 3rd ed.; Wittekind, C., Henson, D.E., Hutter, R.V.P., Sobin, L.H., Eds.; Wiley & Sons: New York, NY, USA, 2003.
7. UICC (International Union of Cancer). *TNM Supplement. A Commentary on Uniform Use*, 4th ed.; Wittekind, C., Henson, D.E., Hutter, R.V.P., Sobin, L.H., Eds.; Wiley-Blackwell: New York, NY, USA, 2012.
8. UICC (International Union of Cancer). *TNM Supplement. A Commentary on Uniform Use*, 5th ed.; Wittekind, C.H., Brierley, J., Lee, A., van Eycken, E., Eds.; Wiley Blackwell: New York, NY, USA, 2019.

9. Hohenberger, W.; Weber, K.; Matzel, K.; Papadopoulos, T.; Merkel, S. Standardized surgery for colonic cancer: Complete mesocolic excision and central ligation–technical notes and outcome. *Colorectal Dis.* **2009**, *11*, 354–364. [CrossRef] [PubMed]
10. Merkel, S.; Weber, K.; Matzel, K.E.; Agaimy, A.; Gohl, J.; Hohenberger, W. Prognosis of patients with colonic carcinoma before, during and after implementation of complete mesocolic excision. *Br. J. Surg.* **2016**, *103*, 1220–1229. [CrossRef] [PubMed]
11. Schmiegel, W.; Buchberger, B.; Follmann, M.; Graeven, U.; Heinemann, V.; Langer, T.; Nothacker, M.; Porschen, R.; Rodel, C.; Rosch, T.; et al. S3-Leitlinie—Kolorektales Karzinom. *Z. Gastroenterol.* **2017**, *55*, 1344–1498. [CrossRef] [PubMed]
12. Greenwood, M. *The Errors of Sampling of the Survivorship Table Reports on Public Health and Medical Subjects*; Her Majesty's Stationery Office: London, UK, 1926; Volume 33.
13. Panarelli, N.C.; Hammer, S.T.G.; Lin, J.; Gopal, P.; Nalbantoglu, I.; Zhao, L.; Cheng, J.; Gersten, A.J.; McHugh, J.B.; Parkash, V.; et al. Reproducibility of AJCC Criteria for Classifying Deeply Invasive Colon Cancers Is Suboptimal for Consistent Cancer Staging. *Am. J. Surg. Pathol.* **2020**, *44*, 1381–1388. [CrossRef] [PubMed]
14. Merkel, S.; Wein, A.; Gunther, K.; Papadopoulos, T.; Hohenberger, W.; Hermanek, P. High-risk groups of patients with Stage II colon carcinoma. *Cancer* **2001**, *92*, 1435–1443. [CrossRef] [PubMed]
15. Burdy, G.; Panis, Y.; Alves, A.; Nemeth, J.; Lavergne-Slove, A.; Valleur, P. Identifying patients with T3-T4 node-negative colon cancer at high risk of recurrence. *Dis. Colon Rectum.* **2001**, *44*, 1682–1688. [CrossRef] [PubMed]
16. Swanson, R.S.; Compton, C.C.; Stewart, A.K.; Bland, K.I. The prognosis of T3N0 colon cancer is dependent on the number of lymph nodes examined. *Ann. Surg. Oncol.* **2003**, *10*, 65–71. [CrossRef] [PubMed]
17. Klingbiel, D.; Saridaki, Z.; Roth, A.D.; Bosman, F.T.; Delorenzi, M.; Tejpar, S. Prognosis of stage II and III colon cancer treated with adjuvant 5-fluorouracil or FOLFIRI in relation to microsatellite status: Results of the PETACC-3 trial. *Ann. Oncol.* **2015**, *26*, 126–132. [CrossRef] [PubMed]
18. Wong, E.M.; Lai, B.M.; Fung, V.K.; Cheung, H.Y.; Ng, W.T.; Law, A.L.; Lai, A.Y.; Khoo, J.L. Limitation of radiological T3 subclassification of rectal cancer due to paucity of mesorectal fat in Chinese patients. *Hong Kong Med. J.* **2014**, *20*, 366–370. [CrossRef] [PubMed]
19. Allen, S.D.; Gada, V.; Blunt, D.M. Variation of mesorectal volume with abdominal fat volume in patients with rectal carcinoma: Assessment with MRI. *Br. J. Radiol.* **2007**, *80*, 242–247. [CrossRef] [PubMed]

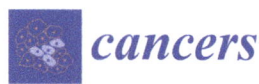 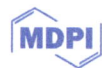

Article

Prognostic Value of Metastatic Lymph Node Ratio and Identification of Factors Influencing the Lymph Node Yield in Patients Undergoing Curative Colon Cancer Resection

Paweł Mroczkowski [1,2,3], Samuel Kim [2,4], Ronny Otto [2], Hans Lippert [2,5], Radosław Zajdel [6,7], Karolina Zajdel [7] and Anna Merecz-Sadowska [6,8,*]

1. Department for General and Colorectal Surgery, Medical University of Lodz, Pl. Hallera 1, 90-647 Lodz, Poland; pawel.mroczkowski@umed.lodz.pl
2. Institute for Quality Assurance in Operative Medicine Ltd., Otto-von-Guericke-University, Leipziger Str. 44, 39120 Magdeburg, Germany; samuel.kim@gmx.net (S.K.); ronny.otto@med.ovgu.de (R.O.); hans.lippert@med.ovgu.de (H.L.)
3. Department for Surgery, University Hospital Knappschaftskrankenhaus, Ruhr-University, In der Schornau 23-25, 44892 Bochum, Germany
4. Sanitätsversorgungszentrum Torgelow, Bundeswehr Neumühler Str. 10b, 17358 Torgelow, Germany
5. Department for General, Visceral and Vascular Surgery, Otto-von-Guericke-University, Leipziger Str. 44, 39120 Magdeburg, Germany
6. Department of Economic and Medical Informatics, University of Lodz, 90-214 Lodz, Poland; radoslaw.zajdel@uni.lodz.pl
7. Department of Medical Informatics and Statistics, Medical University of Lodz, 90-645 Lodz, Poland; karolina.smigiel@umed.lodz.pl
8. Department of Allergology and Respiratory Rehabilitation, Medical University of Lodz, 90-725 Lodz, Poland
* Correspondence: anna.merecz-sadowska@uni.lodz.pl

Simple Summary: In patients with colon cancer, the number of lymph nodes examined during surgery can have a significant impact on their long-term survival. We conducted a study with over 7000 patients and found that those who had at least 12 lymph nodes evaluated had better survival rates. A younger age, specific cancer stages, and a right-sided tumor location were associated with a higher number of lymph nodes examined. Additionally, we discovered that the ratio of metastatic to examined nodes (LNR) was a valuable predictor of survival and provided more precise information than the conventional pN classification system. This research emphasizes the importance of a thorough lymph node evaluation in colon cancer patients for accurate prognosis and treatment decisions.

Abstract: Due to the impact of nodal metastasis on colon cancer prognosis, adequate regional lymph node resection and accurate pathological evaluation are required. The ratio of metastatic to examined nodes may bring an additional prognostic value to the actual staging system. This study analyzes the identification of factors influencing a high lymph node yield and its impact on survival. The lymph node ratio was determined in patients with fewer than 12 or at least 12 evaluated nodes. The study included patients after radical colon cancer resection in UICC stages II and III. For the lymph node ratio (LNR) analysis, node-positive patients were divided into four categories: i.e., LNR 1 (<0.05), LNR 2 ($\geq$0.05; <0.2), LNR 3 ($\geq$0.2; <0.4), and LNR 4 ($\geq$0.4), and classified into two groups: i.e., those with <12 and $\geq$12 evaluated nodes. The study was conducted on 7012 patients who met the set criteria and were included in the data analysis. The mean number of examined lymph nodes was 22.08 (SD 10.64, median 20). Among the study subjects, 94.5% had 12 or more nodes evaluated. These patients were more likely to be younger, women, with a lower ASA classification, pT3 and pN2 categories. Also, they had no risk factors and frequently had a right-sided tumor. In the multivariate analysis, a younger age, ASA classification of II and III, high pT and pN categories, absence of risk factors, and right-sided location remained independent predictors for a lymph node yield $\geq$12. The univariate survival analysis of the entire cohort demonstrated a better five-year overall survival (OS) in patients with at least 12 lymph nodes examined (68% vs. 63%, $p = 0.027$).

Citation: Mroczkowski, P.; Kim, S.; Otto, R.; Lippert, H.; Zajdel, R.; Zajdel, K.; Merecz-Sadowska, A. Prognostic Value of Metastatic Lymph Node Ratio and Identification of Factors Influencing the Lymph Node Yield in Patients Undergoing Curative Colon Cancer Resection. *Cancers* **2024**, *16*, 218. https://doi.org/10.3390/cancers16010218

Academic Editors: Yutaka Midorikawa and Susanne Merkel

Received: 3 November 2023
Revised: 10 December 2023
Accepted: 31 December 2023
Published: 2 January 2024

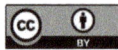

Copyright: © 2024 by the authors. Licensee MDPI, Basel, Switzerland. This article is an open access article distributed under the terms and conditions of the Creative Commons Attribution (CC BY) license (https://creativecommons.org/licenses/by/4.0/).

The LNR groups showed a significant association with OS, reaching from 75.5% for LNR 1 to 33.1% for LNR 4 ($p < 0.001$) in the ≥ 12 cohort, and from 74.8% for LNR2 to 49.3% for LNR4 ($p = 0.007$) in the <12 cohort. This influence remained significant and independent in multivariate analyses. The hazard ratios ranged from 1.016 to 2.698 for patients with less than 12 nodes, and from 1.248 to 3.615 for those with at least 12 nodes. The LNR allowed for a more precise estimation of the OS compared with the pN classification system. The metastatic lymph node ratio is an independent predictor for survival and should be included in current staging and therapeutic decision-making processes.

Keywords: colon cancer; lymph nodes; lymph node yield; lymph node ratio; five-year overall survival

1. Introduction

Colorectal cancer (CRC) is a complex and multifactorial disease with a significant global impact. It ranks as the third most frequently diagnosed cancer and the second leading cause of cancer-related mortality worldwide. Based on the site of onset, rectal cancer comprises 49.66% of cases, whereas colon cancer accounts for 49.09%. When considering both sites together, they collectively represent 1.25% of all cases.

The exact causes of CRC remain uncertain, although they may be associated with various factors such as genetic and dietary elements, as well as noncancerous health conditions. The risk of CRC rises with advancing age. Incidence and mortality rates for CRC are relatively low up to the age of 45; however, later they significantly increase. The highest incidence is observed in the age group over 80 years. Nonetheless, a noteworthy number of cases may still be observed among adolescents.

The epithelial cells of the mucosa in the colon and rectum can go through various stages of development, including hyperplasia, atypical hyperplasia, and adenomas. These adenomas have the potential to progress into carcinomas. In the early stages of CRC, the disease is usually limited to the mucosa and submucosa of the intestinal wall, and lymphatic metastasis is rare at this point. However, when the tumor penetrates the submucosal layer, lymphatic metastasis can occur. CRC usually metastasizes to the liver, lungs, lymph nodes of the abdominal cavity, and the peritoneum [1–4].

CRC is a complex, multi-step disease whose development depends on the accumulation of genetic and epigenetic alterations. These include the loss of tumor suppressor function (including APC and p53) and activation of proto-oncogenes (including KRAS and BRAF). Such molecular derangements ultimately lead to dysregulated cell proliferation, inhibited apoptosis, and the activation of growth-promoting signaling pathways [5–7].

Circulating tumor DNA (ctDNA) refers to fragmented DNA from tumor cells that is released into the bloodstream. In metastatic CRC, ctDNA enables noninvasive molecular profiling to identify actionable biomarkers and guide targeted therapy decisions. Specifically, ctDNA analysis can effectively determine the mutation status, microsatellite instability, and tumor mutational burden. However, tissue biopsy remains the gold standard, with a higher sensitivity for detecting certain genomic alterations. But for CRC, ctDNA has high detection rates nearing 100% in metastatic disease. Ongoing studies continue to evaluate concordance between ctDNA and tissue sequencing across various genomic biomarkers. Overall, ctDNA is becoming an invaluable tool for genotyping and tracking tumor dynamics in CRC [8–10].

Early stages of CRC often give no symptoms. As the disease progresses, patients typically experience symptoms such as hematochezia, intestinal obstruction, abdominal mass, and various systemic symptoms. The five-year overall survival (OS) rate varies depending on the disease stage, with a rate of 90% at stage I, 70–80% at stage II, and 40–65% at stage III. The risk of progression also correlates with the stage of the primary tumor; namely, it is 30% for stage II and 50% for stage III. Additionally, the risk is higher in the first two years following radical surgery [11,12].

This work focuses on colon cancer patients. The management of colon cancer patients is primarily determined by the stage of the disease at diagnosis, underscoring the need for a thorough approach to diagnosing, assessing, and treating the condition. Adequate lymphadenectomy, recently described in the concept of a complete mesocolic excision (CME), remains a crucial element of surgical treatment in nonmetastatic colon cancer [13]. The removal and analysis of lymph nodes play both a therapeutic and prognostic role. The involvement of the lymph nodes determines the stage of the disease, its prognosis and potential indication for adjuvant strategies [11,14].

The current standard of care for stage III colon cancer is immediate resection followed by adjuvant chemotherapy. Adjuvant chemotherapy has been shown to reduce the risk of recurrence and improve the OS in this patient population. Over the past decades, several landmark trials have established the efficacy of various chemotherapeutic regimens in the adjuvant setting [15–17]. Initially, studies demonstrated the efficacy of adjuvant fluorouracil (5-FU) and folinic acid in colon cancer. IMPACT investigators demonstrated the benefits of using 5-FU and folinic acid, increasing the OS from 78% to 83% [18]. The addition of oxaliplatin to 5-FU/folinic acid (FOLFOX regimen) was then validated as more effective than 5-FU regimens alone, becoming the new standard of care. The addition of oxaliplatin was first suggested with the MOSAIC trial, showing a significantly improved six-year OS rate of 78.5% compared to 72.9% with 5-FU alone [19]. More recently, oral fluoropyrimidines like capecitabine combined with oxaliplatin (CAPOX) have shown similar improvements in patient outcomes. The XELOXA trial found that combination therapy with capecitabine and oxaliplatin was superior to 5-FU alone, with a 5-year OS rate of 73% compared to 67% [20]. Thus, an oxaliplatin-based doublet therapy with 5-FU/folinic acid or capecitabine is now the backbone of adjuvant treatment for resected stage III colon cancer [15–17].

Accurate lymph node resection, analysis, and examination (LNE) are crucial in predicting the future outcomes of patients who underwent radical surgery for colon cancer [21]. According to the guidelines issued by the American Joint Committee on Cancer (AJCC), it is recommended to assess a minimum of 12 lymph nodes in order to meet the threshold requirement [22]. In the case of lymph node involvement (stage III colon cancer), there is a risk of misclassification into stages I or II, if the number of LNEs is insufficient. Such misclassification may result in patients not receiving the appropriate adjuvant therapy. Therefore, in recent reports, it has been indicated that an increased number of LNEs correlates with improved prognosis [23–26].

In the seventh edition of classification of malignant tumors (TNM), the AJCC introduced a subdivision of the N parameter for colon cancer, which includes N1a (only 1 metastatic node), N1b (2–3 positive nodes), N2a (4–6 positive lymph nodes), and N2b ($\geq$7 positive lymph nodes). However, the number of LNEs is still not part of the TNM staging system [27,28]. Therefore, there have been suggestions to use the lymph node ratio (LNR) as an improvement in the staging of CRC. The LNR is determined by calculating the ratio of metastatic lymph nodes to the total number of resected lymph nodes. It is believed that the LNR has the potential to serve as a more accurate prognostic factor for CRC compared to the conventional N assessment within the current TNM staging system [29,30].

The present study investigated large real-life population-based cohorts undergoing colectomies for cancer to evaluate factors influencing the achievement of the 12 lymph node limit as well as the prognostic impact of the LNR, in comparison with the actual N-classification within the TNM staging system.

2. Materials and Methods

2.1. Patient Population

The study analyzed the complete data of 7012 patients treated for colon cancer in 122 hospitals that participated in an observational study entitled "Quality Assurance in Colorectal Cancer," managed by the An-Institute at the Otto von Guericke University Magdeburg, Germany in the years 2008–2012. Patients with UICC (Union Internationale Contre le Cancer, Geneva, Switzerland) stage II and III colon adenocarcinoma who underwent radical tumor resection were included. The colon was defined as the segment of the bowel between >16 cm from the anocutaneous line and ileocolic valve. Curative resection was defined as the complete resection of a macroscopic tumor with negative pathological margins, lymphadenectomy, and no evidence of metastases. Patients with rectal cancers, multiple colon cancers, and second primary tumors were excluded from the study.

Since it was an observational study, no ethical approval was required, as confirmed by the local ethics committee of the Otto von Guericke University Magdeburg. Written informed consent was obtained from each patient.

2.2. Data Collection

The hospitals were required to deliver data on every patient treated for colon cancer. The total number of reported patients was cross-checked with the hospital's financial report for insurance companies to avoid a selection bias. The enrolment questionnaire consisted of 68 questions related to personal data, risk factors, reasons for hospitalization, diagnosis prior to surgery, surgical procedure, surgery-related complications, results of pathology tests, and discharge (total: 334 items). Risk factors were defined based on the assessment prior to the surgical treatment and categorized as follows: none, cardiac, respiratory, renal, hepatogenic, nicotine abuse, alcohol abuse, diabetes mellitus, varicosis, and others. Each patient's body mass index (BMI) and American Society of Anesthesiologists (ASA) score were also recorded. The surgical procedures were classified by a surgeon and divided into categories including right hemicolectomy, extended right hemicolectomy, left hemicolectomy, extended left hemicolectomy, and sigmoid resection. The intraoperative course was described by the duration of the surgery, presence and technique of anastomosis, and intraoperative complications (bladder injury, bleeding necessitating > 2 red blood cell concentrates, ureter lesion, iatrogenic tumor perforation, spleen injury, intestinal injury, internal genital injury, problem regarding the capnoperitoneum, and anastomosis complication). The postoperative complications included general and special ones. The general postoperative complications were lung embolism, pulmonary problems (pleural effusion and atelectasis), pneumonia, urinary tract infection, fever (>38 °C, >2 days), cardiac problems, multiple organ failure, thrombosis, and renal problems. The postoperative special complications were bleeding (necessitating surgery), wound abscess, sepsis, anastomosis insufficiency, aseptic wound healing dysfunction, wound infection, intra-abdominal/retrorectal abscess, mechanical ileus (necessitating surgery), fecal fistula, peritonitis, atony lasting longer than three days, peristalsis dysfunction (not necessitating surgery), wound dehiscence, and colostomy complication. The number of resected regional lymph nodes and UICC classification were recorded based on the pathological report. Survival data were collected by review of medical records and comparison with available registers.

2.3. Statistical Analysis

In this analysis, constant variables were used with appropriate measurements and given as the mean with standard deviation, minimum and maximum or as the median, minimum and maximum. Categorical variables were displayed as absolute or relative frequencies. The chi-square test was used to proof the independency of categorical variables. For small sample numbers (<5), cross-tabulation or Fisher's exact test were used. For estimations of systematic differences between the groups, a test of normal distribution was performed (the Shapiro–Wilk test). In the first step, factors influencing lymph node yield (LNY) were analyzed univariately. The independence of the significant factors was verified in a multivariate regression and displayed as an odds ratio (OR) with a 95% confidence interval. For survival analysis, the patient population was divided in two groups: i.e., those with <12 and ≥ 12 examined lymph nodes, in order to exclude potential bias of a low LNY. In univariate survival analysis, the previously identified significant factors influencing LNY were tested according to the Kaplan–Meier method, using the log-rank test. The nodal positive subgroup was divided into four categories: LNR 1 (<0.05), LNR 2 (≥ 0.05; <0.2), LNR 3 (≥ 0.2; <0.4), and LNR 4 (≥ 0.4), as initially proposed by Berger et al. [21]. For multivariate survival analysis, the method of Cox regression was used. The specified hazard ratios (HR) were also given with 95% confidence intervals. All statistical comparisons were performed at the significance level of 5%. Statistical analysis was performed using IBM® SPSS® Statistics, Version 21.0.0, SPSS Inc. (New York, NY, USA).

3. Results

The main data analysis included 7012 patients with UICC stage II and III colon cancer who met the set criteria. The mean number of examined lymph nodes was 22.08 (SD 10.64, median 20). In the study group, 94.5% had 12 or more nodes evaluated. In patients with an LNE < 12, an average of 8.99 (95% CI: 8.78–9.21) nodes were analyzed by the pathologist and 1.14 (95% CI: 0.96–1.32) identified as positive, while in those with an LNE ≥ 12, an average of 22.84 (95% CI: 22.58–23.09) lymph nodes were analyzed and 1.93 (95% CI: 1.83–2.03) were found to be metastatic. Patients with 12 or more nodes were more likely to be younger, women, with a lower ASA classification, pT3 and pN2 categories, and had no risk factors. Additionally, an association with right-sided tumor location was observed as well (Table 1).

Table 1. Univariate analysis of lymph node harvest <12 and ≥12.

	<12 N (%)	≥12 N (%)	p-Value
Age			
<50	3 (0.8)	278 (4.2)	
50–60	44 (11.5)	842 (12.7)	
61–70	101 (26.1)	1643 (24.8)	0.018
71–80	140 (36.3)	2425 (36.6)	
81–90	91 (23.5)	1332 (20.1)	
>90	7 (1.8)	106 (1.6)	
Sex			
Male	225 (58.4)	3472 (52.4)	0.027
Female	161 (41.6)	3154 (47.6)	
ASA Classification			
I	21 (5.4)	417 (6.3)	
II	157 (40.6)	3114 (47.0)	<0.001
III	181 (47.0)	2889 (43.6)	
IV	27 (7.0)	206 (3.1)	
pT Category			
pT1	20 (5.1)	80 (1.2)	
pT2	29 (7.5)	278 (4.2)	<0.001
pT3	264 (68.5)	5036 (76.0)	
pT4	73 (18.9)	1232 (18.6)	
pN Category			
pN0	203 (52.5)	3545 (53.5)	
pN1	147 (38.1)	1955 (29.5)	<0.001
pN2	36 (9.4)	1126 (17.0)	
Risk Factors			
At least one	322 (83.4)	5115 (77.2)	0.004
None	64 (16.6)	1511 (22.8)	
Tumor Location			
Caecum	51 (13.1)	1199 (18.1)	0.011
Colon ascendens	36 (9.4)	1411 (21.3)	<0.001
Colon descendens	36 (9.4)	378 (5.7)	0.005
Colon sigmoideum	187 (48.3)	2319 (35.0)	<0.001
Flexura dextra	16 (4.2)	484 (7.3)	0.019
Flexura sinistra	21 (5.5)	305 (4.6)	0.449
Colon transversum	39 (10.1)	530 (8.0)	0.075

Table 1. Cont.

	<12 N (%)	≥12 N (%)	p-Value
UICC			
II	203 (52.5)	3545 (53.5)	0.682
III	183 (47.5)	3081 (46.5)	
Grading			
G1	8 (2.1)	146 (2.2)	
G2	288 (74.7)	4777 (72.1)	0.490
G3	88 (22.7)	1690 (25.5)	
G4	2 (0.5)	13 (0.2)	
Access			
Laparotomy	331 (85.6)	5599 (84.5)	
Laparoscopy	25 (6.5)	411 (6.2)	0.276
Laparoscopic-assisted	19 (5.0)	477 (7.2)	
conversion	11 (2.9)	139 (2.1)	
Intraoperative Complications			
At least one	11 (2.9)	166 (2.5)	0.661
None	375 (97.1)	6460 (97.5)	

In the multivariate analysis (Table 2), an age < 50, ASA classification of II and III, pT2, pT3, pT4, and pN2 categories, and absence of risk factors remained independent predictors for a LNY ≥ 12, as well as the right-sided location.

Table 2. Multivariate analysis of lymph node harvest ≥12.

	Odds Ratio	95% CI	p-Value
Age			
≥50	Referent		
<50	4.687	1.474–14.900	0.009
ASA Classification			
I	1.982	0.971–4.045	0.060
II	2.335	1.457–3.744	<0.001
III	1.994	1.261–3.152	0.003
IV	Referent		
pT Category			
pT1	Referent		
pT2	2.177	1.134–4.178	0.019
pT3	4.682	2.684–8.166	<0.001
pT4	3.490	1.934–6.297	<0.001
pN Category			
pN0	Referent		
pN1	0.960	0.743–1.241	0.757
pN2	1.788	1.228–2.604	0.002
Risk Factor			
At least one	Referent		
None	1.466	1.030–2.087	0.034
Tumor Location			
Left side	Referent		
Right side	2.309	1.805–2.955	<0.001
Caecum transversum	1.042	0.721–1.508	0.825

A univariate survival analysis of the entire cohort (Table 3) demonstrated a better five-year OS in patients with at least 12 lymph nodes examined (68% vs. 63%, $p = 0.027$, Figure 1). The LNR groups (N = 183 for <12 LNY cohort: N = 85 for LNR 2, N = 56 for LNR

3, and N = 42 for LNR 4; N = 3081 for ≥12 LNY cohort: N = 462 for LNR1, N = 1599 for LNR 2, N = 622 for LNR 3, and N = 398 for LNR 4) showed a significant association with the OS reaching from 75.5% for LNR 1 to 33.1% for LNR 4 ($p < 0.001$) in the ≥12 cohort, and from 74.8% for LNR 2 to 49.3% for LNR 4 ($p = 0.007$) in the <12 cohort (Figures 2 and 3). This influence remained significant and independent from multivariate analyses.

Table 3. Univariate survival analysis for lymph node yield <12 and ≥12. Numbers in percentages.

	<12		≥12	
	5-Years-OS in %	p-Value	5-Years-OS in %	p-Value
LNR				
LNR 1	-		75.5	
LNR 2	74.8	0.007	69.5	<0.001
LNR 3	58.3		54.5	
LNR 4	49.3		33.1	
Sex				
Male	60.9	0.762	67.2	0.591
Female	67.1		68.9	
ASA Classification				
I	64.8		81.6	
II	74.6	0.001	75.5	<0.001
III	53.7		56.7	
IV	42.8		45.7	
pT Category				
pT1	75.8	0.004		
pT2	78.4		92.6	<0.001
pT3	67.0		80.7	
pT4	39.9		71.4	
pN Category				
pN1	68.2	0.005	70.7	<0.001
pN2	46.7		49.0	
Risk Factors				
At least one	60.6	0.046	63.4	<0.001
None	72.5		83.8	
Tumor Location				
Right side	50.3		64.1	
Left side	66.0	0.111	71.5	<0.001
Caecum transversum	73.8		70.8	
Intraoperative Complications				
At least one	53.6	0.492	64.4	0.329
None	63.3		68.1	
Morbidity				
No	67.6	0.049	71.4	<0.001
Yes	55.3		61.3	

The hazard ratios ranged from 1.016 to 2.698 for patients with less than 12 lymph nodes and from 1.248 to 3.615 for those with at least 12 lymph nodes. The LNR allowed a more precise estimation of the OS compared with the pN classification system for LNR 4 in the group with <12 lymph nodes and LNR 3 and LNR 4 in the group with ≥12 lymph nodes (Table 4).

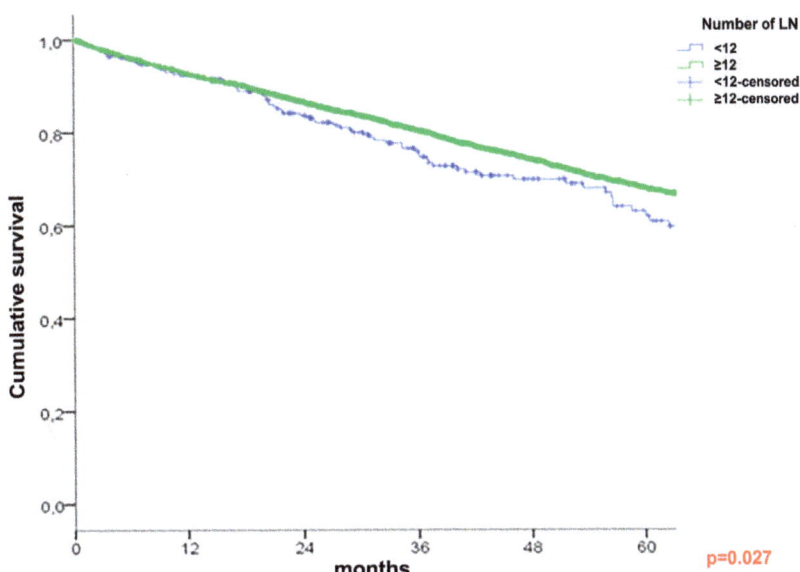

Figure 1. Overall survival in patients with <12 and ≥12 evaluated nodes.

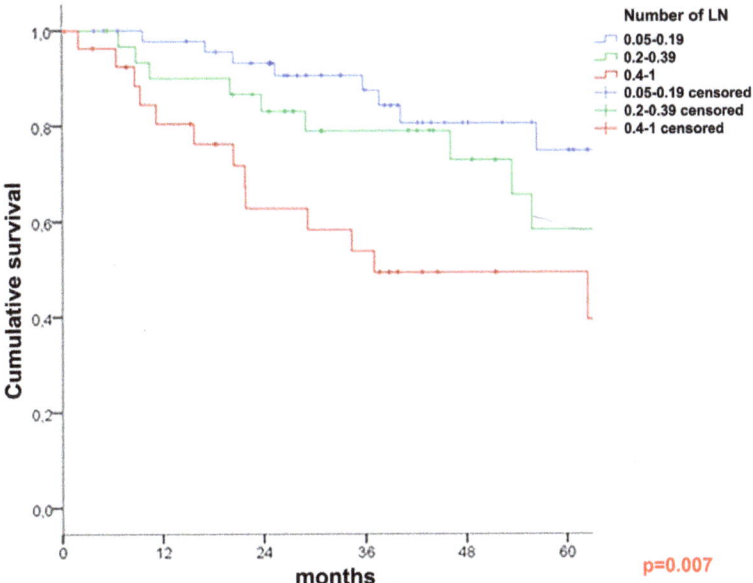

Figure 2. Overall survival in patients with <12 evaluated nodes.

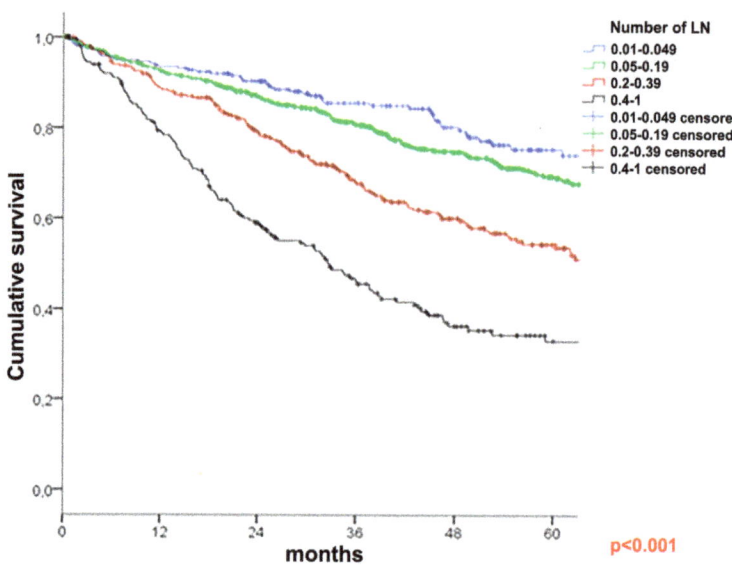

Figure 3. Overall survival in patients with ≥ 12 evaluated nodes.

Table 4. Cox multivariate models for 5-year OS.

	<12 Nodes		≥12 Nodes	
	Hazard Ratio (95% CI)	*p*-Value	Hazard Ratio (95% CI)	*p*-Value
LNR				
LNR 1			Referent	
LNR 2	Referent		1.248 (0.922–1.828)	0.152
LNR 3	1.016 (0.363–2.840)	0.976	1.976 (1.428–2.734)	<0.001
LNR 4	2.698 (1.083–6.718)	0.033	3.615 (2.589–5.047)	<0.001
Age		ns	1.046 (1.036–1.057)	<0.001
ASA Classification				
I	Referent	0.102	Referent	
II	0.273 (0.47–1.571)	0.146	1.120 (0.687–1.828)	0.649
III	0.672 (0.107–4.236)	0.672	1.720 (1.048–2.824)	0.032
IV	0.731 (0.091–5.872)	0.768	2.527 (1.338–4.773)	0.004
pT Category				
pT1	Referent		Referent	
pT2	0.969 (0.164–5.722)	0.972	2.113 (0.639–6.989)	0.220
pT3	0.813 (0.182–3.634)	0.787	3.316 (1.060–10.373)	0.039
pT4	3.578 (0.743–17.223)	0.112	5.997 (1.907–18.861)	0.002
pN Category				
pN1	Referent		Referent	
pN2	2.957 (1.362–6.421)	0.006	1.832 (1.540–2.179)	<0.001
Tumor Location				
Left		ns	Referent	
Right			1.384 (1.151–1.664)	0.001
Caecum transversum			1.177 (0.830–1.670)	0.361
Morbidity		ns	1.324 (1.106–1.585)	0.002

ns = not significant (*p* > 0.05).

4. Discussion

The LNR and pN classification system were independent prognostic factors in both cohorts (<12 and ≥12 nodes). Comparing the HR and OS, the LNR in patients with ≥12 lymph nodes appears to give a more accurate prognosis than the pN categories: HR (LNR 4) = 3.615 vs. HR (pN2) = 1.832, while OS (LNR 4) = 33.1% vs. OS (pN2) = 49.0%. LNR 4 better predicts the OS than the pN2 category when at least 12 nodes are evaluated. These findings are complementary to previous references showing the LNR providing additional staging information to the current staging system. Berger et al., whose cutoffs were adopted in this study, showed the LNR to be a significant prognostic variable in stage II and III if at least 10 nodes were evaluated [31]. However, this initial cohort was significantly smaller (n = 3411) than in the present analysis, and the included patients were part of a randomized controlled trial, not a cohort from a real-life treatment. When analyzing 922 single-center colon cancer patients in stage III, Parnaby et al. demonstrated the superiority of LNR cutoffs of 18%, 42%, and 70% compared to the pN classification system using the Akaike information criterion [32]. In a Danish nationwide study including 8901 patients operated on for nonmetastatic colon cancer (incl. 1263 stage I cases), Lykke et al. showed an association of a high LNY with improved survival, as well as a prognostic advantage of the LNR compared to the pN classification system [33]. Chen et al. analyzed 36,712 colon cancer patients from the administrative National Cancer Institute Surveillance, Epidemiology, and End Results (SEER) database for the years 1992–2004. Similar to our findings, the authors noticed the best prognostic value of LNRs after an LNE ≥ 12, whereas the multivariate analysis suggested the ratio to be a better prognostic factor than the pN classification system [34]. Silva et al. demonstrated that the LNR is a strong predictor for tumor recurrence in stage III colon cancer [35]. Moreover, according to Jang et al., the LNR holds the potential to serve as an autonomous prognostic element for patients with stage IV colon cancer who undergo resection [36]. Additional evidence comes from Mirzaei et al. [37], who demonstrated that LNRs had significant prognostic value for both overall and disease-free survival in stage III colon cancer. Amri et al. [38] reported significant associations of LNRs with cancer-related mortality and recurrence in a cohort of over 1000 patients. Occhionorelli et al. [39] found LNRs to predict the 5-year overall and disease-free survival in emergency colon cancer surgery. In the study by Elbaiomy et al. [40], a high LNR was significantly associated with poorer progression-free and overall survival. Other authors, such as Jakob et al., Schiffman et al., or Mohan et al., could not find any additional prognostic value of LNRs [30,41,42]. However, due to a low number of cases (144–402 patients) and the subdivision of LNRs with only one cutoff, these results have a limited impact.

In our patient cohort with UICC II–III colon cancer, on average, 22.08 (SD 10.645, median 20) lymph nodes were examined. The correlation between LNE and a better OS has already been shown by multiple studies [43]. Foo et al. suggest that the LNY shows a substantial correlation with survival outcomes. A lymph node yield of 20 or more was linked to improved survival. Conversely, a lymph node yield of less than 12 did not demonstrate inferior survival outcomes when compared to those with node yields between 12 and 19 [44]. Lykke et al. propose that in UICC stage I–III colon cancer, a LNY exceeding the recommended 12 lymph nodes was linked to enhanced survival [45]. Our results show a significantly increased survival in patients with ≥12 nodes. Yet, the exact reason for this phenomenon is still uncertain. The evaluation of at least 12 nodes, recommended by numerous guidelines, is supposed to ensure accurate staging and prevent possible understaging and undertreatment. Lykke et al. observed stage migration in UICC III patients with more than 12 nodes evaluated [33]. Our results support this finding: node positive patients were more likely to be ranked into the pN2 category when at least 12 nodes were examined, while the pN1 category was more represented in patients with <12 nodes ($p < 0.001$). Also, the OS in both pN categories was higher in ≥12 nodes. Other authors reject this theory [46–50]. Budde et al. observed no improvement in staging despite the increasing number of examined nodes from 2004 to 2010 [51]. Another theory is that an increased number of nodes is found in patients with a better immunologic response to the tumor, which leads to increased survival [46,48,51–53]. Another additional explanation is that the LNE serves as proxy for quality of surgery and pathology [6,54].

According to our analysis, a younger age was accompanied by OR 4.7 for a LNY $\geq$ 12. Other studies confirmed this finding [55–60]. Chou et al. demonstrated a 9% reduction in LNY for each ten-year interval [59]. Lykke et al. and Nathan et al. observed a decreased OR in older patients (OR 1 to 0.452 and OR 1 to 0.720) [57,58]. This phenomenon results from an insufficient immune response in older patients [57,61]. Another explanation might be the risk reduction of the surgery at the cost of the LNY, prioritizing the minimization of anesthesia thanks to the shorter duration of the surgical procedure in older patients who are often dealing with comorbidities [59]. ASA classifications of II and III were associated with an adequate LNY, while Moro-Valdezate and Nash et al. did not find any statistical correlation [62,63]. In our multivariate analyses, female patients had no statistical benefit for a high LNY. Some authors showed a correlation with the female sex [57,58,61,64], whereas others did not obtain such results [46,63,65–67]. In the present study, no difference was found in the laparotomic and laparoscopic approaches, which confirmed the results of Beccera and Lykke et al. [56,57].

According to our study, a right-sided tumor location was beneficial for a LNY $\geq$ 12 (OR 2.3), which was congruent with other studies [56,57,63,68–72]. The left-sided tumor location was described by Becerra et al. as a risk factor for a yield < 12 (OR 1.158), and with an OR of 5.7–6.7 and even a high-risk factor by Choi et al. [56,64]. Some authors believe it is related to a variable lymphatic anatomy: lymph nodes are more likely to be found along the right-sided ileocolic artery than along the left-sided vessels [57,59,63]. Genetic–immunological causes are considered as well. Microsatellite instability was mainly associated with right-sided tumors. These types of tumors are more amenable to the immune system, resulting in higher yields [73,74].

In multivariate regression, a high pT category was associated with an LNE $\geq$ 12: especially pT3 tumors were found to have an OR of 4.6. Other studies report similar conclusions. Lykke et al. as well as Nathan et al. showed an increasing OR with increasing pT categories for an adequate yield [57,58]. In a Korean study, a low pT category was a risk factor for inadequate yield [64]. A proposed explanation is that tumor necrosis, which is more frequently found in a high pT category, leads to a higher antigen presentation for the immune system, resulting in an increased lymph node yield [57].

This study has several limitations. A multicentric study is based on voluntary participation of hospitals and family physicians, without the discipline and resources of randomized controlled trials. Also, due to the high rate of adequate LNEs, the cases < 12 nodes are low, which must be taken into account when interpreting this part of the results. Our data do not include information about oncological treatments administered after surgery–adjuvant chemotherapy, further resections, or palliative chemotherapy for metastatic disease.

5. Conclusions

The LNR allows for a better estimation of the overall survival compared to the pN status and shows remarkable differences in prognosis within nodal-positive patients. It is unclear why the LNR still remains outside of the UICC stage classification for colon cancer and is not included in the decision-making process concerning adjuvant therapies.

Author Contributions: Conceptualization, P.M. and H.L.; methodology, S.K. and R.O.; software, R.Z., R.O., A.M.-S. and K.Z.; validation, R.O., R.Z. and K.Z.; formal analysis, P.M. and S.K.; investigation, P.M., S.K. and H.L.; data curation, P.M., S.K., H.L., R.O., A.M.-S. and K.Z.; writing—original draft preparation, P.M. and S.K.; writing—review and editing, A.M.-S. and R.Z.; visualization, A.M.-S. and K.Z.; supervision, P.M. and R.Z.; project administration, P.M. All authors have read and agreed to the published version of the manuscript.

Funding: This research received no external funding.

Institutional Review Board Statement: Not applicable.

Informed Consent Statement: Informed consent was obtained from all subjects involved in the study.

Data Availability Statement: Data are contained within the article.

Conflicts of Interest: The authors declare no conflicts of interest.

References

1. Alzahrani, S.M.; Al Doghaither, H.A.; Al-Ghafari, A.B. General insight into cancer: An overview of colorectal cancer (Review). *Mol. Clin. Oncol.* **2021**, *15*, 271. [CrossRef] [PubMed]
2. Mármol, I.; Sánchez-de-Diego, C.; Pradilla Dieste, A.; Cerrada, E.; Rodriguez Yoldi, M.J. Colorectal Carcinoma: A General Overview and Future Perspectives in Colorectal Cancer. *Int. J. Mol. Sci.* **2017**, *18*, 197. [CrossRef] [PubMed]
3. Sung, H.; Ferlay, J.; Siegel, R.L.; Laversanne, M.; Soerjomataram, I.; Jemal, A.; Bray, F. Global Cancer Statistics 2020: GLOBOCAN Estimates of Incidence and Mortality Worldwide for 36 Cancers in 185 Countries. *CA Cancer J. Clin.* **2021**, *71*, 209–249. [CrossRef] [PubMed]
4. Siegel, R.L.; Wagle, N.S.; Cercek, A.; Smith, R.A.; Jemal, A. Colorectal cancer statistics, 2023. *CA Cancer J. Clin.* **2023**, *73*, 233–254. [CrossRef] [PubMed]
5. Labianca, R.; Beretta, G.D.; Kildani, B.; Milesi, L.; Merlin, F.; Mosconi, S.; Pessi, M.A.; Prochilo, T.; Quadri, A.; Gatta, G.; et al. Colon cancer. *Crit. Rev. Oncol. Hematol.* **2010**, *74*, 106–133. [CrossRef] [PubMed]
6. Slattery, M.L.; Herrick, J.S.; Mullany, L.E.; Samowitz, W.S.; Sevens, J.R.; Sakoda, L.; Wolff, R.K. The co-regulatory networks of tumor suppressor genes, oncogenes, and miRNAs in colorectal cancer. *Genes. Chromosomes Cancer.* **2017**, *56*, 769–787. [CrossRef] [PubMed]
7. Armaghany, T.; Wilson, J.D.; Chu, Q.; Mills, G. Genetic alterations in colorectal cancer. *Gastrointest. Cancer Res.* **2012**, *5*, 19–27.
8. de Abreu, A.R.; Op de Beeck, K.; Laurent-Puig, P.; Taly, V.; Benhaim, L. The Position of Circulating Tumor DNA in the Clinical Management of Colorectal Cancer. *Cancers* **2023**, *15*, 1284. [CrossRef]
9. Malla, M.; Loree, J.M.; Kasi, P.M.; Parikh, A.R. Using Circulating Tumor DNA in Colorectal Cancer: Current and Evolving Practices. *J. Clin. Oncol.* **2022**, *40*, 2846–2857. [CrossRef]
10. Dasari, A.; Morris, V.K.; Allegra, C.J.; Atreya, C.; Benson, A.B.; Boland, P.; Chung, K.; Copur, M.S.; Corcoran, R.B.; Deming, D.A.; et al. ctDNA applications and integration in colorectal cancer: An NCI Colon and Rectal-Anal Task Forces whitepaper. *Nat. Rev. Clin. Oncol.* **2020**, *17*, 757–770. [CrossRef]
11. Evdokimova, S.; Kornietskaya, A.; Bolotina, L.; Sidorov, D.; Kaprin, A. Postoperative Chemotherapy After Surgical Resection of Metachronous Metastases of Colorectal Cancer: A Systematic Review. *World J. Oncol.* **2023**, *14*, 26–31. [CrossRef] [PubMed]
12. Holtedahl, K.; Borgquist, L.; Donker, G.A.; Buntinx, F.; Weller, D.; Campbell, C.; Månsson, J.; Hammersley, V.; Braaten, T.; Parajuli, R. Symptoms and signs of colorectal cancer, with differences between proximal and distal colon cancer: A prospective cohort study of diagnostic accuracy in primary care. *BMC Fam. Pract.* **2021**, *22*. [CrossRef] [PubMed]
13. Dimitriou, N.; Griniatsos, J. Complete mesocolic excision: Techniques and outcomes. *World J. Gastrointest. Oncol.* **2015**, *7*, 383–388. [CrossRef] [PubMed]
14. Matsuda, T.; Yamashita, K.; Hasegawa, H.; Oshikiri, T.; Hosono, M.; Higashino, N.; Yamamoto, M.; Matsuda, Y.; Kanaji, S.; Nakamura, T.; et al. Recent updates in the surgical treatment of colorectal cancer. *Ann. Gastroenterol. Surg.* **2018**, *2*, 129–136. [CrossRef] [PubMed]
15. McCleary, N.J.; Benson, A.B.; Dienstmann, R. Personalizing Adjuvant Therapy for Stage II/III Colorectal Cancer. *Am. Soc. Clin. Oncol. Educ. B.* **2017**, *37*, 232–245. [CrossRef]
16. Taieb, J.; Gallois, C. Adjuvant chemotherapy for stage iii colon cancer. *Cancers* **2020**, *12*, 2679. [CrossRef]
17. Gonzalez-Angulo, A.M.; Fuloria, J. The role of chemotherapy in colon cancer. *Ochsner J.* **2002**, *4*, 163–167.
18. Efficacy of adjuvant fluorouracil and folinic acid in colon cancer. International Multicentre Pooled Analysis of Colon Cancer Trials (IMPACT) investigators. *Lancet* **1995**, *345*, 939–944. [CrossRef]
19. André, T.; Boni, C.; Navarro, M.; Tabernero, J.; Hickish, T.; Topham, C.; Bonetti, A.; Clingan, P.; Bridgewater, J.; Rivera, F.; et al. Improved overall survival with oxaliplatin, fluorouracil, and leucovorin as adjuvant treatment in stage II or III colon cancer in the MOSAIC trial. *J. Clin. Oncol.* **2009**, *27*, 3109–3116. [CrossRef]
20. Schmoll, H.J.; Tabernero, J.; Maroun, J.; de Braud, F.; Price, T.; Van Cutsem, E.; Hill, M.; Hoersch, S.; Rittweger, K.; Haller, D.G. Capecitabine Plus Oxaliplatin Compared With Fluorouracil/Folinic Acid As Adjuvant Therapy for Stage III Colon Cancer: Final Results of the NO16968 Randomized Controlled Phase III Trial. *J. Clin. Oncol.* **2015**, *33*, 3733–3740. [CrossRef]
21. Chang, G.J.; Rodriguez-Bigas, M.A.; Skibber, J.M.; Moyer, V.A. Lymph node evaluation and survival after curative resection of colon cancer: Systematic review. *J. Natl. Cancer Inst.* **2007**, *99*, 433–441. [CrossRef] [PubMed]
22. Weiser, M.R. AJCC 8th Edition: Colorectal Cancer. *Ann. Surg. Oncol.* **2018**, *25*, 1454–1455. [CrossRef] [PubMed]
23. Tsai, H.L.; Lu, C.Y.; Hsieh, J.S.; Wu, D.C.; Jan, C.M.; Chai, C.Y.; Chu, K.S.; Chan, H.M.; Wang, J.Y. The prognostic significance of total lymph node harvest in patients with T2-4N0M0 colorectal cancer. *J. Gastrointest. Surg.* **2007**, *11*, 660–665. [CrossRef] [PubMed]
24. Choi, H.K.; Law, W.L.; Poon, J.T.C. The optimal number of lymph nodes examined in stage II colorectal cancer and its impact of on outcomes. *BMC Cancer* **2010**, *10*, 267. [CrossRef]

25. Trepanier, M.; Erkan, A.; Kouyoumdjian, A.; Nassif, G.; Albert, M.; Monson, J.; Lee, L. Examining the relationship between lymph node harvest and survival in patients undergoing colectomy for colon adenocarcinoma. *Surgery* **2019**, *166*, 639–647. [CrossRef]
26. Norderval, S.; Solstad, Ø.B.; Hermansen, M.; Steigen, S.E. Increased lymph node retrieval decreases adjuvant chemotherapy rate for stage II colon cancer. *Scand. J. Gastroenterol.* **2016**, *51*, 949–955. [CrossRef]
27. Hari, D.M.; Leung, A.M.; Lee, J.H.; Sim, M.S.; Vuong, B.; Chiu, C.G.; Bilchik, A.J. AJCC cancer staging manual 7th edition criteria for colon cancer: Do the complex modifications improve prognostic assessment? *J. Am. Coll. Surg.* **2013**, *217*, 181–190. [CrossRef]
28. Brierley, J.D. (Ed.) *TNM Atlas*, 7th ed.; Wiley-Blackwell: Hoboken, NJ, USA, 2021; pp. 112–121.
29. Wang, L.P.; Wang, H.Y.; Cao, R.; Zhu, C.; Wu, X.Z. Proposal of a new classification for stage iii colorectal cancer based on the number and ratio of metastatic lymph nodes. *World J. Surg.* **2013**, *37*, 1094–1102. [CrossRef]
30. Schiffmann, L.; Eiken, A.K.; Gock, M.; Klar, E. Is the lymph node ratio superior to the Union for International Cancer Control (UICC) TNM system in prognosis of colon cancer? *World J. Surg. Oncol.* **2013**, *11*, 79. [CrossRef]
31. Berger, A.C.; Sigurdson, E.R.; LeVoyer, T.; Hanlon, A.; Mayer, R.J.; Macdonald, J.S.; Catalano, P.J.; Haller, D.G. Colon cancer survival is associated with decreasing ratio of metastatic to examined lymph nodes. *J. Clin. Oncol. Off. J. Am. Soc. Clin. Oncol.* **2005**, *23*, 8706–8712. [CrossRef]
32. Parnaby, C.N.; Scott, N.W.; Ramsay, G.; MacKay, C.; Samuel, L.; Murray, G.I.; Loudon, M.A. Prognostic value of lymph node ratio and extramural vascular invasion on survival for patients undergoing curative colon cancer resection. *Br. J. Cancer* **2015**, *113*, 212–219. [CrossRef] [PubMed]
33. Lykke, J.; Roikjaer, O.; Jess, P. The relation between lymph node status and survival in Stage I-III colon cancer: Results from a prospective nationwide cohort study. *Color. Dis.* **2013**, *15*, 559–565. [CrossRef] [PubMed]
34. Chen, S.L.; Steele, S.R.; Eberhardt, J.; Zhu, K.; Bilchik, A.; Stojadinovic, A. Lymph node ratio as a quality and prognostic indicator in stage III colon cancer. *Ann. Surg.* **2011**, *253*, 82–87. [CrossRef] [PubMed]
35. Dedavid e Silva, T.L.; Damin, D.C. Lymph node ratio predicts tumor recurrence in stage III colon cancer. *Rev. Col. Bras. Cir.* **2013**, *40*, 463–470. [CrossRef] [PubMed]
36. Jiang, C.; Wang, F.; Guo, G.; Dong, J.; Liu, S.; He, W.; Zhang, B.; Xia, L. Metastatic lymph node ratio as a prognostic indicator in patients with stage IV colon cancer undergoing resection. *J. Cancer* **2019**, *10*, 2534–2540. [CrossRef] [PubMed]
37. Zare Mirzaei, A.; Abdorrazaghi, F.; Lotfi, M.; Kazemi Nejad, B.; Shayanfar, N. Prognostic Value of Lymph Node Ratio in Comparison to Lymph Node Metastases in Stage III Colon Cancer. *Iran. J. Pathol.* **2015**, *10*, 127–135. [PubMed]
38. Amri, R.; Klos, C.L.; Bordeianou, L.; Berger, D.L. The prognostic value of lymph node ratio in colon cancer is independent of resection length. *Am. J. Surg.* **2016**, *212*, 251–257. [CrossRef]
39. Occhionorelli, S.; Andreotti, D.; Vallese, P.; Morganti, L.; Lacavalla, D.; Forini, E.; Pascale, G. Evaluation on prognostic efficacy of lymph nodes ratio (LNR) and log odds of positive lymph nodes (LODDS) in complicated colon cancer: The first study in emergency surgery. *World J. Surg. Oncol.* **2018**, *16*, 186. [CrossRef]
40. Elbaiomy, M.; Waheed, A.; Elkhodary, T. Prognostic value of lymph node ratio in lymph node-invaded colon cancer. *Ann. Oncol.* **2019**, *30*, IV34. [CrossRef]
41. Jakob, M.O.; Guller, U.; Ochsner, A.; Oertli, D.; Zuber, M.; Viehl, C.T. Lymph node ratio is inferior to pN-stage in predicting outcome in colon cancer patients with high numbers of analyzed lymph nodes. *BMC Surg.* **2018**, *18*, 81. [CrossRef]
42. Mohan, H.M.; Walsh, C.; Kennelly, R.; Ng, C.H.; O'Connell, P.R.; Hyland, J.M.; Hanly, A.; Martin, S.; Gibbons, D.; Sheahan, K.; et al. The lymph node ratio does not provide additional prognostic information compared with the N1/N2 classification in Stage III colon cancer. *Color. Dis.* **2017**, *19*, 165–171. [CrossRef] [PubMed]
43. McDonald, J.R.; Renehan, A.G.; O'Dwyer, S.T.; Haboubi, N.Y. Lymph node harvest in colon and rectal cancer: Current considerations. *World J. Gastrointest. Surg.* **2012**, *4*, 9–19. [CrossRef] [PubMed]
44. Foo, C.C.; Ku, C.; Wei, R.; Yip, J.; Tsang, J.; Chan, T.Y.; Lo, O.; Law, W.L. How does lymph node yield affect survival outcomes of stage I and II colon cancer? *World J. Surg. Oncol.* **2020**, *18*. [CrossRef] [PubMed]
45. Lykke, J.; Rosenberg, J.; Jess, P.; Roikjaer, O. Lymph node yield and tumour subsite are associated with survival in stage I-III colon cancer: Results from a national cohort study. *World J. Surg. Oncol.* **2019**, *17*, 62. [CrossRef] [PubMed]
46. Parsons, H.M.; Tuttle, T.M.; Kuntz, K.M.; Begun, J.W.; McGovern, P.M.; Virnig, B.A. Association Between Lymph Node Evaluation for Colon Cancer and Node Positivity Over the Past 20 Years. *JAMA* **2011**, *306*, 1089–1097. [CrossRef] [PubMed]
47. Van Erning, F.N.; Crolla, R.M.P.H.; Rutten, H.J.T.; Beerepoot, L.V.; van Krieken, J.H.J.M.; Lemmens, V.E.P.P. No change in lymph node positivity rate despite increased lymph node yield and improved survival in colon cancer. *Eur. J. Cancer* **2014**, *50*, 3221–3229. [CrossRef]
48. Bui, L.; Rempel, E.; Reeson, D.; Simunovic, M. Lymph node counts, rates of positive lymph nodes, and patient survival for colon cancer surgery in Ontario, Canada: A population-based study. *J. Surg. Oncol.* **2006**, *93*, 439–445. [CrossRef]
49. Wong, S.L.; Ji, H.; Hollenbeck, B.K.; Morris, A.M.; Baser, O.; Birkmeyer, J.D. Hospital lymph node examination rates and survival after resection for colon cancer. *JAMA* **2007**, *298*, 2149–2154. [CrossRef]
50. Porter, G.A.; Urquhart, R.; Bu, J.; Johnson, P.; Rayson, D.; Grunfeld, E. Improving Nodal Harvest in Colorectal Cancer: So What? *Ann. Surg. Oncol.* **2012**, *19*, 1066–1073. [CrossRef]
51. Budde, C.N.; Tsikitis, V.L.; Deveney, K.E.; Diggs, B.S.; Lu, K.C.; Herzig, D.O. Increasing the number of lymph nodes examined after colectomy does not improve colon cancer staging. *J. Am. Coll. Surg.* **2014**, *218*, 1004–1011. [CrossRef]

52. Hogan, N.M.; Winter, D.C. A nodal positivity constant: New perspectives in lymph node evaluation and colorectal cancer. *World J. Surg.* **2013**, *37*, 878–882. [CrossRef] [PubMed]
53. Simunovic, M.; Baxter, N.N. Lymph node counts in colon cancer surgery: Lessons for users of quality indicators. *JAMA* **2007**, *298*, 2194–2195. [CrossRef]
54. Musselman, R.P.; Xie, M.; McLaughlin, K.; Moloo, H.; Boushey, R.P.; Auer, R.A.C. Should lymph node retrieval be a surgical quality indicator in colon cancer? *J. Clin. Oncol.* **2012**, *30*, 648. [CrossRef]
55. Khan, H.; Olszewski, A.J.; Somasundar, P. Lymph node involvement in colon cancer patients decreases with age; a population based analysis. *Eur. J. Surg. Oncol.* **2014**, *40*, 1474–1480. [CrossRef] [PubMed]
56. Becerra, A.Z.; Aquina, C.T.; Berho, M.; Boscoe, F.P.; Schymura, M.J.; Noyes, K.; Monson, J.R.; Fleming, F.J. Surgeon-, pathologist-, and hospital-level variation in suboptimal lymph node examination after colectomy: Compartmentalizing quality improvement strategies. *Surgery* **2017**, *161*, 1299–1306. [CrossRef] [PubMed]
57. Lykke, J.; Jess, P.; Roikjær, O. A high lymph node yield in colon cancer is associated with age, tumour stage, tumour sub-site and priority of surgery. Results from a prospective national cohort study. *Int. J. Colorectal Dis.* **2016**, *31*, 1299–1305. [CrossRef] [PubMed]
58. Nathan, H.; Shore, A.D.; Anders, R.A.; Wick, E.C.; Gearhart, S.L.; Pawlik, T.M. Variation in Lymph Node Assessment After Colon Cancer Resection: Patient, Surgeon, Pathologist, or Hospital? *J. Gastrointest. Surg.* **2011**, *15*, 471–479. [CrossRef] [PubMed]
59. Chou, J.F.; Row, D.; Gonen, M.; Liu, Y.H.; Schrag, D.; Weiser, M.R. Clinical and pathologic factors that predict lymph node yield from surgical specimens in colorectal cancer: A population-based study. *Cancer* **2010**, *116*, 2560–2570. [CrossRef]
60. Stocchi, L.; Fazio, V.W.; Lavery, I.; Hammel, J. Individual Surgeon, Pathologist, and Other Factors Affecting Lymph Node Harvest in Stage II Colon Carcinoma. Is a Minimum of 12 Examined Lymph Nodes Sufficient? *Ann. Surg. Oncol.* **2011**, *18*, 405–412. [CrossRef]
61. Baxter, N.N.; Virnig, D.J.; Rothenberger, D.A.; Morris, A.M.; Jessurun, J.; Virnig, B.A. Lymph Node Evaluation in Colorectal Cancer Patients: A Population-Based Study. *J. Natl. Cancer Inst.* **2005**, *97*, 219–225. [CrossRef]
62. Moro-Valdezate, D.; Pla-Martí, V.; Martín-Arévalo, J.; Belenguer-Rodrigo, J.; Aragó-Chofre, P.; Ruiz-Carmona, M.D.; Checa-Ayet, F. Factors related to lymph node harvest: Does a recovery of more than 12 improve the outcome of colorectal cancer? *Color. Dis.* **2013**, *15*, 1257–1266. [CrossRef] [PubMed]
63. Nash, G.M.; Row, D.; Weiss, A.; Shia, J.; Guillem, J.G.; Paty, P.B.; Gonen, M.; Weiser, M.R.; Temple, L.K.; Fitzmaurice, G.; et al. A predictive model for lymph node yield in colon cancer resection specimens. *Ann. Surg.* **2011**, *253*, 318–322. [CrossRef] [PubMed]
64. Choi, J.P.; Park, I.J.; Lee, B.C.; Hong, S.M.; Lee, J.L.; Yoon, Y.S.; Kim, C.W.; Lim, S.-B.; Lee, J.B.; Yu, C.S.; et al. Variability in the lymph node retrieval after resection of colon cancer: Influence of operative period and process. *Medicine* **2016**, *95*, e4199. [CrossRef] [PubMed]
65. Yacoub, M.; Swistak, S.; Chan, S.; Chichester, T.; Dawood, S.; Berri, R.; Hawasli, A. Factors that influence lymph node retrieval in the surgical treatment of colorectal cancer: A comparison of the laparoscopic versus open approach. *Am. J. Surg.* **2013**, *205*, 339–342, discussion 342. [CrossRef] [PubMed]
66. Morikawa, T.; Tanaka, N.; Kuchiba, A.; Nosho, K.; Yamauchi, M.; Hornick, J.L.; Swanson, R.S.; Chan, A.T.; Meyerhardt, J.A.; Huttenhower, C.; et al. Predictors of Lymph Node Count in Colorectal Cancer Resections Data From. *Arch. Surg.* **2012**, *147*, 715–723. [CrossRef] [PubMed]
67. Betge, J.; Harbaum, L.; Pollheimer, M.J.; Lindtner, R.A.; Kornprat, P.; Ebert, M.P.; Langner, C. Lymph node retrieval in colorectal cancer: Determining factors and prognostic significance. *Int. J. Colorectal Dis.* **2017**, *32*, 991–998. [CrossRef]
68. Rajput, A.; Romanus, D.; Weiser, M.R.; Ter Veer, A.; Niland, J.; Wilson, J.; Skibber, J.M.; Wong, Y.-N.; Benson, A.; Earle, C.C.; et al. Meeting the 12 lymph node (LN) benchmark in colon cancer. *J. Surg. Oncol.* **2010**, *102*, 3–9. [CrossRef]
69. Valsecchi, M.E.; Leighton, J.; Tester, W. Modifiable Factors That Influence Colon Cancer Lymph Node Sampling and Examination. *Clin. Colorectal Cancer.* **2010**, *9*, 162–167. [CrossRef]
70. Nedrebø, B.S.; Søreide, K.; Nesbakken, A.; Eriksen, M.T.; Søreide, J.A.; Kørner, H. Risk factors associated with poor lymph node harvest after colon cancer surgery in a national cohort. *Color. Dis.* **2013**, *15*, e301–e308. [CrossRef]
71. Scabini, S.; Rimini, E.; Romairone, E.; Scordamaglia, R.; Pertile, D.; Testino, G.; Ferrando, V. Factors that influence 12 or more harvested lymph nodes in resective R0 colorectal cancer. *Hepatogastroenterology* **2010**, *57*, 728–733.
72. Pappas, A.V.; Lagoudianakis, E.E.; Dallianoudis, I.G.; Kotzadimitriou, K.T.; Koronakis, N.E.; Chrysikos, I.D.; Koukoutsi, I.D.; Markogiannakis, H.E.; Antonakis, P.T.; Manouras, A.J. Differences in colorectal cancer patterns between right and left sided colorectal cancer lesions. *J. BUON* **2010**, *15*, 509–513. [PubMed]
73. Belt, E.J.T.; te Velde, E.A.; Krijgsman, O.; Brosens, R.P.M.; Tijssen, M.; van Essen, H.F.; Stockmann, H.B.A.C.; Bril, H.; Carvalho, B.; Ylstra, B.; et al. High Lymph Node Yield is Related to Microsatellite Instability in Colon Cancer. *Ann. Surg. Oncol.* **2012**, *19*, 1222–1230. [CrossRef] [PubMed]
74. Vilar, E.; Gruber, S.B. Microsatellite instability in colorectal cancer-the stable evidence. *Nat. Rev. Clin. Oncol.* **2010**, *7*, 153–162. [CrossRef] [PubMed]

Disclaimer/Publisher's Note: The statements, opinions and data contained in all publications are solely those of the individual author(s) and contributor(s) and not of MDPI and/or the editor(s). MDPI and/or the editor(s) disclaim responsibility for any injury to people or property resulting from any ideas, methods, instructions or products referred to in the content.

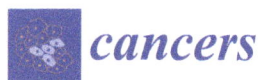 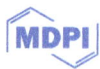

Review

Blood Vessel-Targeted Therapy in Colorectal Cancer: Current Strategies and Future Perspectives

Anne Jacobsen [1,2,3], Jürgen Siebler [2,4], Robert Grützmann [2,3], Michael Stürzl [1,2] and Elisabeth Naschberger [1,2,*]

[1] Division of Molecular and Experimental Surgery, Translational Research Center, Universitätsklinikum Erlangen, Friedrich-Alexander-Universität Erlangen-Nürnberg (FAU), Kussmaulallee 12, D-91054 Erlangen, Germany; anne.jacobsen@uk-erlangen.de (A.J.); michael.stuerzl@uk-erlangen.de (M.S.)

[2] Comprehensive Cancer Center Erlangen-EMN (CCC ER-EMN), D-91054 Erlangen, Germany; juergen.siebler@uk-erlangen.de (J.S.); robert.gruetzmann@uk-erlangen.de (R.G.)

[3] Department of General and Visceral Surgery, Universitätsklinikum Erlangen, Friedrich-Alexander-University Erlangen-Nürnberg (FAU), D-91054 Erlangen, Germany

[4] Department of Medicine 1—Gastroenterology, Universitätsklinikum Erlangen, Friedrich-Alexander-University Erlangen-Nürnberg (FAU), D-91054 Erlangen, Germany

* Correspondence: elisabeth.naschberger@uk-erlangen.de; Tel.: +49-9131-85-39524

Simple Summary: This review summarizes the history and current clinical applications of antiangiogenic treatment. It specifically discusses current challenges of the treatment and opportunities for optimization, including normalization of the tumor vasculature, modulation of milieu-dependent heterogeneity of the vasculature, and targeting of angiocrine protein functions.

Abstract: The vasculature is a key player and regulatory component in the multicellular microenvironment of solid tumors and, consequently, a therapeutic target. In colorectal carcinoma (CRC), antiangiogenic treatment was approved almost 20 years ago, but there are still no valid predictors of response. In addition, treatment resistance has become a problem. Vascular heterogeneity and plasticity due to species-, organ-, and milieu-dependent phenotypic and functional differences of blood vascular cells reduced the hope of being able to apply a standard approach of antiangiogenic therapy to all patients. In addition, the pathological vasculature in CRC is characterized by heterogeneous perfusion, impaired barrier function, immunosuppressive endothelial cell anergy, and metabolic competition-induced microenvironmental stress. Only recently, angiocrine proteins have been identified that are specifically released from vascular cells and can regulate tumor initiation and progression in an autocrine and paracrine manner. In this review, we summarize the history and current strategies for applying antiangiogenic treatment and discuss the associated challenges and opportunities, including normalizing the tumor vasculature, modulating milieu-dependent vascular heterogeneity, and targeting functions of angiocrine proteins. These new strategies could open perspectives for future vascular-targeted and patient-tailored therapy selection in CRC.

Keywords: antiangiogenic treatment; cancer; colorectal cancer; endothelial cells; tumor microenvironment; bevacizumab; ramucirumab; aflibercept; regorafenib; fruquintinib; angiocrine; vasculature; vascular heterogeneity

Citation: Jacobsen, A.; Siebler, J.; Grützmann, R.; Stürzl, M.; Naschberger, E. Blood Vessel-Targeted Therapy in Colorectal Cancer: Current Strategies and Future Perspectives. *Cancers* **2024**, *16*, 890. https://doi.org/10.3390/cancers16050890

Academic Editor: Alain P. Gobert

Received: 20 November 2023
Revised: 6 February 2024
Accepted: 10 February 2024
Published: 22 February 2024

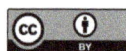

Copyright: © 2024 by the authors. Licensee MDPI, Basel, Switzerland. This article is an open access article distributed under the terms and conditions of the Creative Commons Attribution (CC BY) license (https://creativecommons.org/licenses/by/4.0/).

1. History and Development of Antiangiogenic Treatment for Cancer

Colorectal cancer (CRC) is the third most common cancer and accounts for approximately 10% of cancer cases worldwide [1]. CRC incidence rates remain high in highly developed countries such as Canada and Northern Europe and are rising rapidly in many less developed countries, particularly in Eastern Europe, Asia and South America [2]. The established risk factors for CRC include high intake of processed meats and low intake of fruits and vegetables, a sedentary lifestyle, obesity, smoking, and excessive alcohol consumption [1]. The introduction of population-based screening in a growing number of countries likely contributed to decreasing mortality rates in some regions [2]. Since the 1990s, despite an overall downward trend, particularly in high-income countries, there has been an increase in digestive tract cancers in adults under the age of 50 [3]. Despite these recent observations, CRC remains significantly more common in older people. Considering the steadily increasing global life expectancy at birth, a doubling of the incidence of CRC in old world regions by 2035 has been predicted [2].

Although the prognosis for CRC has improved in recent decades, this disease is still responsible for 880,000 deaths globally [2]. Approximately 15–30% of patients present with metastases at the time of diagnosis, and more than 20% of patients with initially localized disease will develop metastases over time [4]. These high numbers require continued intense and relentless efforts to combat the disease. The most urgent targets for improvement are the expansion of prescreening programs, education about a tumor-preventing lifestyle, the availability of healthy food to the global population and improved forms of therapy in association with specific approaches to predetermine therapy responses.

In accordance with the clinical need for improvement in treatment regimens, we will focus here on the status of CRC therapy, specifically by analyzing the role of the vascular system as a therapeutic target. With the appreciation of the important role of the microenvironment in carcinogenesis approximately 15 years ago, it became clear that not only tumor cells alone but also the interplay of tumor cells with the different cell types in the surrounding stroma mediated by many different cytokines and growth factors is a paramount denominator of tumor progression and therapeutic responses [5]. In this framework, it is highly remarkable that more than 50 years ago, Judah Folkman had already recognized the importance of the vasculature as a stromal-derived component for tumor therapy. His hypothesis was that vessels are needed for the delivery of nutrients to tumor cells and that blocking vessel growth into tumors may consequently reduce tumor progression [6]. In comparison to tumor cell-directed cancer therapy, this approach is thought to have several advantages, including (i) reduced resistance achieved by targeting genetically stable tumor vessel endothelial cells (TECs) instead of tumor cells, where genetic instability is an important driver of resistance. (ii) Furthermore, the endothelium is considered to be easily accessible to drugs applied through the blood circulation. (iii) Finally, it was shown that approximately one endothelial cell delivers nutrients to up to 100 tumor cells, and accordingly, amplification effects are expected in endothelial cell-directed therapy [7].

These findings initiated a series of fascinating experimental approaches in animal models, which convincingly supported the important role of the vascular system in tumor therapy. All of these findings have been comprehensively reviewed in the literature [8,9]. Consequently, only some of the most important results are highlighted in the following section.

One of the first requirements for antiangiogenic therapy was the availability of the respective inhibitors. In the first step, these substances directly inhibit endothelial cell proliferation or migration. Among these substances was fumagillin, which was first isolated from *Aspergillus fumigatus* in 1949 as an antiphage agent [10,11]. Fumagillin was shown to be an antiangiogenic agent when Folkman's coworker revealed that it inhibited capillary endothelial cell proliferation in *Aspergillus fumigatus*-contaminated cell cultures [12]. To reduce its nonspecific toxicity, derivatives of fumagillin were synthesized, and these substances significantly inhibited tumor growth in preclinical experimental tumor models [12]. A further key development was based on two important points: first, the observation that the growth of metastases dramatically increased after surgical removal of the primary tumor in certain rodent carcinoma models; second, the hypothesis that inhibitors of angiogenesis may be enriched in the primary tumors but trumped by stimulators; and that this balance may be shifted distantly in the circulation when inhibitors are more stable and stimulators are rapidly cleared [9]. These conditions specifically inhibit angiogenesis, which is needed for distant metastasis formation in the presence of the primary tumor. Based on these considerations, two angiogenesis inhibitors that are released in proteolytically active primary tumors as cleavage products of other proteins were identified. These inhibitors were named angiostatin, a cleavage product of the blood protein plasminogen involved in fibrolyis, and endostatin, a cleavage product of the extracellular matrix protein collagen XVIII [13,14]. Both proteins specifically inhibited endothelial cell proliferation but had no effect on resting endothelial cells or other cell types [9,13,14]. Moreover, endostatin and angiostatin strongly inhibited the growth of many different tumors, including breast, colorectal and lung cancer, in different mouse models [15]. Most importantly, for endostatin, this drug did not lead to acquired drug resistance after several cycles of treatment or tumor regrowth during phases where treatment ceased [16]. These results led to great euphoria and high hopes in researchers, medical doctors and patient populations with respect to antiangiogenic cancer therapy in humans. This culminated when *The New York Times* headlined these findings in 1998 and cited the codiscoverer of the DNA structure and Nobel laureate James D. Watson with the sentence "Judah Folkman is going to cure cancer in two years" [17]. This expression is often used to demonstrate excitement in the field but was quickly contradicted by Watson himself, who stated that he was misquoted and instead referred to the urgent need for clinical trials, which would show within the year whether the substances are effective [18]. Folkman's statements were more focused on the actual facts when he was cited: "If you have cancer and you are a mouse, we can take good care of you" [17]. In fact, in the effort to translate the preclinical results to clinical therapy, severe pitfalls arose, and altogether, there was less excitement when these substances were examined in clinical studies. It took several years until 2004 when antiangiogenic therapy was successfully applied to a human cancer, namely, CRC, for the first time [19]. In the following paragraphs, we will specifically discuss the present standing of antiangiogenic therapy in CRC and summarize putative reasons for therapy failure in humans as well as putative perspectives.

2. Clinical Application of Antiangiogenic Treatment in Colorectal Cancer

The vasculature plays an essential role in CRC therapy. First, angiogenesis is the target of antiangiogenic therapy, as explained above. Second, the vasculature also determines the extent of surgical resection of CRC (Figure 1). Two groups of antiangiogenic drugs are currently used to treat metastatic CRC (mCRC): monoclonal antibodies and small molecules, specifically tyrosine kinase inhibitors (TKIs) [20] (Table 1).

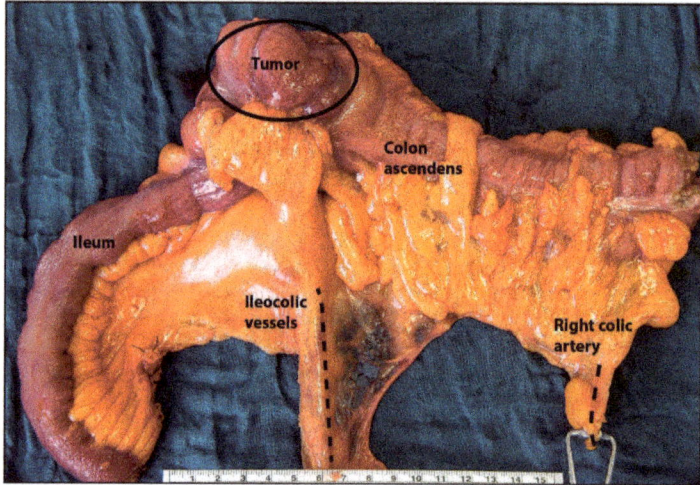

Figure 1. The tumor-related vascular structure and hierarchy determine the surgical resection strategy used for colorectal cancer. Surgical preparation after right hemicolectomy with complete mesocolic excision because of cecal carcinoma (circle). Central ligation of the ileocolic vessels (artery and vein) and the right colic artery (dashed lines) ensures resection of the regional lymph nodes, which is well known to improve survival.

Table 1. Pivotal phase III clinical trials of antiangiogenic agents in treatment of mCRC.

Clinical Trial	Treatment	Indication	mOS, Months (95%CI)	mPFS, Months (95% CI)	ORR, %	HR (OS) (95%CI)	Ref.
AVF2107g	Beva + IFL Beva + placebo	1st line	20.3 (n.r.) 15.6 (n.r.)	10.6 (n.r.) 6.2 (n.r.)	44.8 34.8	0.66 (n.r.), $p < 0.001$	[19]
ITACa	Beva + FOLFOX/FOLFIRI FOLFOX/FOLFIRI	1st line	20.8 (15.9–23.2) 21.3 (19.9–24.1)	9.6 (8.2–10.3) 8.4 (7.2–9.0)	50.6 50	1.13 (0.89–1.43), $p = 0.304$	[21]
ML18147	Beva+FOLFOX/FOLFIRI FOLFOX/FOLFIRI	2nd line	11.2 (10.4–12.2) 9.8 (8.9–10.7)	5.7 (5.2–6.2) 4.1 (3.7–4.4)	5 4	0.81 (0.69–0.94), $p = 0.0062$	[22]
VELOUR	Aflibercept + FOLFIRI FOLFIRI	2nd line	13.5 (12.52–14.95) 12.6 (11.07–13.11)	6.9 (6.51–7.2) 4.67 (4.21–5.36)	19.8 11.1	0.817 (0.713–0.937), $p = 0.0032$	[23]
RAISE	Ramucirumab + FOLFIRI FOLFIRI	2nd line	13.3 (12.4–14.5) 11.7 (10.8–12–7)	5.7 (5.5–6.2) 4.5 (4.2–5.4)	13.4 12.5	0.844 (0.73–0.976), $p = 0.0219$	[24]
CORRECT	Regorafenib Placebo	refractory	6.4 (CI n.r.) 5.0 (CI n.r.)	1.9 (CI n.r.) 1.7 (CI n.r.)	1 0.4	0.77 (0.64–0.94), $p = 0.0052$	[25]
FRESCO II	Fruquintinib Placebo	3rd/later line	7.4 (6.7–8.2) 4.8 (4.0–5.8)	3.7 (3.5–3.8) 1.8 (1.8–1.9)	5 0	0.66 (0.55–0.80), $p < 0.0001$	[26]

mOS: median overall survival. mPFS: median progression-free survival. ORR: objective response rate. HR (OS): hazard ratio of overall survival. CI: confidence interval. Beva: bevacizumab. FOLFOX: 5-fluorouracil, leucovorin, oxaliplatin. FOLFIRI: 5-fluorouracil, leucovorin, irinotecan. IFL: irinotecan, bolus fluorouracil, leucovorin. n.r.: not reported.

2.1. Monoclonal Antibodies

Currently, clinically used monoclonal antibodies block the VEGF-VEGFR2 axis and, accordingly, the activation of VEGF signaling pathways. Bevacizumab, the first approved antiangiogenic drug, binds to VEGF-A and prevents its binding to the corresponding receptors [27]. Aflibercept is a soluble VEGF receptor that also captures VEGF before it can bind to the respective cellular receptors. Ramucirumab binds directly to VEGFR2, thereby inhibiting its activation [20]. All three antibodies are used globally in combination with chemotherapy in standard second-line therapy for unresectable CRC. However, only bevacizumab is recommended in first-line setting [4,28,29]. Toxicity and adverse effects, including hypertension, proteinuria, hemorrhage, GI perforation, wound complications, and thromboembolic events, are mostly modest and manageable [30–33].

2.1.1. Bevacizumab

Bevacizumab was the first antiangiogenic drug approved for clinical application, and it is still the most widely used [27]. In mCRC, bevacizumab was established in first and later lines of therapy in combination with chemotherapy, as monotherapy has no relevant impact in mCRC [20]. In the first clinical trials, bevacizumab seemed to improve the response rate (RR), progression-free survival (PFS), and overall survival (OS) in combination with chemotherapy. Kabbinavar et al. [34] reported a dose-dependent positive effect of bevacizumab in combination with 5-FU/leucovorin on the RR, PFS and OS in a phase II trial in patients with mCRC. Hurwitz et al. [19] also reported better outcomes for all three parameters for patients treated with bevacizumab in combination with bolus 5-FU/leucovorin/irinotecan than for patients treated with the same chemotherapeutic regimen plus placebo in first-line therapy for untreated mCRC. These outcomes resulted in the approval of bevacizumab for the first-line treatment of metastatic colorectal disease.

In the following years, different combinations of bevacizumab and chemotherapeutic regimens were tested in many clinical trials. Although some of the studies reported improved PFS, the OS did not improve by adding bevacizumab [21,35–38].

Bevacizumab in first-line therapy seems to improve both OS and PFS when combined with fluoropyrimidine monotherapy, for example for patients with reduced general health, but only PFS when combined with commonly recommended combined chemotherapies based on infusional 5-FU (FOLFOX, FOLFIRI) [39].

Several clinical trials have compared bevacizumab to anti-EGFR agents, such as cetuximab or panitumumab, in first-line therapies. Heinemann et al. compared FOLFIRI/cetuximab versus FOLFIRI/bevacizumab as first-line treatment for patients with KRAS wild-type (wt) mCRC in a randomized phase III trial (FIRE-3) and reported a significantly prolonged OS in the cetuximab group (28.7 vs. 25.0 months in the bevacizumab group), although RR and PFS did not significantly differ [40]. Venook et al. conducted a similar trial (CALGB/SWOG 80405) to test either FOLFIRI or FOLFOX plus cetuximab or bevacizumab and found no differences in OS, PFS and RR between bevacizumab and cetuximab [41]. In the phase II PEAK study, when comparing FOLFOX plus panitumumab or bevacizumab as first-line therapy in patients with unresectable KRAS-wt mCRC, a prolonged OS and a similar PFS were found for the panitumumab group with KRAS-wt exon 2 [42]. Today, it is well known that right-sided and left-sided CRC differ clinically and molecularly, so sidedness is essential for clinical trials and therapeutic decisions. Holch et al. analyzed the primary tumor location in relation to the response to anti-EGFR therapy versus anti-VEGFR therapy in a meta-analysis of the three abovementioned studies (FIRE-3, CALGB/SWOG 80405, PEAK). The authors concluded that patients with left-sided RAS-wt mCRC benefit from treatment with an anti-EGFR antibody, whereas bevacizumab should be preferred for right-sided mCRC [43]. Sidedness was also addressed in a retrospective subgroup analysis of the two pivotal first-line bevacizumab trials of Hurwitz et al. (2004) [19] and Saltz et al. (2008) [37] mentioned above. This retrospective analysis revealed that bevacizumab had an effect independent of tumor sidedness in mCRC [44].

Currently, bevacizumab is regularly used in combination with different first-line chemotherapies for the treatment of mCRC. Its combination with FOLFOX, FOLFIRI or the triplet FOLFOXIRI is recommended for right-sided RAS- and BRAF-wt mCRC but also for RAS-mut and BRAF-mut mCRC, independent of the sidedness [4,28], although its efficacy, in particular in combination with potent chemotherapies as FOLFOX, FOLFIRI or FOLFOXIRI is still unclear.

The efficacy of bevacizumab was also analyzed for maintenance and second-line treatment. The CAIRO3 trial demonstrated capecitabine plus bevacizumab, and the AIO 0207 trial demonstrated fluoropyrimidine plus bevacizumab as preferable options for maintenance therapy in mCRC [45]. In second-line treatment, the combination of chemotherapy and bevacizumab compared to chemotherapy alone improved OS and PFS in different phase III trials, although the absolute benefit was only 1–2 months in terms of the median OS [46].

Today, bevacizumab is regularly used in combination with first- and second-line chemotherapy as well as maintenance therapy in the treatment of mCRC. Moreover, starting in 2023, bevacizumab has been used in last-line therapy in combination with trifluridine-tipiracil, as the SUNLIGHT trial showed a relevant improvement in OS (10.8 versus 7.5 months) and PFS (5.6 versus 2.4 months) for patients treated with trifluridine-tipiracil plus bevacizumab compared to those treated with trifluridine-tipiracil alone [47].

2.1.2. Ramucirumab

Ramucirumab is a human immunoglobulin G1 (IgG 1) monoclonal antibody that blocks VEGF receptor 2 (VEGFR-2), thereby preventing its activation [24]. In the RAISE study, a phase III clinical trial, ramucirumab was tested in a second-line setting with FOLFIRI in patients with mCRC who had disease progression during or within six months after first-line therapy with bevacizumab, oxaliplatin and a fluoropyrimidine. Patients treated with ramucirumab/FOLFIRI had a significantly longer OS (13.3 months) than patients treated with placebo/FOLFIRI (11.7 months) and a significantly longer PFS [24].

2.1.3. Aflibercept

Aflibercept is a fusion protein of the VEGF-binding domain of VEGFR1 and VEGFR2 with an Fc fragment of a human IgG1 antibody. This protein is a high-affinity ligand trap for VEGFA, VEGFB, and placental growth factor (PlGF), thereby preventing the binding of these proteins to VEGFR [23]. In a phase III clinical trial, patients treated with aflibercept in combination with FOLFIRI had significantly better OS (13.5 vs. 12.6 months) and PFS (6.9 vs. 4.7 months) than did patients treated with FOLFIRI/placebo in second-line therapy after previous treatment with oxaliplatin [23].

It is unclear which of the three antibodies should be preferred in the second-line treatment of mCRC [48]. To address this question, Hashimoto et al. initiated the ongoing prospective randomized phase II clinical trial (JCOG2004) to compare bevacizumab with ramucirumab and aflibercept, each in combination with FOLFIRI, in second-line treatment for unresectable CRC after first-line therapy with fluoropyrimidine and oxaliplatin [49].

2.2. Tyrosine Kinase Inhibitors

Antiangiogenic tyrosine kinase inhibitors (TKIs) are small molecules that traditionally affect a wide range of tyrosine and serine-threonine kinases in addition to the intended VEGFR signaling pathway [50]. Due to this low selectivity, TKIs often cause serious toxicity, making their clinical use challenging, particularly in combination with chemotherapy [51]. Moreover, the combination of TKIs with chemotherapy in mCRC patients has been disappointing [20]. In monotherapy, the typical adverse effects of the TKIs regorafenib and fruquintinib, used in mCRC therapy, include hypertension, hand-foot skin reaction, diarrhea, fatigue and dysphonia [25,52].

2.2.1. Regorafenib

Until recently, the only TKI used in the clinical treatment of mCRC was regorafenib, an oral multikinase inhibitor with activity against VEGFR-2, VEGFR-3, TIE-2, platelet-derived growth factor receptor (PDGFR), fibroblast growth factor receptor (FGFR), rearranged during transfection (RET) and c-Kit, as well as a signal transduction inhibitor of the RAF/MEK/ERK pathway [33]. Regorafenib had a statistically significant, but only moderate, effect on OS (6.4 vs. 5.0 months) as monotherapy for chemorefractory patients with mCRC compared to placebo in the phase III multicenter CORRECT trial [25].

2.2.1.1. Fruquintinib

Fruquintinib is a new antiangiogenic TKI that targets VEGFR. It is a small molecule that is orally applied and, in contrast to regorafenib, exhibits high selectivity for VEGFR-1, -2 and -3 [52]. Its effectiveness in mCRC was evaluated in the pivotal FRESCO trial, a randomized, double-blinded, multicenter phase III clinical trial in China that compared fruquintinib monotherapy versus placebo in patients with mCRC and progression after two lines of chemotherapy without VEGFR inhibitors. Median overall survival (9.3 vs. 6.6 months) and PFS (3.7 vs. 1.8 months) were significantly better in the fruquintinib group than in the placebo group [53]. These results led to the approval of fruquintinib for third- or later-line therapy for mCRC in China [54]. The authors state that the results may not be applicable to the Western population, as the standard treatment for mCRC in China does not include anti-VEGF therapy in prior therapy lines [53]. This phenomenon has been addressed in the global FRESCO-2 trial (NCT04322539), which included almost 700 patients from the United States, Europe, Japan and Australia [26]. The results showed a promising effect of fruquintinib in the treatment of patients with advanced, chemotherapy-refractory mCRC, with an OS of 7.4 months in the fruquintinib group versus 4.8 months in the placebo group [26]. These outcomes resulted in the recent FDA approval of fruquintinib for previously treated mCRC in November 2023.

Several additional monoclonal antibodies, a peptibody and many TKIs that target tumor angiogenesis through multiple pathways have been tested in mCRC patients in recent decades. Unfortunately, most of these agents showed no relevant efficacy in therapy of mCRC or had unfavorable toxicity. An overview of some of these regimens that have reached randomized phase II/III clinical trials but did not obtain approval for clinical application in mCRC is given in Table 2. Notably, some of those regimens are still under evaluation in combination with other therapies.

Table 2. Selection of antiangiogenic drugs in phase II/III trials in the last decade not receiving clinical approval.

Drug	Target	Regimen	Phase	Indication	Results in CRC	Ref.
TKI						
Brivanib	VEGFR-2, -3, FGFR-1, -2, -3	Brivanib/cetuximab Placebo/cetuximab	III	Refractory	No improvement of OS, significant improvement of ORR and PFS, increased toxicity	[55]
Cediranib	VEGFR-1, -2, -3, PDGFRβ, KIT	Cediranib/FOLFOX Beva/FOLFOX	II	2nd line	No improvement of PFS or OS	[56]
		Cediranib/FOLFOX or CAPOX Placebo/FOLFOX or CAPOX	III	1st line	Modest PFS prolongation, no impact on OS	[57]
		Cediranib/FOLFOX Beva/FOLFOX	II/III	1st line	PFS and OS comparable to those of beva, less favorable profile of adverse events	[58]
Linifanib	VEGFR-1, -2, -3, PDGFRβ	Linifanib/FOLFOX Beva/FOLFOX	II	2nd line	PFS and OS comparable to those of beva, more adverse events	[59]
Tivozanib	VEGFR-1, -2, -3, KIT, PDGFRβ	Tivozanib/FOLFOX Beva/FOLFOX	II	1st line	Efficacy comparable to that of beva	[60]
Vandetanib	EGFR, VEGFR-2, RET, BRK, TIE-2	Vandetanib/FOLFOX Placebo/FOLFOX	II	2nd line	No efficacy	[61]
Vatalanib	VEGFR-1, -2, -3	Vatalanib/FOLFOX Placebo/FOLFOX	III	1st line	No efficacy in OS, PFS, ORR	[62]
		Vatalanib/FOLFOX Placebo/FOLFOX	III	2nd line	Improvement of PFS, but not OS	[63]
Famitinib	VEGFR-2, -3, KIT, PDGFR, RET	Famitinib Placebo	II	3rd or later line	Prolongation of PFS, no improvement of OS	[64]
Nintedanib	VEGFR-1, -2, -3, FGFR-1, -2, -3, PDGFRα/β	Nintedanib/FOLFOX Beva/FOLFOX	I/II	1st line	Similar PFS	[65]
		Nintedanib/FOLFOX Placebo/FOLFOX	II	2nd line	Nonsignificant trend for improved PFS, OS, DCR	[66]
		Nintedanib Placebo	III	Refractory	No improvement of OS, modest increase of PFS	[67]
Monoclonal antibodies						
Axitinib	VEGFR-1, -2, -3	Axitinib/FOLFOX Beva/FOLFO Axitinib/Beva/FOLFOX	II	1st line	No improvement of ORR, PFS or OS by addition of axitinib or combination with beva	[68]
		Axitinib vs. placebo	II	Maintenance	Significantly longer PFS with axitinib	[69]
		Axitinib/FOLFOX Beva/FOLFOX Axitinib/FOLFIRI Beva/FOLFIRI	II	2nd line	No improvement of PFS and OR, but more adverse events with axitinib	[70]
Parsatuzumab	EGFL7	Parsatuzumab/FOLFOX/beva Placebo/FOLFOX/beva	II	1st line	No improvement of ORR, PFS, OS	[71]
Vanucizumab	VEGF-A, Ang-2	Vanucizumab/FOLFOX Placebo/FOLFOX	II	1st line	No improvement of PFS, increased toxicity	[72]
Peptibody						
Trebananib	Ang-1, -2	Trebananib/FOLFIRI Placebo/FOLFIRI	II	2nd line	No improvement of OS or PFS	[73]

CRC: colorectal cancer. VEGFR: vascular endothelial growth factor receptor. FGFR: fibroblast growth factor receptor. FOLFOX: 5-fluorouracil, leucovorin, oxaliplatin. FOLFIRI: 5-fluorouracil, leucovorin, irinotecan. OS: overall survival. ORR: objective response rate. PDGFRβ: platelet-derived growth factor β. Beva: bevacizumab. CAPOX: capecitabine, oxaliplatin. PFS: progression-free survival. KIT: tyrosine protein kinase KIT. EGFR: epidermal growth factor receptor. RET: rearranged during transfection. BRK: breast tumor kinase. TIE-2: EGFL7: Ang: angiopoietin.

3. Challenges in Antiangiogenic Treatment of CRC

To discuss the current challenges of antiangiogenic treatment in CRC, we need to rethink the original aims of the treatment. Initially, antiangiogenic treatment was thought to completely cut off the tumor from its blood supply to induce starvation of the tumor cells, thereby stopping tumor growth and inducing tumor cell death and tumor regression. However, it soon became evident that a superior therapeutic effect is observed by "normalization" of the tumor vasculature [51]. In the context of tumor vessel normalization, also defined as vessel pruning and regression, oxygenation and perfusion of the tumor improve in association with a reduction in tumor vessel size and tortuosity [74]. This results in the restoration of vascular maturation, increased capacity to sustain tissue pressure and normalization of the basement membrane [75]. This approach ultimately allows improved delivery and efficacy of chemotherapeutic drugs given in combination with antiangiogenic treatment [74]. This concept is supported by the observation that cytotoxic therapy results in a better outcome within the window of tumor vessel normalization than did cytotoxic therapy before or after [76]. Unfortunately, as detailed in the previous section, antiangiogenic treatment combined with chemotherapy causes only mild increases in survival, low response rates and moderate efficacy [19]. Notably, even partial progression of disease under treatment or treatment resistance occurs together with a lack of bio-markers for stratifying patients [51,77–79]. Based on these issues, we discuss below the predominant challenges in the antiangiogenic treatment of colorectal cancer.

3.1. Dosing and Timing of Antiangiogenic Treatment

The dosing and timing of the current treatment schedule are parameters that impact the outcome of antiangiogenic treatment. This issue was addressed by comparing conventional schedules of chemotherapy with the maximum tolerated dose (MTD) combined with antiangiogenic treatment to alternative metronomic dosing schedules. Metronomic treatment regimens are characterized by the administration of lower doses than the MTD but at a greater frequency. The application of such metronomic schedules showed an increased clinical benefit, particularly in the metastatic disease setting, together with the advantage of lower overall toxicity [80]. This finding has the potential to update the current application schemes accordingly in the future. However, it should be noted that the high frequency of drug administration is challenging for patients, and reports of a lacking advantage of this metronomic therapy schedule also exist [81]. Moreover, overdosing is known to hamper the efficacy of antiangiogenic treatment, as it has been reported that low-dose anti-VEGF treatment sensitizes patients more efficiently to PD-1 blockade than does the conventional dose [82].

3.2. Combination of Antiangiogenic Treatment with Alternative Drugs

Many studies currently in progress aim to overcome the limitations of antiangiogenic treatment by combining antiangiogenic agents with alternative regimens, such as novel immunomodulatory drugs. The most common treatment regimens are anti-VEGF therapy in combination with PD-1 blockade, for example, the addition of atezolizumab (an anti-PD-L1 antibody) to capecitabine and bevacizumab [83]. Additionally, the combination of angiopoietin-2 (ANG2) blockade and VEGF plus immunotherapy is currently being investigated and has shown promising results [82,84–86]. Interestingly, in this context, triple blockade of PD-1, ANG2 and VEGF resulted in increased CTL levels and global tumor vessel normalization, which was greatest in the triple therapy scheme [86]. Accordingly, the combination of antiangiogenic treatment with immunomodulatory drugs has great additional potential by overcoming milieu-dependent immunosuppressive functions and further increasing therapeutic efficacy by fostering vessel normalization [86,87]. Notably, efforts are also underway to optimize the combination schedules of different drugs by developing algorithms that predict optimal low-dose drug combinations to improve the outcome of antiangiogenic treatment, and these algorithms have shown beneficial effects [85,88].

3.3. Heterogeneity of ECs According to Vessel Type, Organ, Disease, Patient, EC Hierarchy and Activation State

Initially, compared with tumor cells, tumor endothelial cells were believed to be a superior therapeutic target because they are a more uniform, genetically stable and homogenous cell population. However, there is reasonable heterogeneity of endothelial cells in human tumor patients. First, tumor vessels differ from normal vessels, and within a single tumor, different types of vessels can be detected, such as blood and lymphatic vessels, arteries, veins and capillaries, together with vessels that regulate their function and protein expression in a milieu-dependent manner (Figure 2). Moreover, vessels may harbor different states of maturation and angiogenic activation and are composed of different types of ECs within a single vessel. For example, the hierarchical organization of angiogenically active vessels in tip and stalk cells with different phenotypes and functions is well accepted [89]. Therefore, it is obvious that specific targeting of the TEC population may be difficult. As an example of the therapeutic consequences of EC heterogeneity, it can be noted that the normal vasculature regresses along with the tumor vasculature upon treatment, indicating that not even TECs as a whole can be specifically targeted, not considering that different TEC populations exist [90]. Another example is vessel-associated pericytes/mural cells that contribute to vascular maturation and may protect vessels from antiangiogenic treatment, thereby fostering therapeutic resistance [77]. Moreover, compensatory functions of the lymphatic vessel system must be considered [91]. Notably, in preclinical studies, differentiating therapeutic responses with respect to different types of vessels or EC activation states has mostly not been considered. Disease- and patient-dependent heterogeneity of tumor endothelial cells has clearly been demonstrated by multiregion sequencing of renal carcinoma [92], and this approach may similarly apply to CRC. The abovementioned examples of EC heterogeneity, organ-dependent heterogeneity and the function of TECs are considered causes of differential responses to antiangiogenic treatment [93,94]. Finally, tumor vessel invasion may arise through different mechanisms, such as vessel co-option or vascular mimicry, which are not necessarily dependent on active angiogenesis and, accordingly, may result in resistance to antiangiogenic treatment approaches [95]. In conclusion, both TEC heterogeneity and the different mechanisms through which tumor cells arrange their supply of oxygen and nutrients cause the tumor vasculature to be a more complex target, as initially appreciated [77,78,96].

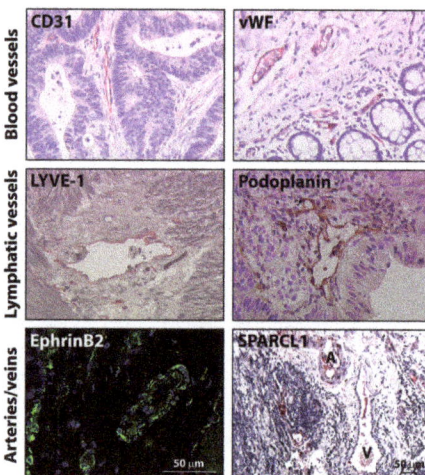

Figure 2. Different types of vessels are present in human colorectal cancer tissues. In human CRC, blood vessels can be labeled using the markers CD31 or vWF. Lymphatic vessels may be stained with LYVE-1 or podoplanin. Arteries and veins can be differentiated by labeling using the artery marker ephrinB2. This may be complemented by morphological differentiation of arteries (A) and veins (V) together with analysis of milieu-dependent expression of vessel markers such as SPARCL1. CD31, vWF, LYVE-1 and podoplanin panels: 25× objective; ephrinB2 and SPARCL1 panels: scale bars corresponding to 50 µm. The vWF panel is modified from Schellerer et al., Lab Invest 2007 [97].

3.4. Tumor Microenvironment (TME)-Dependent Plasticity of ECs Involving Angiocrine Mediators

Moreover, in recent years, it has become clear that ECs in tumors are not just passive conduits of blood that deliver oxygen, nutrients and circulating cells or remove waste products from tissues. Endothelial cells are part of the tumor microenvironment (TME), which is defined by direct or indirect interactions through paracrine mediators of tumor cells with their surrounding stromal cells. These interactions can alter the phenotypes and functions of the involved cell populations, including TECs. It was shown that TECs in CRC are epigenetically imprinted in a TME-dependent manner, resulting in stably maintained differential phenotypes with an impact on patient prognosis [98].

Notably, the vasculature can release so-called "angiocrine" molecules that act on neighboring cells, including tumor cells, which may promote or counteract tumor growth. Tumor-supporting angiocrine activities were described for vascular-derived IL-6 in glioblastoma (GBM), which induces TME-dependent alternative macrophage polarization by activating HIF-2α and arginase-1, resulting in GBM progression [99], or for TEC-derived jagged-1, which induces B-cell lymphoma invasiveness and chemoresistance [79]. Specifically, the antitumorigenic functions of angiocrine tumor vessel activities may have an unappreciated clinical impact on the outcome of antiangiogenic therapy [100]. Thrombospondin-1 is an angiocrine molecule with antitumorigenic functions that has been shown to induce tumor dormancy in the perivascular niche in breast cancer [101]. Similarly, in CRC, the TEC-derived matricellular protein SPARCL1 is associated with a positive prognosis in patients and is suspected to mediate the antitumorigenic functions of tumor vessels [99,102]. Notably, two other angiocrine mediators, ANG2 and BMP2, have recently gained attention as novel targets because of the consideration of ANG2 inhibitors and Tie2 activators in the ANG/Tie pathway as drug candidates [103] or BMP2 as a target in the calcineurin/NFAT-axis [104]. These initial observations indicate that under certain conditions, not only inhibiting but also supporting tumor vessels may be advantageous for patients. Whether angiocrine antitumorigenic functions of tumor vessels also contribute to the positive effects of vessel normalization strategies warrants further investigation [105].

3.5. Induction of EC Anergy

In recent years, modulation of the immune response by induction of endothelial cell anergy has attracted increased amounts of attention. This lack of responsiveness to inflammatory signals termed "endothelial cell anergy" is associated with immune cell exclusion and the downregulation of adhesion molecules such as ICAM-1/VCAM-1, which enable tissue extravasation of immune cells [106]. The presence of EC anergy renders tumors less responsive to immunotherapy given in combination with antiangiogenic treatment. An immunosuppressive function of the endothelial barrier has been reported for galectin-1-driven T-cell exclusion in the tumor endothelium, promoting immunotherapy resistance [107]. Another molecule involved in this context is the death mediator Fas L, which is specifically detected in the tumor vasculature and cooperatively induced by VEGF and PGE_2, resulting in a tumor endothelial death barrier that promotes immune tolerance associated with low CD8+ T-cell levels. Immune tolerance can be pharmacologically attenuated by VEGF and PGE_2 inhibition [108]. In conclusion, the presence of EC anergy under certain conditions in human patients results in immune tolerance, and immune cell exclusion is an issue hampering the response to antiangiogenic therapy.

3.6. Genomic Instability of TECs

Several reports have challenged the initial assumption that TECs are genetically stable. For example, in B-cell lymphoma patients, tumor cell-specific genetic alterations have been detected in microvascular endothelial cells [109]. Furthermore, vascular mimicry is presently defined as the autonomous formation of tumor vessels through tumor cells without the presence of a tumor endothelium. Vascular mimicry may coexist with mosaic vessels where the tumor endothelium is still partially integrated into the vessel wall [110]. Both types of tumor vasculature formation have implications for therapy by fostering resistance, as observed for vessels assembled by melanoma and endothelial cells [111]. Moreover, tumor cell differentiation into "endothelial-like" cells may occur and are considered an additional mode of therapeutic resistance. This was highlighted for GBM patients, in which endothelial cell-like cells were found to transdifferentiate from GBM stem-like cells [112–114]. Furthermore, increased aneuploidy was detected in TECs in human renal carcinoma [115] and in mouse melanoma models with high and low metastatic potential [116]. The potential genomic instability of TECs themselves or vessel walls made of tumor cells could be an issue as an escape and resistance mechanism limiting antiangiogenic treatment. However, this potential mode of resistance may be less relevant for CRC specifically. This assumption is based on the findings of a recent study in which potential genetic alterations in TECs were analyzed via systematic omics analyses in human CRC patients. Compared with their normal colon endothelial counterparts, corresponding PBMCs or tumor cells were found to be genetically stable from TECs isolated from these patients [98]. Furthermore, genetic drift of tumor-specific alterations to endothelial cells could not be detected, but the high load of mutations in MSI-positive patients warrants further investigation [97].

3.7. Imbalance of Intracellular Signaling Molecules (ROS, Calcium)

For a summary on the role of intracellular signaling and regulation in endothelial cells via the classical VEGFR/VEGF, FGFR/FGF, Tie2/Ang2, Notch/DLL4/Jagged1 and EphB/Ephrin B axes, we refer to a comprehensive review published recently [51]. In addition to these mainstream factors, altered concentrations of calcium and reactive oxygen species (ROS) may contribute to therapy resistance and side effects. ROS and calcium are two closely interconnected signaling molecules in eukaryotic cells, and calcium is known to modulate ROS homeostasis [117]. In CRC liver metastasis of bevacizumab-resistant patients, increased matrix stiffness was detected, which resulted in lipid metabolic cross-talk between the tumor and stromal cells characterized by increased levels of ROS and free fatty acids and a higher fatty acid oxidation rate, all of which contributed to bevacizumab resistance [118]. A ROS imbalance in HUVECs after anti-VEGF treatment was also reported by others [119]. Anti-VEGF treatment may increase calcium and ROS levels in parallel with decreased ATP production and increased cell damage, as has been observed in renal cells [120]. The addition of the calcium channel blocker benidipine to antiangiogenic treatment reduced renal toxicity, a known side effect of bevacizumab treatment [120]. Accordingly, modulating intracellular ROS and calcium imbalances during antiangiogenic treatment may help to overcome therapeutic resistance or side effects in the future.

3.8. Inadequate Preclinical Models and/or Limited Analysis

Until recently, for colorectal cancer, no or only very limited in vivo animal models existed that exhibit spontaneous distant metastasis similar to that of human patients. Considering that metastasis is the major cause of death in CRC patients and that the vasculature plays a key role in regulating tumor cell dissemination, optimizing antiangiogenic therapy regimens in appropriate model systems with distant metastasis is key. Meanwhile, novel organoid-based in vivo animal models that recapitulate spontaneous distant metastasis similar to that observed in human patients have been established; therefore, these models have great potential for improving preclinical screening [121,122]. In the future, novel targets are expected to be identified using such advanced models, and novel drug candidates can be evaluated in the preclinical setting, including distant metastasis. Furthermore, in the preclinical animal models used to date, the different types or activation states of ECs present in tumors have mostly not been analyzed with respect to differential treatment responses. This is a substantial issue that hampers the understanding of a potential milieu-dependent EC response to treatment and should be addressed in the future.

4. Conclusions and Future Opportunities for Antiangiogenic Tumor Therapy in CRC

After the first euphoria and the subsequent challenges in translating experimental results into clinical application, angiogenic inhibitors are currently an inherent part of therapy not only for mCRC but also for multiple other benign and malignant diseases. Nonetheless, almost 20 years after the first approval of bevacizumab for mCRC treatment, the results of antiangiogenic therapy for mCRC have been inconsistent, the effects have been less than initially expected and only five drugs have been approved. These are, within the class of monoclonal antibodies, bevacizumab, ramucirumab and aflibercept and, within the class of tyrosine kinase inhibitors, regorafenib and the new, promising TKI fruquintinib.

The prevailing challenges, which are complex and not adequately addressed yet, include the design of the therapy schedule, heterogeneity and TME-dependent plasticity of endothelial cells, the induction of immunosuppressive EC anergy, a low number of drug targets, deregulated intracellular signal mediators, a lack of stratification and response biomarkers, and the continued use of limited preclinical animal models lacking sporadic distant metastasis, the latter representing the major issue during disease progression and management.

Opportunities to overcome these challenges in the future include the integration of novel combinations of antiangiogenic drugs with immunotherapy, such as combined PD-1/VEGF blockade; novel application modes, such as metronomic dosing; or optimized low-dose combinations. Moreover, novel targets originating mostly from the pool of angiocrine proteins, such as those targeting the Tie2/Ang2 or Notch1/DLL4 axes, are promising for improving the efficacy of antiangiogenic treatment; these drugs are either in development or are already in clinical trials. Moreover, other angiocrine modulators, such as thrombospondin or SPARCL1, could be used as future therapeutic targets or biomarkers and may warrant further investigation in preclinical studies. Drugs targeting intracellular signal mediators deregulated during antiangiogenic treatment, such as calcium in combination with VEGF blockade, may also help to overcome therapeutic resistance or reduce side effects. Notably, improved tailored pretherapeutic drug testing with advanced tools, such as organoid-based animal models able to spontaneously metastasize in the periphery or the use of patient-derived organoids to individualized therapy, may help to overcome current issues. Most importantly, it will be necessary to consider, analyze and differentiate the impact of EC heterogeneity and the milieu-dependent plasticity of TECs in response to antiangiogenic therapy in more detail. This has to be considered in improved preclinical models with spontaneous distant metastasis to ultimately translate this aspect successfully into later clinical application.

Author Contributions: Conceptualization, M.S. and E.N.; investigation, A.J., E.N., M.S.; resources, M.S. and R.G.; data curation, M.S. and E.N.; writing—original draft preparation, A.J., M.S. and E.N.; writing—review and editing, A.J., J.S., M.S. and E.N.; visualization, A.J. and E.N.; supervision, M.S. and E.N.; project administration, M.S. and E.N.; funding acquisition, M.S. and E.N. All authors have read and agreed to the published version of the manuscript.

Funding: The work of the authors was supported by grants from the German Research Foundation (DFG) FOR 2438, subproject 2 (project ID 280163318) to E.N./M.S.; by the DFG SFB/TRR 241, subproject A06 (project ID 375876048) to M.S.; by the DFG STU 238/10-1 (project ID 437201724) to M.S.; by the DFG TRR 305, subproject B08 (project ID 429280966) to E.N.; by the DFG-NOTICE program (project ID 493624887) to E.N. and R.G.; by the W. Lutz Stiftung to M.S.; and by the Forschungsstiftung Medizin am Universitätsklinikum Erlangen to M.S.

Conflicts of Interest: The authors declare no competing interests.

References

1. World Health Organization. Colorectal Cancer. 2023. Available online: https://www.who.int/news-room/fact-sheets/detail/colorectal-cancer (accessed on 15 December 2023).
2. Arnold, M.; Abnet, C.C.; Neale, R.E.; Vignat, J.; Giovannucci, E.L.; McGlynn, K.A.; Bray, F. Global Burden of 5 Major Types of Gastrointestinal Cancer. *Gastroenterology* **2020**, *159*, 335–349.e15. [CrossRef]
3. Ugai, T.; Sasamoto, N.; Lee, H.-Y.; Ando, M.; Song, M.; Tamimi, R.M.; Kawachi, I.; Campbell, P.T.; Giovannucci, E.L.; Weiderpass, E.; et al. Is early-onset cancer an emerging global epidemic? Current evidence and future implications. *Nat. Rev. Clin. Oncol.* **2022**, *19*, 656–673. [CrossRef]
4. Cervantes, A.; Adam, R.; Roselló, S.; Arnold, D.; Normanno, N.; Taïeb, J.; Seligmann, J.; De Baere, T.; Osterlund, P.; Yoshino, T.; et al. Metastatic colorectal cancer: ESMO Clinical Practice Guideline for di-agnosis, treatment and follow-up. *Ann. Oncol.* **2022**, *34*, 10–32. [CrossRef]
5. Hanahan, D.; Weinberg, R.A. Hallmarks of cancer: The next generation. *Cell* **2011**, *144*, 646–674. [CrossRef]
6. Folkman, J. Tumor angiogenesis: Therapeutic implications. *N. Engl. J. Med.* **1971**, *285*, 1182–1186.
7. Folkman, J. *Antiangiogenesis Agents, in Cancer: Principles and Practice of Oncology*; Vincent, S.H., De Vita, T., Jr., Rosenberg, S.A., Eds.; Lippincott Williams & Wilkins Publishers: Baltimore, MD, USA, 2001.
8. Cao, Y.; Langer, R. A review of Judah Folkman's remarkable achievements in biomedicine. *Proc. Natl. Acad. Sci. USA* **2008**, *105*, 13203–13205. [CrossRef]
9. Ribatti, D. Judah Folkman, a pioneer in the study of angiogenesis. *Angiogenesis* **2008**, *11*, 3–10. [CrossRef]
10. Hanson, F.R.; Eble, T.E. An Antiphage Agent Isolated from *Aspergillus* sp. *J. Bacteriol.* **1949**, *58*, 527–529. [CrossRef]
11. Guruceaga, X.; Perez-Cuesta, U.; Cerio, A.D.D.; Gonzalez, O.; Rementeria, A. Fumagillin, a Mycotoxin of Aspergillus fumigatus: Biosynthesis, Biological Activities, Detection, and Ap-plications. *Toxins* **2019**, *12*, 7. [CrossRef]
12. Ingber, D.; Fujita, T.; Kishimoto, S.; Sudo, K.; Kanamaru, T.; Brem, H.; Folkman, J. Synthetic analogues of fumagillin that inhibit angiogenesis and suppress tumour growth. *Nature* **1990**, *348*, 555–557. [CrossRef]
13. O'Reilly, M.S.; Boehm, T.; Shing, Y.; Fukai, N.; Vasios, G.; Lane, W.S.; Flynn, E.; Birkhead, J.R.; Olsen, B.R.; Folkman, J. Endostatin: An Endogenous Inhibitor of Angiogenesis and Tumor Growth. *Cell* **1997**, *88*, 277–285. [CrossRef]
14. O'Reilly, M.S.; Holmgren, L.; Shing, Y.; Chen, C.; Rosenthal, R.A.; Moses, M.; Lane, W.S.; Cao, Y.; Sage, E.; Folkman, J. Angiostatin: A novel angiogenesis inhibitor that mediates the suppression of metastases by a lewis lung carcinoma. *Cell* **1994**, *79*, 315–328. [CrossRef]
15. O'Reilly, M.S.; Holmgren, L.; Chen, C.; Folkman, J. Angiostatin induces and sustains dormancy of human primary tumors in mice. *Nat. Med.* **1996**, *2*, 689–692. [CrossRef]
16. Boehm, T.; Folkman, J.; Browder, T.; O'Reilly, M.S. Antiangiogenic therapy of experimental cancer does not induce acquired drug resistance. *Nature* **1997**, *390*, 404–407. [CrossRef]
17. Kolata, G. Hope in the Lab: A Special Report; A Cautious Awe Greets Drugs That Eradicate Tumors in Mice. *The New York Times*, 3 May 1998.
18. Watson, J.D. Opinion, High Hopes on Cancer, Letter to the Editor. *The New York Times*, 1998.
19. Hurwitz, H.; Fehrenbacher, L.; Novotny, W.; Cartwright, T.; Hainsworth, J.; Heim, W.; Berlin, J.; Baron, A.; Griffing, S.; Holmgren, E.; et al. Bevacizumab plus Irinotecan, Fluorouracil, and Leucovorin for Metastatic Colorectal Cancer. *N. Engl. J. Med.* **2004**, *350*, 2335–2342. [CrossRef]
20. Hansen, T.F.; Qvortrup, C.; Pfeiffer, P. Angiogenesis Inhibitors for Colorectal Cancer. A Review of the Clinical Data. *Cancers* **2021**, *13*, 1031. [CrossRef]
21. Passardi, A.; Nanni, O.; Tassinari, D.; Turci, D.; Cavanna, L.; Fontana, A.; Ruscelli, S.; Mucciarini, C.; Lorusso, V.; Ragazzini, A.; et al. Effectiveness of bevacizumab added to standard chemotherapy in metastatic colorectal cancer: Final results for first-line treatment from the ITACa randomized clinical trial. *Ann. Oncol.* **2015**, *26*, 1201–1207. [CrossRef]
22. Bennouna, J.; Sastre, J.; Arnold, D.; Österlund, P.; Greil, R.; Van Cutsem, E.; von Moos, R.; Viéitez, J.M.; Bouché, O.; Borg, C.; et al. Continuation of bevacizumab after first progression in metastatic colorectal cancer (ML18147): A randomised phase 3 trial. *Lancet Oncol.* **2013**, *14*, 29–37. [CrossRef]
23. Van Cutsem, E.; Tabernero, J.; Lakomy, R.; Prenen, H.; Prausová, J.; Macarulla, T.; Ruff, P.; van Hazel, G.A.; Moiseyenko, V.; Ferry, D.; et al. Addition of Aflibercept to Fluorouracil, Leucovorin, and Irinotecan Improves Survival in a Phase III Randomized Trial in Patients with Metastatic Colorectal Cancer Previously Treated With an Oxaliplatin-Based Regimen. *J. Clin. Oncol.* **2012**, *30*, 3499–3506. [CrossRef]
24. Tabernero, J.; Yoshino, T.; Cohn, A.L.; Obermannova, R.; Bodoky, G.; Garcia-Carbonero, R.; Ciuleanu, T.E.; Portnoy, D.C.; Cutsem, E.V.; Grothey, A.; et al. Ramucirumab versus placebo in combination with second-line FOLFIRI in patients with metastatic colo-rectal carcinoma that progressed during or after first-line therapy with bevacizumab, oxaliplatin, and a fluoropyrimidine (RAISE): A randomised, double-blind, multicentre, phase 3 study. *Lancet Oncol.* **2015**, *16*, 499–508. [CrossRef]
25. Grothey, A.; Van Cutsem, E.; Sobrero, A.; Siena, S.; Falcone, A.; Ychou, M.; Humblet, Y.; Bouché, O.; Mineur, L.; Barone, C.; et al. Regorafenib monotherapy for previously treated metastatic colorectal cancer (CORRECT): An international, multicentre, randomised, placebo-controlled, phase 3 trial. *Lancet* **2013**, *381*, 303–312. [CrossRef]

26. Dasari, A.; Lonardi, S.; Garcia-Carbonero, R.; Elez, E.; Yoshino, T.; Sobrero, A.; Yao, J.; García-Alfonso, P.; Kocsis, J.; Gracian, A.C.; et al. Fruquintinib versus placebo in patients with refractory metastatic colorectal cancer (FRESCO-2): An interna-tional, multicentre, randomised, double-blind, phase 3 study. *Lancet* **2023**, *402*, 41–53. [CrossRef]
27. Garcia, J.; Hurwitz, H.I.; Sandler, A.B.; Miles, D.; Coleman, R.L.; Deurloo, R.; Chinot, O.L. Bevacizumab (Avastin®) in cancer treatment: A review of 15 years of clinical experience and future outlook. *Cancer Treat. Rev.* **2020**, *86*, 102017. [CrossRef]
28. Watanabe, T.; Itabashi, M.; Shimada, Y.; Tanaka, S.; Ito, Y.; Ajioka, Y.; Hamaguchi, T.; Hyodo, I.; Igarashi, M.; Ishida, H.; et al. Japanese Society for Cancer of the Colon and Rectum (JSCCR) guidelines 2019 for the treatment of colorectal cancer. *Int. J. Clin. Oncol.* **2020**, *25*, 1–42.
29. Benson, A.B.; Venook, A.P.; Al-Hawary, M.M.; Arain, M.A.; Chen, Y.J.; Ciombor, K.K.; Cohen, S.; Cooper, H.S.; Deming, D.; Farkas, L. Colon Cancer, Version 2.2021, NCCN Clinical Practice Guidelines in Oncology. *J. Natl. Compr. Cancer Netw.* **2021**, *19*, 329–359. [CrossRef]
30. Chen, H.X.; Cleck, J.N. Adverse effects of anticancer agents that target the VEGF pathway. *Nat. Rev. Clin. Oncol.* **2009**, *6*, 465–477. [CrossRef]
31. Souglakos, J.; Ziras, N.; Kakolyris, S.; Boukovinas, I.; Kentepozidis, N.; Makrantonakis, P.; Xynogalos, S.; Christophyllakis, C.; Kouroussis, C.; Vamvakas, L.; et al. Randomised phase-II trial of CAPIRI (capecitabine, irinotecan) plus bevacizumab vs FOLFIRI (folinic acid, 5-fluorouracil, irinotecan) plus bevacizumab as first-line treatment of patients with unresectable/metastatic colorectal cancer (mCRC). *Br. J. Cancer* **2012**, *106*, 453–459. [CrossRef]
32. Van Cutsem, E.; Rivera, F.; Berry, S.; Kretzschmar, A.; Michael, M.; DiBartolomeo, M.; Mazier, M.-A.; Canon, J.-L.; Georgoulias, V.; Peeters, M.; et al. Safety and efficacy of first-line bevacizumab with FOLFOX, XELOX, FOLFIRI and fluoropyrimidines in metastatic colorectal cancer: The BEAT study. *Ann. Oncol.* **2009**, *20*, 1842–1847. [CrossRef]
33. Tampellini, M.; Sonetto, C.; Scagliotti, G.V. Novel anti-angiogenic therapeutic strategies in colorectal cancer. *Expert Opin. Investig. Drugs* **2016**, *25*, 507–520. [CrossRef]
34. Kabbinavar, F. Phase II, randomized trial comparing bevacizumab plus fluorouracil (FU)/leucovorin (LV) with FU/LV alone in patients with metastatic colorectal cancer. *J. Clin. Oncol.* **2003**, *21*, 60–65. [CrossRef]
35. Cunningham, D.; Lang, I.; Marcuello, E.; Lorusso, V.; Ocvirk, J.; Shin, D.B.; Jonker, D.; Osborne, S.; Andre, N.; Waterkamp, D.; et al. Bevacizumab plus capecitabine versus capecitabine alone in elderly patients with previously untreated metastatic colorectal cancer (AVEX): An open-label, randomised phase 3 trial. *Lancet Oncol.* **2013**, *14*, 1077–1085. [CrossRef]
36. Kabbinavar, F.F.; Schulz, J.; McCleod, M.; Patel, T.; Hamm, J.T.; Hecht, J.R.; Mass, R.; Perrou, B.; Nelson, B.; Novotny, W.F. Addition of Bevacizumab to Bolus Fluorouracil and Leucovorin in First-Line Metastatic Colorectal Cancer: Results of a Randomized Phase II Trial. *J. Clin. Oncol.* **2005**, *23*, 3697–3705. [CrossRef]
37. Saltz, L.B.; Clarke, S.; Diaz-Rubio, E.; Scheithauer, W.; Figer, A.; Wong, R.; Koski, S.; Lichinitser, M.; Yang, T.-S.; Rivera, F.; et al. Bevacizumab in Combination With Oxaliplatin-Based Chemotherapy As First-Line Therapy in Metastatic Colorectal Cancer: A Randomized Phase III Study. *J. Clin. Oncol.* **2008**, *26*, 2013–2019. [CrossRef]
38. Tebbutt, N.C.; Wilson, K.; Gebski, V.J.; Cummins, M.M.; Zannino, D.; van Hazel, G.A.; Robinson, B.; Broad, A.; Ganju, V.; Ackland, S.P.; et al. Capecitabine, Bevacizumab, and Mitomycin in First-Line Treatment of Metastatic Colorectal Cancer: Results of the Australasian Gastrointestinal Trials Group Randomized Phase III MAX Study. *J. Clin. Oncol.* **2010**, *28*, 3191–3198. [CrossRef]
39. Baraniskin, A.; Buchberger, B.; Pox, C.; Graeven, U.; Holch, J.W.; Schmiegel, W.; Heinemann, V. Efficacy of bevacizumab in first-line treatment of metastatic colorectal cancer: A systematic review and meta-analysis. *Eur. J. Cancer* **2019**, *106*, 37–44. [CrossRef]
40. Heinemann, V.; von Weikersthal, L.F.; Decker, T.; Kiani, A.; Vehling-Kaiser, U.; Al-Batran, S.E.; Heintges, T.; Lerchenmüller, C.; Kahl, C.; Seipelt, G.; et al. FOLFIRI plus cetuximab versus FOLFIRI plus bevacizumab as first-line treatment for patients with metastatic colorectal cancer (FIRE-3): A randomised, open-label, phase 3 trial. *Lancet Oncol.* **2014**, *15*, 1065–1075. [CrossRef]
41. Venook, A.P.; Niedzwiecki, D.; Lenz, H.J.; Innocenti, F.; Fruth, B.; Meyerhardt, J.A.; Schrag, D.; Greene, C.; O'Neil, B.H.; Atkins, J.N.; et al. Effect of First-Line Chemotherapy Combined with Cetuximab or Bevacizumab on Overall Survival in Patients with KRAS Wild-Type Advanced or Metastatic Colorectal Cancer: A Randomized Clinical Trial. *JAMA* **2017**, *317*, 2392–2401. [CrossRef]
42. Schwartzberg, L.S.; Rivera, F.; Karthaus, M.; Fasola, G.; Canon, J.-L.; Hecht, J.R.; Yu, H.; Oliner, K.S.; Go, W.Y. PEAK: A Randomized, Multicenter Phase II Study of Panitumumab Plus Modified Fluorouracil, Leucovorin, and Oxaliplatin (mFOLFOX6) or Bevacizumab Plus mFOLFOX6 in Patients with Previously Untreated, Unresectable, Wild-Type *KRAS* Exon 2 Metastatic Colorectal Cancer. *J. Clin. Oncol.* **2014**, *32*, 2240–2247. [CrossRef]
43. Holch, J.W.; Ricard, I.; Stintzing, S.; Modest, D.P.; Heinemann, V. The relevance of primary tumour location in patients with metastatic colorectal cancer: A meta-analysis of first-line clinical trials. *Eur. J. Cancer* **2016**, *70*, 87–98. [CrossRef]
44. Loupakis, F.; Hurwitz, H.I.; Saltz, L.; Arnold, D.; Grothey, A.; Nguyen, Q.L.; Osborne, S.; Talbot, J.; Srock, S.; Lenz, H.-J. Impact of primary tumour location on efficacy of bevacizumab plus chemotherapy in metastatic colorectal cancer. *Br. J. Cancer* **2018**, *119*, 1451–1455. [CrossRef]
45. Hegewisch-Becker, S.; Graeven, U.; A Lerchenmüller, C.; Killing, B.; Depenbusch, R.; Steffens, C.-C.; Al-Batran, S.-E.; Lange, T.; Dietrich, G.; Stoehlmacher, J.; et al. Maintenance strategies after first-line oxaliplatin plus fluoropyrimidine plus bevacizumab for patients with metastatic colorectal cancer (AIO 0207): A randomised, non-inferiority, open-label, phase 3 trial. *Lancet Oncol.* **2015**, *16*, 1355–1369. [CrossRef]

46. Masi, G.; Salvatore, L.; Boni, L.; Loupakis, F.; Cremolini, C.; Fornaro, L.; Schirripa, M.; Cupini, S.; Barbara, C.; Safina, V.; et al. Continuation or reintroduction of bevacizumab beyond progression to first-line therapy in metastatic colorectal cancer: Final results of the randomized BEBYP trial. *Ann. Oncol.* **2015**, *26*, 724–730. [CrossRef]
47. Prager, G.W.; Taieb, J.; Fakih, M.; Ciardiello, F.; Van Cutsem, E.; Elez, E.; Cruz, F.M.; Wyrwicz, L.; Stroyakovskiy, D.; Pápai, Z.; et al. Trifluridine–Tipiracil and Bevacizumab in Refractory Metastatic Colorectal Cancer. *N. Engl. J. Med.* **2023**, *388*, 1657–1667. [CrossRef]
48. Otsu, S.; Hironaka, S. Current Status of Angiogenesis Inhibitors as Second-Line Treatment for Unresectable Colorectal Cancer. *Cancers* **2023**, *15*, 4564. [CrossRef]
49. Hashimoto, T.; Otsu, S.; Hironaka, S.; Takashima, A.; Mizusawa, J.; Kataoka, T.; Fukuda, H.; Tsukamoto, S.; Hamaguchi, T.; Kanemitsu, Y. Phase II biomarker identification study of anti-VEGF agents with FOLFIRI for pretreated metastatic colorectal cancer. *Future Oncol.* **2023**, *19*, 1593–1600. [CrossRef]
50. Kumar, R.; Crouthamel, M.-C.; Rominger, D.H.; Gontarek, R.R.; Tummino, P.J.; A Levin, R.; King, A.G. Myelosuppression and kinase selectivity of multikinase angiogenesis inhibitors. *Br. J. Cancer* **2009**, *101*, 1717–1723. [CrossRef]
51. Cao, Y.; Langer, R.; Ferrara, N. Targeting angiogenesis in oncology, ophthalmology and beyond. *Nat. Rev. Drug Discov.* **2023**, *22*, 476–495. [CrossRef]
52. Zhang, Y.; Zou, J.Y.; Wang, Z.; Wang, Y. Fruquintinib: A novel antivascular endothelial growth factor receptor tyrosine kinase inhibitor for the treatment of metastatic colorectal cancer. *Cancer Manag. Res.* **2019**, *11*, 7787–7803. [CrossRef]
53. Li, J.; Qin, S.; Xu, R.H.; Shen, L.; Xu, J.; Bai, Y.; Yang, L.; Deng, Y.; Chen, Z.D.; Zhong, H.; et al. Effect of Fruquintinib vs Placebo on Overall Survival in Patients with Previously Treated Metastatic Colorectal Cancer: The FRESCO Randomized Clinical Trial. *JAMA* **2018**, *319*, 2486–2496. [CrossRef]
54. Shirley, M. Fruquintinib: First Global Approval. *Drugs* **2018**, *78*, 1757–1761. [CrossRef]
55. Siu, L.L.; Shapiro, J.D.; Jonker, D.J.; Karapetis, C.S.; Zalcberg, J.R.; Simes, J.; Couture, F.; Moore, M.J.; Price, T.J.; Siddiqui, J.; et al. Phase III Randomized, Placebo-Controlled Study of Cetuximab Plus Brivanib Alaninate Versus Cetuximab Plus Placebo in Patients With Metastatic, Chemotherapy-Refractory, Wild-Type *K-RAS* Colorectal Carcinoma: The NCIC Clinical Trials Group and AGITG CO.20 Trial. *J. Clin. Oncol.* **2013**, *31*, 2477–2484.
56. Cunningham, D.; Wong, R.P.; D'Haens, G.; Douillard, J.Y.; Robertson, J.; Stone, A.M.; Van Cutsem, E. Cediranib with mFOLFOX6 vs bevacizumab with mFOLFOX6 in previously treated metastatic colo-rectal cancer. *Br. J. Cancer* **2013**, *108*, 493–502. [CrossRef]
57. Hoff, P.M.; Hochhaus, A.; Pestalozzi, B.C.; Tebbutt, N.C.; Li, J.; Kim, T.W.; Koynov, K.D.; Kurteva, G.; Pintér, T.; Cheng, Y.; et al. Cediranib Plus FOLFOX/CAPOX Versus Placebo Plus FOLFOX/CAPOX in Patients with Previously Untreated Metastatic Colorectal Cancer: A Randomized, Double-Blind, Phase III Study (HORIZON II). *J. Clin. Oncol.* **2012**, *30*, 3596–3603. [CrossRef]
58. Schmoll, H.-J.; Cunningham, D.; Sobrero, A.; Karapetis, C.S.; Rougier, P.; Koski, S.L.; Kocakova, I.; Bondarenko, I.; Bodoky, G.; Mainwaring, P.; et al. Cediranib With mFOLFOX6 Versus Bevacizumab With mFOLFOX6 As First-Line Treatment for Patients with Advanced Colorectal Cancer: A Double-Blind, Randomized Phase III Study (HORIZON III). *J. Clin. Oncol.* **2012**, *30*, 3588–3595. [CrossRef]
59. O'Neil, B.H.; Cainap, C.; Van Cutsem, E.; Gorbunova, V.; Karapetis, C.S.; Berlin, J.; Goldberg, R.M.; Qin, Q.; Qian, J.; Ricker, J.L.; et al. Randomized Phase II Open-Label Study of mFOLFOX6 in Combination with Linifanib or Bevacizumab for Metastatic Colorectal Cancer. *Clin. Color. Cancer* **2014**, *13*, 156–163.e2. [CrossRef]
60. Benson, A.B., 3rd; Kiss, I.; Bridgewater, J.; Eskens, F.A.; Sasse, C.; Vossen, S.; Chen, J.; Van Sant, C.; Ball, H.A.; Keating, A.; et al. BATON-CRC: A Phase II Randomized Trial Comparing Tivozanib Plus mFOLFOX6 with Bevacizumab Plus mFOLFOX6 in Stage IV Metastatic Colorectal Cancer. *Clin. Cancer Res.* **2016**, *22*, 5058–5067. [CrossRef]
61. Yang, T.S.; Oh, D.Y.; Guimbaud, R.; Szanto, J.; Salek, T.; Thurzo, L.; Vieitez, J.M.; Pover, G.M.; Kim, T.W. Vandetanib plus mFOLFOX6 in patients with advanced colorectal cancer (CRC): A randomized, double-blind, placebo-controlled phase II study. *J. Clin. Oncol.* **2009**, *27*, 4084. [CrossRef]
62. Hecht, J.R.; Trarbach, T.; Hainsworth, J.D.; Major, P.; Jäger, E.; Wolff, R.A.; Lloyd-Salvant, K.; Bodoky, G.; Pendergrass, K.; Berg, W.; et al. Randomized, placebo-controlled, phase III study of first-line oxaliplatin-based chemotherapy plus PTK787/ZK 222584, an oral vascular endothelial growth factor receptor inhibitor, in patients with metastatic colorectal adenocarcinoma. *J. Clin. Oncol.* **2011**, *29*, 1997–2003. [CrossRef]
63. Van Cutsem, E.; Bajetta, E.; Valle, J.; Köhne, C.H.; Hecht, J.R.; Moore, M.; Germond, C.; Berg, W.; Chen, B.L.; Jalava, T.; et al. Randomized, placebo-controlled, phase III study of oxaliplatin, fluorouracil, and leucovorin with or without PTK787/ZK 222584 in patients with previously treated metastatic colorectal adenocarcinoma. *J. Clin. Oncol.* **2011**, *29*, 2004–2010. [CrossRef]
64. Xu, R.-H.; Shen, L.; Wang, K.-M.; Wu, G.; Shi, C.-M.; Ding, K.-F.; Lin, L.-Z.; Wang, J.-W.; Xiong, J.-P.; Wu, C.-P.; et al. Famitinib versus placebo in the treatment of refractory metastatic colorectal cancer: A multicenter, randomized, double-blinded, placebo-controlled, phase II clinical trial. *Chin. J. Cancer* **2017**, *36*, 97. [CrossRef]
65. Van Cutsem, E.; Prenen, H.; D'Haens, G.; Bennouna, J.; Carrato, A.; Ducreux, M.; Bouché, O.; Sobrero, A.; Latini, L.; Staines, H.; et al. A phase I/II, open-label, randomised study of nintedanib plus mFOLFOX6 versus bevacizumab plus mFOLFOX6 in first-line metastatic colorectal cancer patients. *Ann. Oncol.* **2015**, *26*, 2085–2091. [CrossRef]
66. Ettrich, T.J.; Perkhofer, L.; Decker, T.; Hofheinz, R.D.; Heinemann, V.; Hoffmann, T.; Hebart, H.F.; Herrmann, T.; Hannig, C.V.; Büchner-Steudel, P.; et al. Nintedanib plus mFOLFOX6 as second-line treatment of metastatic, chemorefractory colorectal cancer: The randomised, placebo-controlled, phase II TRICC-C study (AIO-KRK-0111). *Int. J. Cancer* **2021**, *148*, 1428–1437. [CrossRef]

67. Van Cutsem, E.; Yoshino, T.; Lenz, H.; Lonardi, S.; Falcone, A.; Limón, M.; Saunders, M.; Sobrero, A.; Park, Y.; Ferreiro, R.; et al. Nintedanib for the treatment of patients with refractory metastatic colorectal cancer (LUME-Colon 1): A phase III, international, randomized, placebo-controlled study. *Ann. Oncol.* **2018**, *29*, 1955–1963. [CrossRef]
68. Infante, J.R.; Reid, T.R.; Cohn, A.L.; Edenfield, W.J.; Cescon, T.P.; Hamm, J.T.; Malik, I.A.; Rado, T.A.; McGee, P.J.; Richards, D.A.; et al. Axitinib and/or bevacizumab with modified FOLFOX-6 as first-line therapy for metastatic colorectal cancer: A randomized phase 2 study. *Cancer* **2013**, *119*, 2555–2563. [CrossRef]
69. Grávalos, C.; Carrato, A.; Tobeña, M.; Rodriguez-Garrote, M.; Soler, G.; Vieitez, J.M.; Robles, L.; Valladares-Ayerbes, M.; Polo, E.; Limón, M.L.; et al. A Randomized Phase II Study of Axitinib as Maintenance Therapy After First-line Treatment for Metastatic Colorectal Cancer. *Clin. Color. Cancer* **2018**, *17*, e323–e329. [CrossRef]
70. Bendell, J.C.; Tournigand, C.; Swieboda-Sadlej, A.; Barone, C.; Wainberg, Z.A.; Kim, J.G.; Pericay, C.; Pastorelli, D.; Tarazi, J.; Rosbrook, B.; et al. Axitinib or Bevacizumab Plus FOLFIRI or Modified FOLFOX-6 After Failure of First-Line Therapy for Metastatic Colorectal Cancer: A Randomized Phase II Study. *Clin. Color. Cancer* **2013**, *12*, 239–247. [CrossRef]
71. García-Carbonero, R.; van Cutsem, E.; Rivera, F.; Jassem, J.; Gore, I., Jr.; Tebbutt, N.; Braiteh, F.; Argiles, G.; Wainberg, Z.; Funke, R.; et al. Randomized Phase II Trial of Parsatuzumab (Anti-EGFL7) or Placebo in Combination with FOLFOX and Bevacizumab for First-Line Metastatic Colorectal Cancer. *Oncologist* **2017**, *22*, 1281. [CrossRef]
72. Bendell, J.C.; Sauri, T.; Gracián, A.C.; Alvarez, R.; Lopez, C.L.; García-Alfonso, P.; Hussein, M.; Miron, M.L.; Cervantes, A.; Montagut, C.; et al. The McCAVE Trial: Vanucizumab plus mFOLFOX-6 Versus Bevacizumab plus mFOLFOX-6 in Patients with Previously Untreated Metastatic Colorectal Carcinoma (mCRC). *Oncologist* **2019**, *25*, e451–e459. [CrossRef]
73. Peeters, M.; Strickland, A.H.; Lichinitser, M.; Suresh, A.V.S.; Manikhas, G.; Shapiro, J.; Rogowski, W.; Huang, X.; Wu, B.; Warner, D.; et al. A randomised, double-blind, placebo-controlled phase 2 study of trebananib (AMG 386) in combination with FOLFIRI in patients with previously treated metastatic colorectal carcinoma. *Br. J. Cancer* **2013**, *108*, 503–511. [CrossRef]
74. Martin, J.D.; Seano, G.; Jain, R.K. Normalizing Function of Tumor Vessels: Progress, Opportunities, and Challenges. *Annu. Rev. Physiol.* **2019**, *81*, 505–534. [CrossRef]
75. Jain, R.K. Normalization of Tumor Vasculature: An Emerging Concept in Antiangiogenic Therapy. *Science* **2005**, *307*, 58–62. [CrossRef]
76. Winkler, F.; Kozin, S.V.; Tong, R.T.; Chae, S.-S.; Booth, M.F.; Garkavtsev, I.; Xu, L.; Hicklin, D.J.; Fukumura, D.; di Tomaso, E.; et al. Kinetics of vascular normalization by VEGFR2 blockade governs brain tumor response to radiation: Role of oxygenation, angiopoietin-1, and matrix metalloproteinases. *Cancer Cell* **2004**, *6*, 553–563.
77. Helfrich, I.; Scheffrahn, I.; Bartling, S.; Weis, J.; von Felbert, V.; Middleton, M.; Kato, M.; Ergün, S.; Augustin, H.G.; Schadendorf, D. Resistance to antiangiogenic therapy is directed by vascular phenotype, vessel stabilization, and maturation in malignant melanoma. *J. Exp. Med.* **2010**, *207*, 491–503. [CrossRef]
78. Frentzas, S.; Simoneau, E.; Bridgeman, V.L.; Vermeulen, P.B.; Foo, S.; Kostaras, E.; Nathan, M.R.; Wotherspoon, A.; Gao, Z.-H.; Shi, Y.; et al. Vessel co-option mediates resistance to anti-angiogenic therapy in liver metastases. *Nat. Med.* **2016**, *22*, 1294–1302. [CrossRef]
79. Cao, Z.; Ding, B.-S.; Guo, P.; Lee, S.B.; Butler, J.M.; Casey, S.C.; Simons, M.; Tam, W.; Felsher, D.W.; Shido, K.; et al. Angiocrine Factors Deployed by Tumor Vascular Niche Induce B Cell Lymphoma Invasiveness and Chemoresistance. *Cancer Cell* **2014**, *25*, 350–365. [CrossRef]
80. Kerbel, R.S.; Shaked, Y. The potential clinical promise of 'multimodality' metronomic chemotherapy revealed by preclinical studies of metastatic disease. *Cancer Lett.* **2017**, *400*, 293–304. [CrossRef]
81. Cremolini, C.; Marmorino, F.; Bergamo, F.; Aprile, G.; Salvatore, L.; Masi, G.; Dell'aquila, E.; Antoniotti, C.; Murgioni, S.; Allegrini, G.; et al. Phase II randomised study of maintenance treatment with bevacizumab or bevacizumab plus metronomic chemotherapy after first-line induction with FOLFOXIRI plus Bevacizumab for metastatic colorectal cancer patients: The MOMA trial. *Eur. J. Cancer* **2019**, *109*, 175–182. [CrossRef]
82. Li, Q.; Wang, Y.; Jia, W.; Deng, H.; Li, G.; Deng, W.; Chen, J.; Kim, B.Y.; Jiang, W.; Liu, Q.; et al. Low-Dose Anti-Angiogenic Therapy Sensitizes Breast Cancer to PD-1 Blockade. *Clin. Cancer Res.* **2020**, *26*, 1712–1724. [CrossRef]
83. Mettu, N.B.; Ou, F.S.; Zemla, T.J.; Halfdanarson, T.R.; Lenz, H.J.; Breakstone, R.A.; Boland, P.M.; Crysler, O.V.; Wu, C.; Nixon, A.B. Assessment of Capecitabine and Bevacizumab with or Without Atezolizumab for the Treatment of Refractory Metastatic Colorectal Cancer: A Randomized Clinical Trial. *JAMA Netw. Open* **2022**, *5*, e2149040. [CrossRef]
84. Lamplugh, Z.; Fan, Y. Vascular Microenvironment, Tumor Immunity and Immunotherapy. *Front. Immunol.* **2021**, *12*, 811485. [CrossRef]
85. Schmittnaegel, M.; Rigamonti, N.; Kadioglu, E.; Cassará, A.; Rmili, C.W.; Kiialainen, A.; Kienast, Y.; Mueller, H.-J.; Ooi, C.-H.; Laoui, D.; et al. Dual angiopoietin-2 and VEGFA inhibition elicits antitumor immunity that is enhanced by PD-1 checkpoint blockade. *Sci. Transl. Med.* **2017**, *9*, eaak9670. [CrossRef]
86. Di Tacchio, M.; Macas, J.; Weissenberger, J.; Sommer, K.; Bahr, O.; Steinbach, J.P.; Senft, C.; Seifert, V.; Glas, M.; Herrlinger, U.; et al. Tumor Vessel Normalization, Immunostimulatory Reprogramming, and Improved Survival in Glio-blastoma with Combined Inhibition of PD-1, Angiopoietin-2, and VEGF. *Cancer Immunol. Res.* **2019**, *7*, 1910–1927. [CrossRef]

87. Shigeta, K.; Datta, M.; Hato, T.; Kitahara, S.; Chen, I.X.; Matsui, A.; Kikuchi, H.; Mamessier, E.; Aoki, S.; Ramjiawan, R.R.; et al. Dual Programmed Death Receptor-1 and Vascular Endothelial Growth Factor Receptor-2 Blockade Promotes Vascular Normalization and Enhances Antitumor Immune Responses in Hepatocellular Carcinoma. *Hepatology* **2019**, *71*, 1247–1261. [CrossRef]
88. Weiss, A.; Ding, X.; van Beijnum, J.R.; Wong, I.; Wong, T.J.; Berndsen, R.H.; Dormond, O.; Dallinga, M.; Shen, L.; Schlingemann, R.O.; et al. Rapid optimization of drug combinations for the optimal angiostatic treatment of cancer. *Angiogenesis* **2015**, *18*, 233–244. [CrossRef]
89. Gerhardt, H.; Golding, M.; Fruttiger, M.; Ruhrberg, C.; Lundkvist, A.; Abramsson, A.; Jeltsch, M.; Mitchell, C.; Alitalo, K.; Shima, D.; et al. VEGF guides angiogenic sprouting utilizing endothelial tip cell filopodia. *J. Cell Biol.* **2003**, *161*, 1163–1177. [CrossRef]
90. Yang, Y.; Zhang, Y.; Cao, Z.; Ji, H.; Yang, X.; Iwamoto, H.; Wahlberg, E.; Länne, T.; Sun, B.; Cao, Y. Anti-VEGF– and anti-VEGF receptor–induced vascular alteration in mouse healthy tissues. *Proc. Natl. Acad. Sci. USA* **2013**, *110*, 12018–12023. [CrossRef]
91. Huang, X.; Bai, X.; Cao, Y.; Wu, J.; Huang, M.; Tang, D.; Tao, S.; Zhu, T.; Liu, Y.; Yang, Y.; et al. Lymphoma endothelium preferentially expresses Tim-3 and facilitates the progression of lymphoma by me-diating immune evasion. *J. Exp. Med.* **2010**, *207*, 505–520. [CrossRef]
92. Gerlinger, M.; Rowan, A.J.; Horswell, S.; Math, M.; Larkin, J.; Endesfelder, D.; Gronroos, E.; Martinez, P.; Matthews, N.; Stewart, A.; et al. Intratumor heterogeneity and branched evolution revealed by multiregion sequencing. *N. Engl. J. Med.* **2012**, *366*, 883–892. [CrossRef]
93. Nolan, D.J.; Ginsberg, M.; Israely, E.; Palikuqi, B.; Poulos, M.G.; James, D.; Ding, B.-S.; Schachterle, W.; Liu, Y.; Rosenwaks, Z.; et al. Molecular Signatures of Tissue-Specific Microvascular Endothelial Cell Heterogeneity in Organ Maintenance and Regeneration. *Dev. Cell* **2013**, *26*, 204–219. [CrossRef]
94. Zhao, Q.; Eichten, A.; Parveen, A.; Adler, C.; Huang, Y.; Wang, W.; Ding, Y.; Adler, A.; Nevins, T.; Ni, M.; et al. Single-Cell Transcriptome Analyses Reveal Endothelial Cell Heterogeneity in Tumors and Changes following Antiangiogenic Treatment. *Cancer Res.* **2018**, *78*, 2370–2382. [CrossRef]
95. Van Beijnum, J.R.; Nowak-Sliwinska, P.; Huijbers, E.J.; Thijssen, V.L.; Griffioen, A.W. The great escape; the hallmarks of resistance to antiangiogenic therapy. *Pharmacol. Rev.* **2015**, *67*, 441–461. [CrossRef]
96. Bridgeman, V.L.; Vermeulen, P.B.; Foo, S.; Bilecz, A.; Daley, F.; Kostaras, E.; Nathan, M.R.; Wan, E.; Frentzas, S.; Schweiger, T.; et al. Vessel co-option is common in human lung metastases and mediates resistance to anti-angiogenic therapy in preclinical lung metastasis models. *J. Pathol.* **2016**, *241*, 362–374. [CrossRef]
97. Schellerer, V.S.; Croner, R.S.; Weinländer, K.; Hohenberger, W.; Stürzl, M.; Naschberger, E. Endothelial cells of human colorectal cancer and healthy colon reveal phenotypic differences in culture. *Lab Investig.* **2007**, *87*, 1159–1170. [CrossRef]
98. Naschberger, E.; Fuchs, M.; Dickel, N.; Kunz, M.; Popp, B.; Anchang, C.G.; Demmler, R.; Lyu, Y.; Uebe, S.; Ekici, A.B.; et al. Tumor microenvironment-dependent epigenetic imprinting in the vasculature predicts colon cancer outcome. *Cancer Commun.* **2023**, *43*, 1280–1285. [CrossRef]
99. Wang, Q.; He, Z.; Huang, M.; Liu, T.; Wang, Y.; Xu, H.; Duan, H.; Ma, P.; Zhang, L.; Zamvil, S.S.; et al. Vascular niche IL-6 induces alternative macrophage activation in glioblastoma through HIF-2α. *Nat. Commun.* **2018**, *9*, 559. [CrossRef]
100. Naschberger, E.; Liebl, A.; Schellerer, V.S.; Schütz, M.; Britzen-Laurent, N.; Kölbel, P.; Schaal, U.; Haep, L.; Regensburger, D.; Wittmann, T.; et al. Matricellular protein SPARCL1 regulates tumor microenvironment-dependent endothelial cell heterogeneity in colorectal carcinoma. *J. Clin. Investig.* **2016**, *126*, 4187–4204. [CrossRef]
101. Ghajar, C.M.; Peinado, H.; Mori, H.; Matei, I.R.; Evason, K.J.; Brazier, H.; Almeida, D.; Koller, A.; Hajjar, K.A.; Stainier, D.Y.; et al. The perivascular niche regulates breast tumour dormancy. *Nat. Cell Biol.* **2013**, *15*, 807–817. [CrossRef]
102. Hu, H.; Zhang, H.; Ge, W.; Liu, X.; Loera, S.; Chu, P.; Chen, H.; Peng, J.; Zhou, L.; Yu, S.; et al. Secreted protein acidic and rich in cysteines-like 1 suppresses aggressiveness and predicts better survival in colorectal cancers. *Clin. Cancer Res.* **2012**, *18*, 5438–5448. [CrossRef]
103. Khan, A.K.; Wu, F.T.; Cruz-Munoz, W.; Kerbel, R.S. Ang2 inhibitors and Tie2 activators: Potential therapeutics in perioperative treatment of early stage cancer. *EMBO Mol. Med.* **2021**, *13*, e08253. [CrossRef]
104. Hendrikx, S.; Coso, S.; Prat-Luri, B.; Wetterwald, L.; Sabine, A.; Franco, C.A.; Nassiri, S.; Zangger, N.; Gerhardt, H.; Delorenzi, M.; et al. Endothelial Calcineurin Signaling Restrains Metastatic Outgrowth by Regulating Bmp2. *Cell Rep.* **2019**, *26*, 1227–1241.e6. [CrossRef]
105. Thomas, H. Colorectal cancer: CRC endothelial regulation. *Nat. Rev. Gastroenterol. Hepatol.* **2016**, *13*, 682.
106. Dirkx, A.E.M.; Egbrink, M.G.A.O.; E Kuijpers, M.J.; Van Der Niet, S.T.; Heijnen, V.V.T.; Steege, J.C.A.B.-T.; Wagstaff, J.; Griffioen, A.W. Tumor angiogenesis modulates leukocyte-vessel wall interactions in vivo by reducing endothelial adhesion molecule expression. *Cancer Res.* **2003**, *63*, 2322–2329.
107. Nambiar, D.K.; Aguilera, T.; Cao, H.; Kwok, S.; Kong, C.; Bloomstein, J.; Wang, Z.; Rangan, V.S.; Jiang, D.; von Eyben, R.; et al. Galectin-1–driven T cell exclusion in the tumor endothelium promotes immunotherapy resistance. *J. Clin. Investig.* **2019**, *129*, 5553–5567. [CrossRef]
108. Motz, G.T.; Santoro, S.P.; Wang, L.-P.; Garrabrant, T.; Lastra, R.R.; Hagemann, I.S.; Lal, P.; Feldman, M.D.; Benencia, F.; Coukos, G. Tumor endothelium FasL establishes a selective immune barrier promoting tolerance in tumors. *Nat. Med.* **2014**, *20*, 607–615. [CrossRef]

109. Streubel, B.; Chott, A.; Huber, D.; Exner, M.; Jäger, U.; Wagner, O.; Schwarzinger, I. Lymphoma-Specific Genetic Aberrations in Microvascular Endothelial Cells in B-Cell Lymphomas. *N. Engl. J. Med.* **2004**, *351*, 250–259. [CrossRef]
110. Dunleavey, J.M.; Dudley, A.C. Vascular Mimicry: Concepts and Implications for Anti-Angiogenic Therapy. *Curr. Angiogenesis* **2012**, *1*, 133–138. [CrossRef]
111. Van der Schaft, D.W.; Seftor, R.E.; Seftor, E.A.; Hess, A.R.; Gruman, L.M.; Kirschmann, D.A.; Yokoyama, Y.; Griffioen, A.W.; Hendrix, M.J. Effects of angiogenesis inhibitors on vascular network formation by human endothelial and melanoma cells. *J. Natl. Cancer Inst.* **2004**, *96*, 1473–1477. [CrossRef]
112. Zhao, C.; Gomez, G.A.; Zhao, Y.; Yang, Y.; Cao, D.; Lu, J.; Yang, H.; Lin, S. ETV2 mediates endothelial transdifferentiation of glioblastoma. *Signal Transduct. Target. Ther.* **2018**, *3*, 4. [CrossRef]
113. Ricci-Vitiani, L.; Pallini, R.; Biffoni, M.; Todaro, M.; Invernici, G.; Cenci, T.; Maira, G.; Parati, E.A.; Stassi, G.; Larocca, L.M.; et al. Tumor vascularization via endothelial differentiation of glioblastoma stem-like cells. *Nature* **2010**, *468*, 824–828. [CrossRef]
114. Wang, R.; Chadalavada, K.; Wilshire, J.; Kowalik, U.; Hovinga, K.E.; Geber, A.; Fligelman, B.; Leversha, M.; Brennan, C.; Tabar, V. Glioblastoma stem-like cells give rise to tumour endothelium. *Nature* **2010**, *468*, 829–833. [CrossRef]
115. Akino, T.; Hida, K.; Hida, Y.; Tsuchiya, K.; Freedman, D.; Muraki, C.; Ohga, N.; Matsuda, K.; Akiyama, K.; Harabayashi, T.; et al. Cytogenetic Abnormalities of Tumor-Associated Endothelial Cells in Human Malignant Tumors. *Am. J. Pathol.* **2009**, *175*, 2657–2667. [CrossRef]
116. Ohga, N.; Ishikawa, S.; Maishi, N.; Akiyama, K.; Hida, Y.; Kawamoto, T.; Sadamoto, Y.; Osawa, T.; Yamamoto, K.; Kondoh, M.; et al. Heterogeneity of tumor endothelial cells: Comparison between tumor endothelial cells isolated from high- and low-metastatic tumors. *Am. J. Pathol.* **2012**, *180*, 1294–1307. [CrossRef]
117. Yan, Y.; Wei, C.-L.; Zhang, W.-R.; Cheng, H.-P.; Liu, J. Cross-talk between calcium and reactive oxygen species signaling. *Acta Pharmacol. Sin.* **2006**, *27*, 821–826. [CrossRef]
118. Zheng, Y.; Zhou, R.; Cai, J.; Yang, N.; Wen, Z.; Zhang, Z.; Sun, H.; Huang, G.; Guan, Y.; Huang, N.; et al. Matrix Stiffness Triggers Lipid Metabolic Cross-talk between Tumor and Stromal Cells to Mediate Bevacizumab Resistance in Colorectal Cancer Liver Metastases. *Cancer Res.* **2023**, *83*, 3577–3592. [CrossRef]
119. Sun, Y.; Wen, F.; Yan, C.; Su, L.; Luo, J.; Chi, W.; Zhang, S. Mitophagy Protects the Retina Against Anti-Vascular Endothelial Growth Factor Therapy-Driven Hypoxia via Hypoxia-Inducible Factor-1α Signaling. *Front. Cell Dev. Biol.* **2021**, *9*, 727822. [CrossRef]
120. Suleyman, H.; Kocaturk, H.; Bedir, F.; Turangezli, O.; Arslan, R.; Coban, T.; Altuner, D. Effect of adenosine triphosphate, benidipine and their combinations on bevacizumab-induced kidney damage in rats. *Adv. Clin. Exp. Med.* **2021**, *30*, 1175–1183. [CrossRef]
121. Jackstadt, R.; van Hooff, S.R.; Leach, J.D.; Cortes-Lavaud, X.; Lohuis, J.O.; Ridgway, R.A.; Wouters, V.M.; Roper, J.; Kendall, T.J.; Roxburgh, C.S.; et al. Epithelial NOTCH Signaling Rewires the Tumor Microenvironment of Colorectal Cancer to Drive Poor-Prognosis Subtypes and Metastasis. *Cancer Cell* **2019**, *36*, 319–336.e7. [CrossRef]
122. Varga, J.; Nicolas, A.; Petrocelli, V.; Pesic, M.; Mahmoud, A.; Michels, B.E.; Etlioglu, E.; Yepes, D.; Häupl, B.; Ziegler, P.K.; et al. AKT-dependent NOTCH3 activation drives tumor progression in a model of mesenchymal colorectal cancer. *J. Exp. Med.* **2020**, *217*, e20191515. [CrossRef]

Disclaimer/Publisher's Note: The statements, opinions and data contained in all publications are solely those of the individual author(s) and contributor(s) and not of MDPI and/or the editor(s). MDPI and/or the editor(s) disclaim responsibility for any injury to people or property resulting from any ideas, methods, instructions or products referred to in the content.

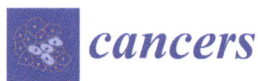

Article

A Novel m7G-Related Gene Signature Predicts the Prognosis of Colon Cancer

Jing Chen [1,2,†], Yi-Wen Song [3,†], Guan-Zhan Liang [1,2], Zong-Jin Zhang [1,2], Xiao-Feng Wen [1,2], Rui-Bing Li [1,2], Yong-Le Chen [1,2], Wei-Dong Pan [4], Xiao-Wen He [1,2], Tuo Hu [1,2,*] and Zhen-Yu Xian [1,2,*]

[1] Department of Colorectal Surgery, The Sixth Affiliated Hospital, Sun Yat-sen University, Guangzhou 510655, China
[2] Guangdong Provincial Key Laboratory of Colorectal and Pelvic Floor Diseases, The Sixth Affiliated Hospital, Sun Yat-sen University, Guangzhou 510655, China
[3] Department of Radiotherapy, The Sixth Affiliated Hospital, Sun Yat-sen University, Guangzhou 510655, China
[4] Department of Pancreatic Hepatobiliary Surgery, The Sixth Affiliated Hospital, Sun Yat-sen University, Guangzhou 510655, China
* Correspondence: hutuo3@mail.sysu.edu.cn (T.H.); xianzhy@mail2.sysu.edu.cn (Z.-Y.X.); Tel.: +86-020-38254009 (Z.-Y.X.)
† These authors contributed equally to this work.

Simple Summary: N7-methylguanosine (m7G) plays an important role in the tumorigenesis and progression of colon cancer (CC). According to the capability of m7G-related genes, they are classified into three types: methyltransferases, binding proteins and demethylases. Hence, m7G-related genes could promote cancers by regulating RNAs. To further explore the functions of m7G, 29 m7G-related genes were selected and then 15 of them were utilized to construct a novel signature, termed the m7G score. Altogether, we found that the prognosis of CC patients with distinct m7G scores were significantly different. Furthermore, we applied various experiments and bioinformatics analyses to validate our results. We expect that the m7G score could indicate the correct clinical situation, which might optimize our treatments for CC patients.

Abstract: Colon cancer (CC), one of the most common malignancies worldwide, lacks an effective prognostic prediction biomarker. N7-methylguanosine (m7G) methylation is a common RNA modification type and has been proven to influence tumorigenesis. However, the correlation between m7G-related genes and CC remains unclear. The gene expression levels and clinical information of CC patients were downloaded from public databases. Twenty-nine m7G-related genes were obtained from the published literature. Via unsupervised clustering based on the expression levels of m7G-related genes, CC patients were divided into three m7G clusters. Based on differentially expressed genes (DEGs) from the above three groups, CC patients were further divided into three gene clusters. The m7G score, a prognostic model, was established using principal component analysis (PCA) based on 15 prognosis-associated m7G genes. KM curve analysis demonstrated that the overall survival rate was remarkably higher in the high-m7G score group, which was much more significant in advanced CC patients as confirmed by subgroup analysis. Correlation analysis indicated that the m7G score was associated with tumor mutational burden (TMB), PD-L1 expression, immune infiltration, and drug sensitivity. The expression level of prognosis-related m7G genes was further confirmed in human CC cell lines and samples. This study established an m7G gene-based prognostic model (m7G score), which demonstrated the important roles of m7G-related genes during CC initiation and progression. The m7G score could be a practical biomarker to predict immunotherapy response and prognosis in CC patients.

Keywords: N7-methylguanosine (m7G) methylation; m7G-related genes; colon cancer; prognostic model

Citation: Chen, J.; Song, Y.-W.; Liang, G.-Z.; Zhang, Z.-J.; Wen, X.-F.; Li, R.-B.; Chen, Y.-L.; Pan, W.-D.; He, X.-W.; Hu, T.; et al. A Novel m7G-Related Gene Signature Predicts the Prognosis of Colon Cancer. *Cancers* 2022, 14, 5527. https://doi.org/10.3390/cancers14225527

Academic Editor: Susanne Merkel

Received: 11 October 2022
Accepted: 8 November 2022
Published: 10 November 2022

Publisher's Note: MDPI stays neutral with regard to jurisdictional claims in published maps and institutional affiliations.

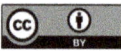

Copyright: © 2022 by the authors. Licensee MDPI, Basel, Switzerland. This article is an open access article distributed under the terms and conditions of the Creative Commons Attribution (CC BY) license (https://creativecommons.org/licenses/by/4.0/).

1. Introduction

CC is one of the most common cancer types with relatively high mortality. Recently, with the rapid development of colonoscopy and CC therapy, the morbidity and mortality of CC patients have gradually decreased in some developed countries [1,2]. However, effective prognostic biomarkers are still lacking, which could improve the clinical management of CC patients. Hence, the exploration of new biomarkers with prognostic value is especially important.

N7-methylguanosine (m7G), an important post-transcriptional modification, occurs at the N7 atom of RNA guanine by addition of a methyl group [3]. The m7G modification has been reported to promote cancer progression by modifying tRNA, miRNA and lncRNA, including the progression of intrahepatic cholangiocarcinoma, breast cancer, and lung adenocarcinoma [4–6]. Based on their functions in biological processes, m7G-related genes are classified into three types: writers (methyltransferases), readers (binding proteins), and erasers (demethylases) [3,7,8]. In human beings, methyltransferase-like 1 (METTL1) and the WD repeat domain 4 (WDR4) are the most well-studied regulators of m7G, and have been reported to participate in tumor progression by regulating tumor immunity, metabolic reprogramming, and drug resistance [9–13].

As demonstrated in the published literature, several genes are involved in the regulation of the m7G process. AGO2 has been reported to inhibit stable translation by binding to the cap located on target mRNA [14]. Additionally, translation efficiency and mRNA nuclear export are regulated by eIF4E, which could bind to the m7G cap directly [15]. Wang et al. demonstrated that DCP2 plays a vital role in decapping m7G caps on mRNA [16]. Although the above research has demonstrated the biological characteristics of m7G in detail, the prognostic value of m7G in CC patients remains elusive.

Our study constructed a m7G gene-based prognostic model (the m7G score) for CC patients based on the data from the TCGA and GEO public databases. The predictive capability of the m7G score was evaluated by KM survival curve analysis. Moreover, we have validated the expression of 15 prognosis-related m7G genes in cell lines and CC tissues from our institution. Altogether, our study identified the m7G score as a useful tool for prognosis prediction and clinical treatment guidance for CC patients.

2. Materials and Methods

2.1. Data Collection

The gene expression data, clinical characteristics, and mutational information of CC samples were obtained from The Cancer Genome Atlas (TCGA) and Gene Expression Omnibus (GEO). TCGA-COAD (n = 514) was downloaded from https://portal.gdc.cancer.gov up to 5 July 2022 and converted from FTPM into TPM. GSE39582 (n = 585) was downloaded from https://www.ncbi.nlm.nih.gov/geo/ up to 5 July 2022. Copy number variations (CNVs) of CC patients were downloaded from http://xena.ucsc.edu, accessed on 5 July 2022. The data from TCGA-COAD and GSE39582 were merged to form a new dataset via an R package for subsequent analysis. As illustrated in Supplementary Table S1, a total of 29 m7G-related genes were extracted from the published literature [5].

2.2. Unsupervised Clustering of 29 m7G-Related Genes

Among 29 m7G-related genes, there were 3 writers (METTL1, WDR4, and NSUN2), 8 erasers (DCP2, DCPS, NUDT10, NUDT11, NUDT16, NUDT3, NUDT4, and NUDT4B), and 18 readers (AGO2, CYFIP1, EIF4E, EIF4E1B, EIF4E2, EIF4E3, GEMIN5, LARP1, NCBP1, NCBP2, NCBP3, EIF3D, EIF4A1, EIF4G3, IFIT5, LSM1, NCBP2L, and SNUPN). The STRING database (http://www.db.org/ (accessed on 7 November 2022)) was utilized to analyze the interactive network of these m7G-related genes. Unsupervised clustering analysis was conducted via the Consensus Cluster Plus package (version 1.58.0) based on the k-means algorithm to evaluate the distinct expression of m7G-related genes or prognostic genes [17]. Then, CC patients were divided into three m7G clusters based on the expression level of m7G-related genes.

2.3. Gene Set Variation Analysis (GSVA)

Gene set variation analysis (GSVA) was performed to identify the distinct biological processes between expression signatures of m7G-related genes from different clusters via the GSVA R package (version 1.42.1). The c2.cp.kegg.V7.2.symbols gene set, downloaded from the Molecular Signatures Database, was used for GSVA. A p value less than 0.05 was considered statistically significant in the GSVA analysis [18].

2.4. Differentially Expressed Genes (DEGs)

Based on the expression level of m7G-related genes, CC patients were divided into 3 different m7G clusters. Then, DEGs among these three m7G clusters were evaluated via the R package "limma" (version 3.50.3) [19].

2.5. Gene Ontology (GO)

GO was used for enrichment analyses via the R package "cluster Profiler" (version 4.2.2). Differentially expressed genes with a p value < 0.05 were selected for GO enrichment pathway analysis [20].

2.6. Construction of Gene Clusters and m7G Score

A random forest was selected to delete redundant DEGs obtained from the previous step. Then, the prognostic significance of remaining genes was assessed via univariate cox regression analysis. CC patients were divided into 3 different gene clusters for subsequent analysis based on DEGs with prognostic significance using unsupervised clustering analysis. Then, principal component analysis (PCA) was conducted to quantify the expression signature of 15 DEGs with prognostic significance, termed the m7G score. The m7G score was established and formulated as follows:

$$\text{m7G score} = \sum PC1i + \sum PC2i$$

PC1 and PC2 are principal component 1 and principal component 2 respectively, while i means the expression level of DEGs with prognostic significance among three gene clusters. The optimal cutoff was selected to divide CC patients into high- and low-m7G score groups.

2.7. Single Sample Gene Set Enrichment Analysis (ssGSEA)

ssGSEA was used to evaluate the infiltration of immunocytes in CC patients among different m7G clusters, which demonstrated the correlation between m7G-related gene expression and immunotherapy response.

2.8. RNA Extraction and Quantitative Polymerase Chain Reaction (qPCR)

To further validate the prognostic value of the m7G score, we assessed the expression level of 15 m7G-related genes in human CC cell lines and tissue samples. CC tissues and adjacent normal tissues were obtained from the tissue bank of Sixth Affiliated Hospital, Sun Yat-sen University. An RNA extraction process was performed using TRIzol to collect the total RNA from cell lines and tissue specimens. The reverse transcription reaction was performed using a ReverTra Ace qPCR RT Kit (Toyobo, Japan). The real-time PCR was conducted based on cDNA obtained from the above reverse transcription reaction using ABI QuantStudio™ 7 Flex Real Time PCR Systems. The expression level of m7G-related genes was normalized to β-actin using the $2^{-\Delta\Delta Ct}$ method. The primer sequences of the indicated genes were listed in Supplementary Table S5.

3. Results

3.1. The Alterations and Biological Characteristics of 29 m7G-Related Genes in CC Patients

A total of 29 m7G-related genes were ultimately selected based on previous studies and the expression matrices of 29 m7G-related genes were obtained from the TCGA and GEO databases (Supplementary Table S1). The regulation network diagram of these m7G-related genes is exhibited in Figure 1A. As visualized by the loop graph, the m7G-related genes were scattered across most chromosomes except for chromosomes 7, 13, 14, 18, 19, and 20 (Figure 1B). The mutation information of m7G-related genes in CC samples are displayed in Figure 1C. Overall, 102 out of 454 (22.47%) samples harbored different types of mutations, with EIF4G3 as the most common mutated m7G-related gene. Meanwhile, no mutation was identified in NUDT16, NUDT4, and NUDT4B, and missense mutations were found in EIF4E, EIF4A1, and SNUPN. Among all mutation types, missense mutation was the most frequent mutation type found in CC patients. Copy number amplification was demonstrated in 13 m7G-related genes (AGO2, LSM1, NCBP2, NSUN2, NUDT3, EIF4E1B, EIF3D, METTL1, EIF4E3, NUDT16, LARP1, GEMIN5, and NCBP3), while copy number deletion was found in 11 m7G-related genes (EIF4E2, SNUPN, IFIT5, DCPS, NCBP1, EIF4G3, EIF4E, NUDT4, DCP2, CYFIP1, and EIF4A1) (Figure 1D). As illustrated in Figure 1E, the expression levels of the indicated m7G-related genes were significantly different between CC and normal samples except for NUDT4B, CYFIP1, NCBP3, and IFIT5. Moreover, the differential expression levels of m7G-related genes in CC patients with wild EIF4G3 and mutated EIF4G3 are demonstrated in Figure S1A–E. Taken together, these data indicate that copy number variation might be one of the regulatory mechanisms for m7G-related genes' expression.

3.2. The m7G-Related Colon Cancer Subtype and Clinical Prognosis

Data from TCGA-COAD and GSE39582 were merged to form a new dataset via an R package for subsequent analysis. Based on the expression level of 29 m7G-related genes, k-means clustering was performed with different k values (k = 2–5). The best clustering effect was obtained with a k value of three (Figures 2A,B and S1F–K). CC patients were divided into three groups based on the expression level of 29 m7G-related genes, named m7G cluster A, B, and C. Moreover, based on the expression level of DEGs among the above three m7G clusters, 1535 intersecting genes were obtained and displayed in a Venn diagram (Figure 2C, Supplementary Table S2). PCA results demonstrated that the clustering result was significantly different and effective (Figure 2D). Kaplan–Meier (KM) curves demonstrated that the overall survival (OS) of CC patients in m7G clusters A and B was much better than that in m7G cluster C (Figure 2E). The heatmap illustrated m7G-related gene expression levels in CC patients with different clinical characteristics and m7G clusters (Figure 2F).

3.3. Biological Differences among CC Patients from Three m7G Clusters

To further identify the biological difference among CC patients in different m7G clusters, GO, GSVA, and ssGSEA analyses were performed. GO analysis results revealed that DEGs among m7G clusters were mainly enriched in the following pathways: organelle fission and nuclear division (Biological Process); chromosomal region and centromeric region (Cellular Component); and GTPase regulator activity and nucleoside-triphosphatase regulator activity (Molecular Function, Figure 3A,B). These results suggested that the DEGs among the three m7G clusters might be involved in metabolic reprogramming of CC cells.

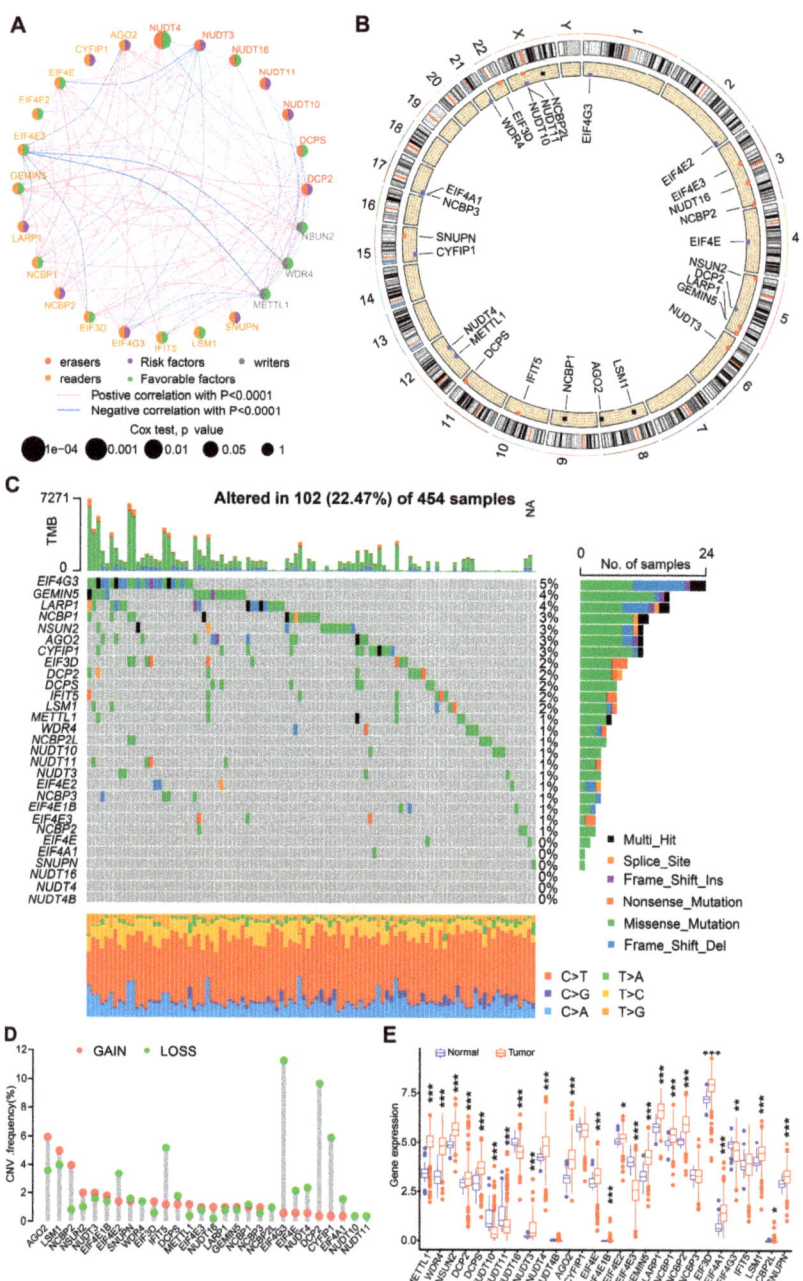

Figure 1. Genetic alterations and expression of the 29 m7G-related genes in CC patients. (**A**) Expression modification of m7G-related genes and their effect on regulation. (**B**) Gene location on chromosome with mutation information. Blue dots indicate deletion and red dots mean amplification. (**C**) Copy number variation (CNV) of m7G-related genes in CC samples; the mutation frequency is listed on the right. (**D**) Copy number of each m7G-related gene in detail. GAIN refers to copy number amplification and LOSS means copy number deletion. (**E**) The boxplot for the differentially expressed m7G-related genes between normal and CC samples. * $p < 0.05$, ** $p < 0.01$, *** $p < 0.001$.

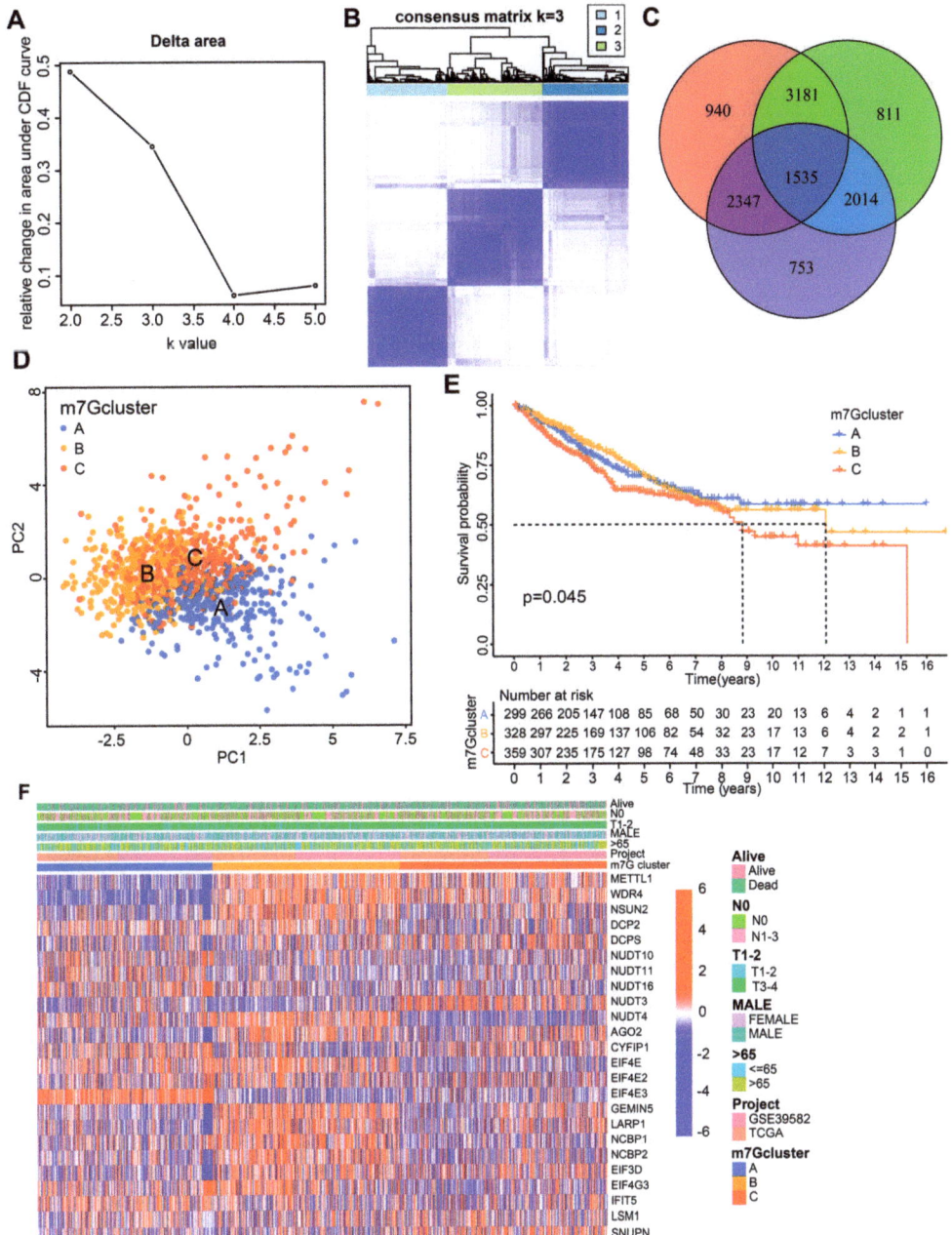

Figure 2. The construction of m7G-related subtype clusters. (**A**) Cumulative distribution function curve illustrates the most effective way of m7G clustering. (**B**) The consensus matrix of the clustering analysis based on m7G expression profiles via k-means clustering (k = 3). (**C**) The Venn diagram depicted the intersection of differentially expressed genes among different m7G clusters. (**D**) The principal component analysis (PCA) for m7G clusters. (**E**) Kaplan–Meier (KM) curves for the overall survival (OS) of CC patients among different m7G groups. (**F**) Heatmap of m7G-associated genes' expression in CC patients with different clinical characteristics, data sources and m7G clusters.

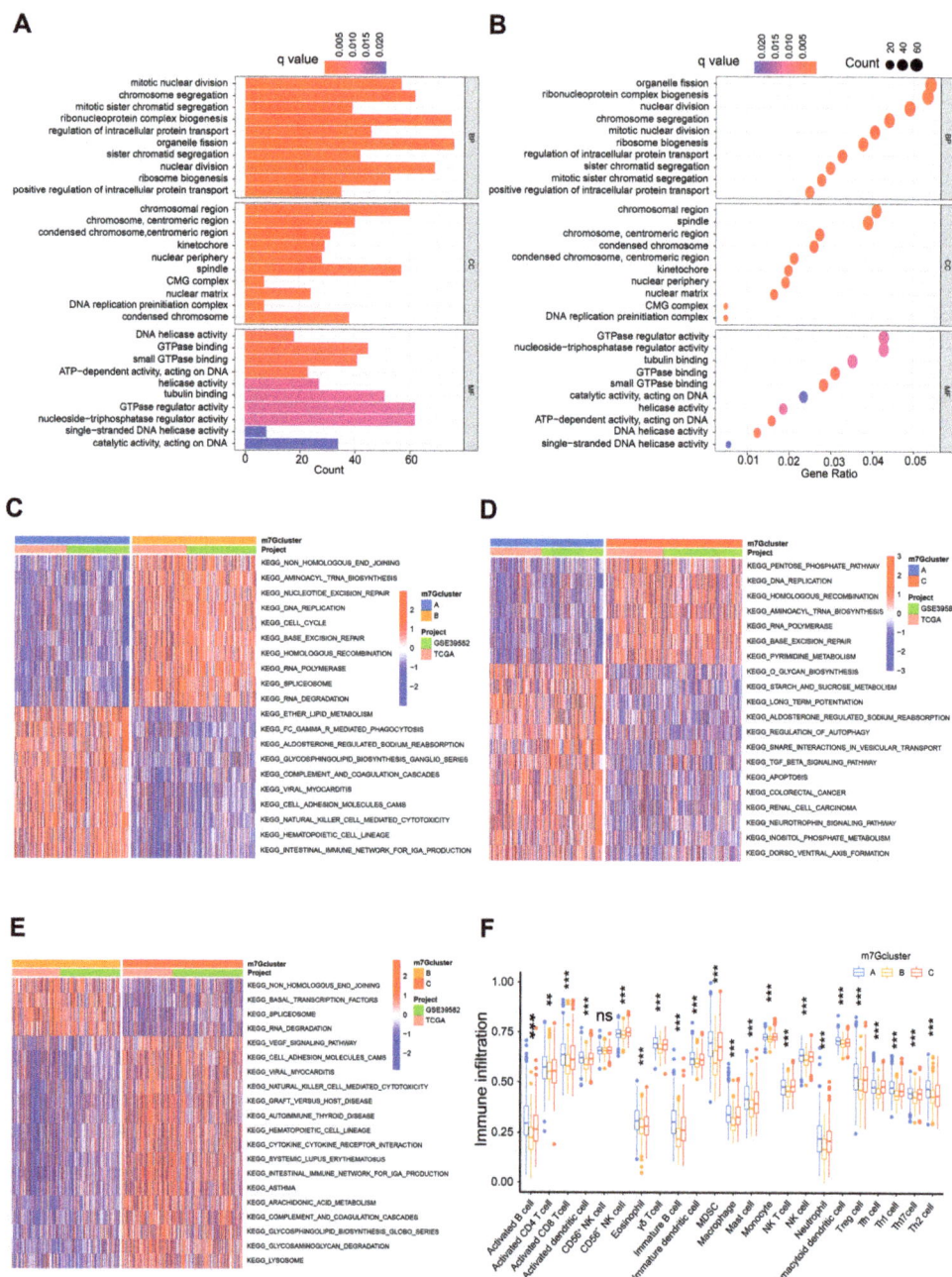

Figure 3. Biological characteristics and immunocyte infiltration information of three m7G Clusters. (**A**,**B**) GO analysis for the differentially expressed genes from different m7G clusters. (**C**–**E**) Heatmaps of the remarkably different pathways among different m7G groups by GSVA analysis. (**F**) The boxplot for immune infiltration among CC patients from different m7G groups. * $p < 0.05$, ** $p < 0.01$, *** $p < 0.001$.

As shown in Figure 3C–E, the significantly dysregulated pathways between CC patients from different m7G clusters are listed. Among them, cell proliferation and metastasis-associated pathways like DNA replication, cell adhesion, and VEGF signaling were significantly enriched in m7G Cluster C. In addition, some metabolic reprogramming pathways, such as arachidonic acid metabolism, glycosphingolipid biosynthesis, and pyrimidine metabolism were remarkably upregulated in m7G Cluster C. The immune cell infiltration level was estimated by ssGSEA to further explore the difference in tumor microenvironment (TME) among CC patients from three m7G clusters. As shown in Figure 3F, infiltration of 23 immunocyte subtypes was remarkably different among CC patients from different m7G clusters.

3.4. Identification of Prognostic DEGs and Construction of Gene Clusters

Based on the DEGs among the three m7G clusters obtained above (Figure 2C), univariate cox analysis was performed and identified 211 DEGs with prognostic significance in CC patients (Supplementary Table S3). Based on the expression level of 211 prognostic DEGs, k-means clustering was conducted with k value ranging from two to nine. The best grouping effect was obtained with a k value of three (Figures 4A,B and S2). Therefore, the CC patients were divided into three groups, termed gene clusters A, B and C. As with the survival analysis results based on the m7G clusters, KM curves indicated that the OS of CC patients in gene cluster C was much worse than those in the other two groups (Figure 4C). Moreover, the expression level of m7G-related genes was significantly different among the three gene clusters (Figure 4D). The heatmap illustrated expression levels of prognostic DEGs in CC patients with different m7G clusters and gene clusters (Figure 4E). These results validly demonstrated the remarkable effectiveness of the prognostic DEGs-based clustering.

3.5. Construction and Validation of the m7G Score Prognostic Risk Model

3.5.1. Construction and Bioinformatic Verification of the m7G Score Prognostic Model

To further investigate the prognostic value of m7G genes, we constructed the m7G score based on the above m7G Clusters. The Sankey diagram was constructed to illustrate the modeling process (Figure 5A). Multivariate Cox regression analysis was utilized for 211 prognostic DEGs identified by univariate cox analysis in Supplementary Table S3. Furthermore, AGO2, CYFIP1, EIF4E, EIF4E2, EIF4E3, GEMIN5, METTL1, NCBP1, NSUN2, NUDT10, NUDT11, NUDT3, NUDT4, SNUPN, and WDR4 (Figure S3, Supplementary Table S4) were chosen for m7G prognostic model construction by the formula: m7G score = $\sum PC1_i + \sum PC2_i$.

As demonstrated in Figure 5B,C, the m7G score was remarkably different in CC patients among different m7G clusters and gene clusters, which indicated the significant effectiveness of m7G score construction. Then, CC patients were divided into high- and low-m7G score groups by an optimal cutoff. The OS of CC patients in the high-m7G score group was much better than that of the low group (Figure 5D). Furthermore, subgroup analysis results revealed that the survival rate difference was much more significant in CC patients with T3–T4 cancer, which illustrated that the prognostic prediction power of the m7G score was stronger in advanced CC patients (Figure 5E,F).

More importantly, the performance of the m7G score was further validated in another external GEO cohort (GSE31595). CC patients were divided into high-m7G score and low-m7G score groups utilizing the same grouping method. As shown in Figure 5G, the survival rate of CC patients with a high m7G score was much higher than that of low-m7G score patients. Taken together, the m7G score is a robust prognostic model with excellent predictive power for CC patients.

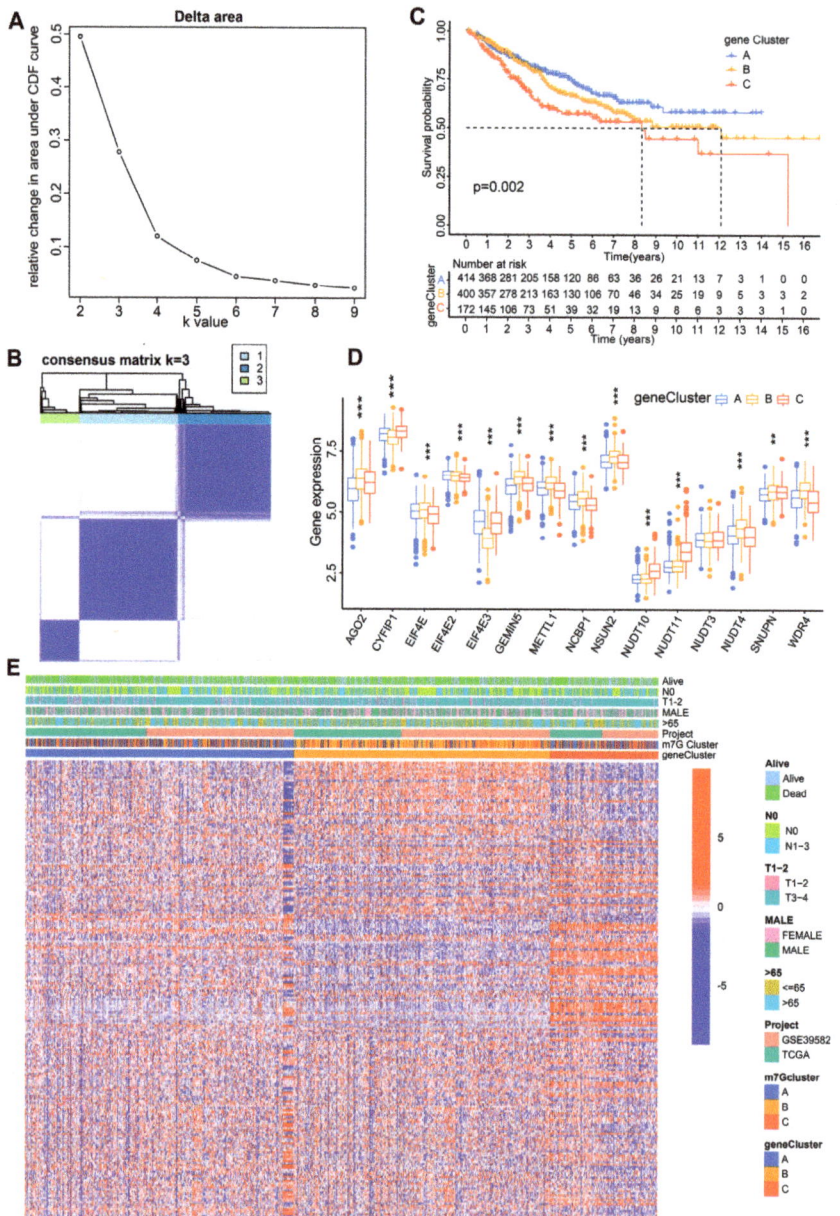

Figure 4. Gene clustering based on prognostic m7G-related DEGs in CC patients. (**A**) Cumulative distribution function curve demonstrates the most effective way of gene clustering. (**B**) The consensus matrix of the clustering analysis based on prognostic m7G-related gene expression profiles via k-means clustering (k = 3). (**C**) KM curves of OS among CC patients from different gene clusters. (**D**) The boxplot for m7G-related genes' expression levels among CC patients from different gene clusters. (**E**) Heatmap depicting expression levels of prognostic m7G-related genes in CC patients with different clinical characteristics, data sources, m7G clusters, and gene clusters. * $p < 0.05$, ** $p < 0.01$, *** $p < 0.001$.

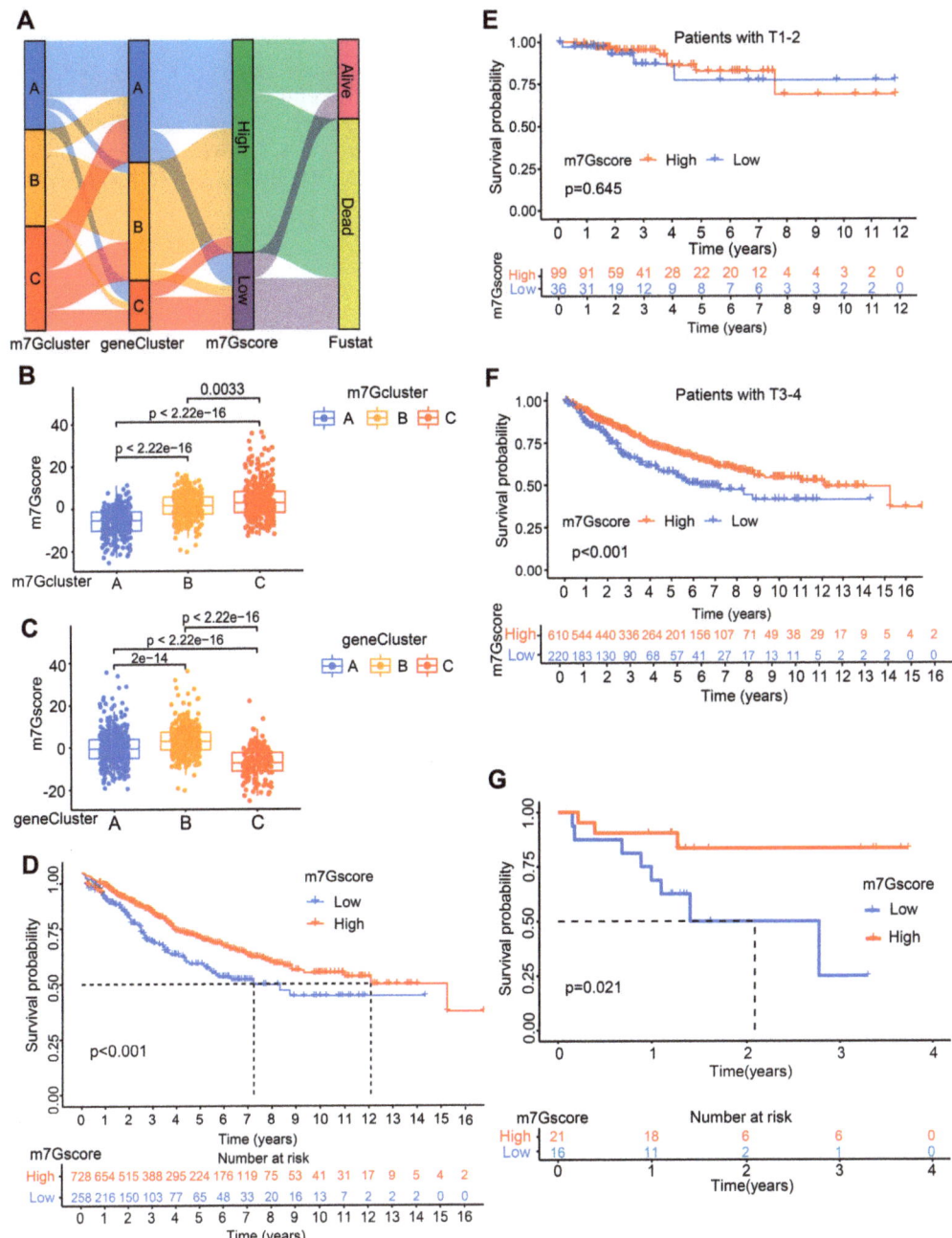

Figure 5. Construction and verification of the m7G score prognostic model. (**A**) Sankey diagram for the modeling process. (**B**) The m7G score level in CC patients from different m7G clusters. (**C**) The m7G score level in CC patients from different gene clusters. (**D**) KM curves for the OS of CC patients from high- and low-m7G score groups. (**E**,**F**) KM survival analysis based on m7G score in CC patients at different T stages. (**G**) KM survival curves based on m7G scores in CC patients from the GSE31595 validated cohort.

3.5.2. Validation in Human CC Cell Lines by qPCR Assay

We further evaluated the expression level of 15 m7G prognostic genes used for m7G score construction in human CC cell lines and tissues using a qPCR assay. As demonstrated in Figure 6A–O, the mRNA levels of AGO2, CYFIP1, EIF4E, METTL1, NSUN2, NUDT3, SNUPN, NUDT4, GEMIN5, EIF4E2, NCBP1, and WDR4 were remarkably higher in CC cell lines (HCT15, DLD1, RKO, HCT8, HCT116, SW48, and WiDr) than those in the normal cell line HIEC6. By contrast, the expression levels of EIF4E3, NUDT10 and NUDT11 were significantly lower in CC cell lines.

3.5.3. Validation in Human CC Tissues by qPCR Assay

More importantly, the mRNA levels of 15 m7G prognostic genes were assessed in 15 matched CC and normal tissues from our tissue bank. Similar expression patterns for these m7G prognostic genes were obtained in human CC tissues by qPCR results (Figure 7A–O). These results further validated the robust efficiency of the m7G score.

3.6. Drug Sensitivity in High- and Low-m7G Score Groups

To further explore differences in drug resistance in CC patients with high and low m7G scores, we assessed the estimated IC50 levels of chemotherapy drugs or inhibitors in the above two groups. As demonstrated in Figure 8, CC patients with a high m7G score were found to be more sensitive to Vinblastine, BIBW2992, Cytarabine, Docetaxel, Erlotinib, Paclitaxel and Rapamycin, while patients with a low m7G score responded better to AP.24534, Bleomycin, Cisplatin, Doxorubicin, Embelin, Gefitinib, Meformin and Pazopanib. Altogether, these data revealed that the m7G score could also be a potential indicator for drug sensitivity in CC patients.

3.7. Tumor Microenvironment in High- and Low-m7G Score Groups

Since the m7G score was associated with the prognosis of CC patients, the correlation between m7G score and tumor microenvironment was further assessed. The tumor mutation burden (TMB) was found to be negatively correlated with m7G score in CC patients ($R = -0.13$, $p = 0.0085$; Figure 9A). More importantly, the PD-L1 expression level of CC patients in the low-m7G score group was significantly higher than that in the high group, which demonstrated that the m7G score could serve as an indicator for predicting anti-PD1/PD-L1 immunotherapy response (Figure 9B).

The CIBERSORT algorithm was applied to further identify the correlation between immune infiltration and m7G score. Negative correlations between m7G score and immune infiltration were identified in several immunocytes, including B cells, naive B cells, Macrophages, M1 Macrophages, M2 Macrophages, Myeloid dendritic cells, Neutrophils, CD4+ T cells and CD4+ memory resting T cells. Meanwhile, positive correlations between m7G score and immune infiltration were observed in plasma B cells, CD8+ T cells and regulatory T cells (Figure 9C–N). Therefore, the m7G score was significantly associated with immune cell infiltration in CC patients.

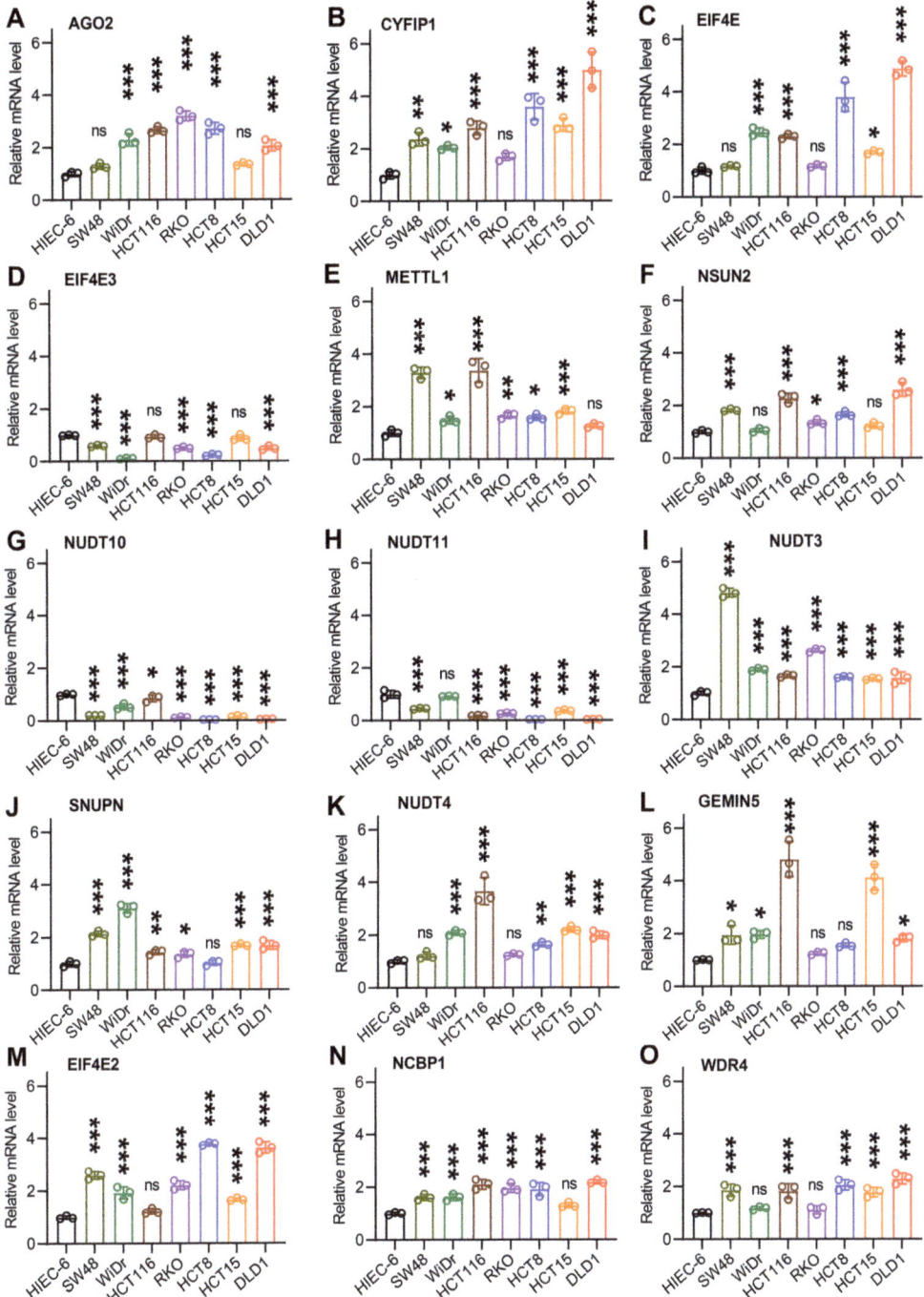

Figure 6. Validation for the expression level of 15 prognostic m7G-related genes in human CC cell lines. (**A–O**) Expression level of 15 prognosis-associated m7G genes in 7 human CC cell lines (RKO, HCT8, HCT116, SW48, WiDr, HCT15, and DLD1) and normal human intestinal epithelial cells (HIEC6). * $p < 0.05$, ** $p < 0.01$, *** $p < 0.001$.

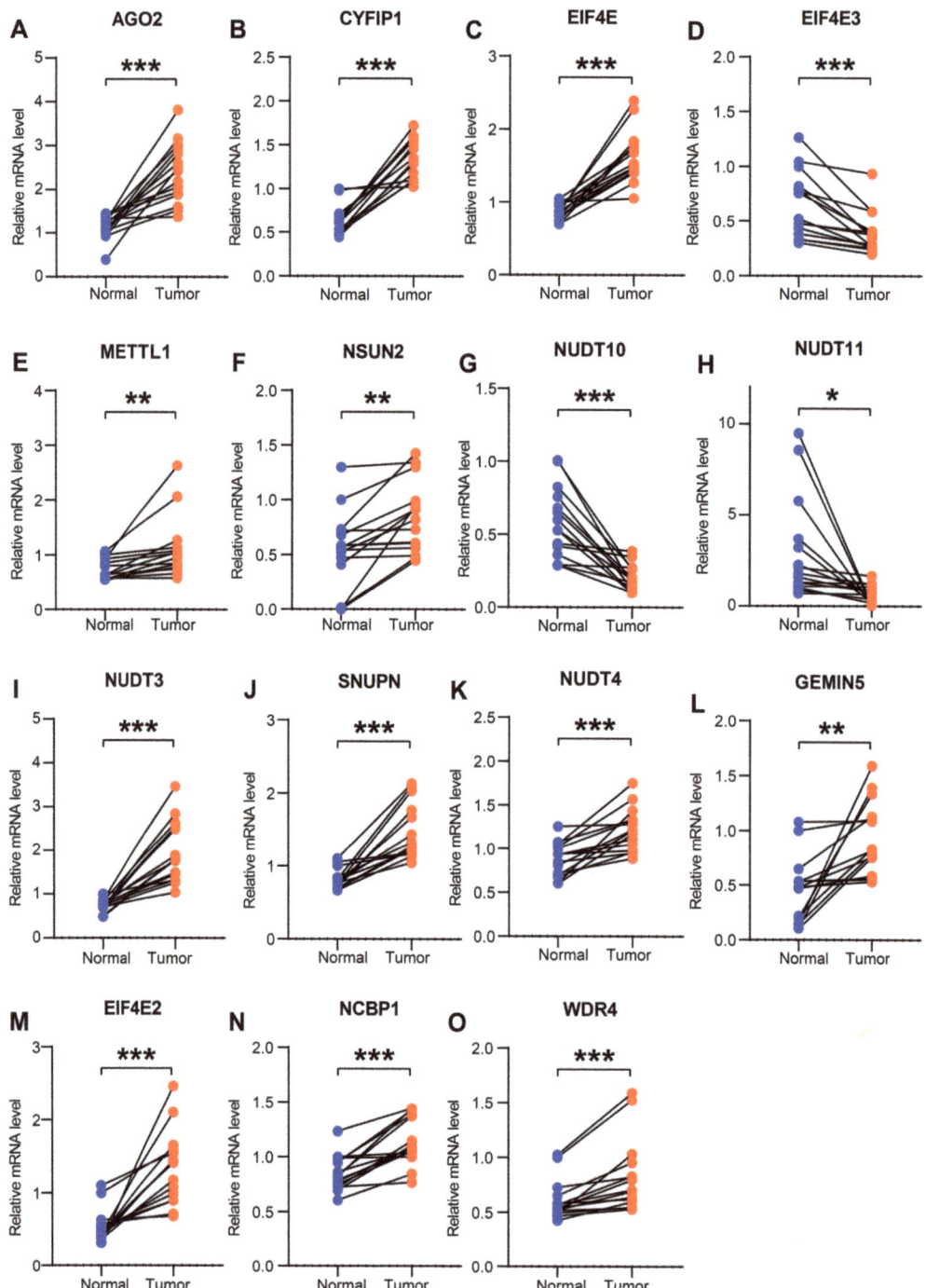

Figure 7. Validation of the expression level 15 prognostic m7G-related genes in human CC tissues. (**A–O**) Expression level of prognostic m7G-related genes in 15 paired human CC and adjacent normal tissues. * $p < 0.05$, ** $p < 0.01$, *** $p < 0.001$.

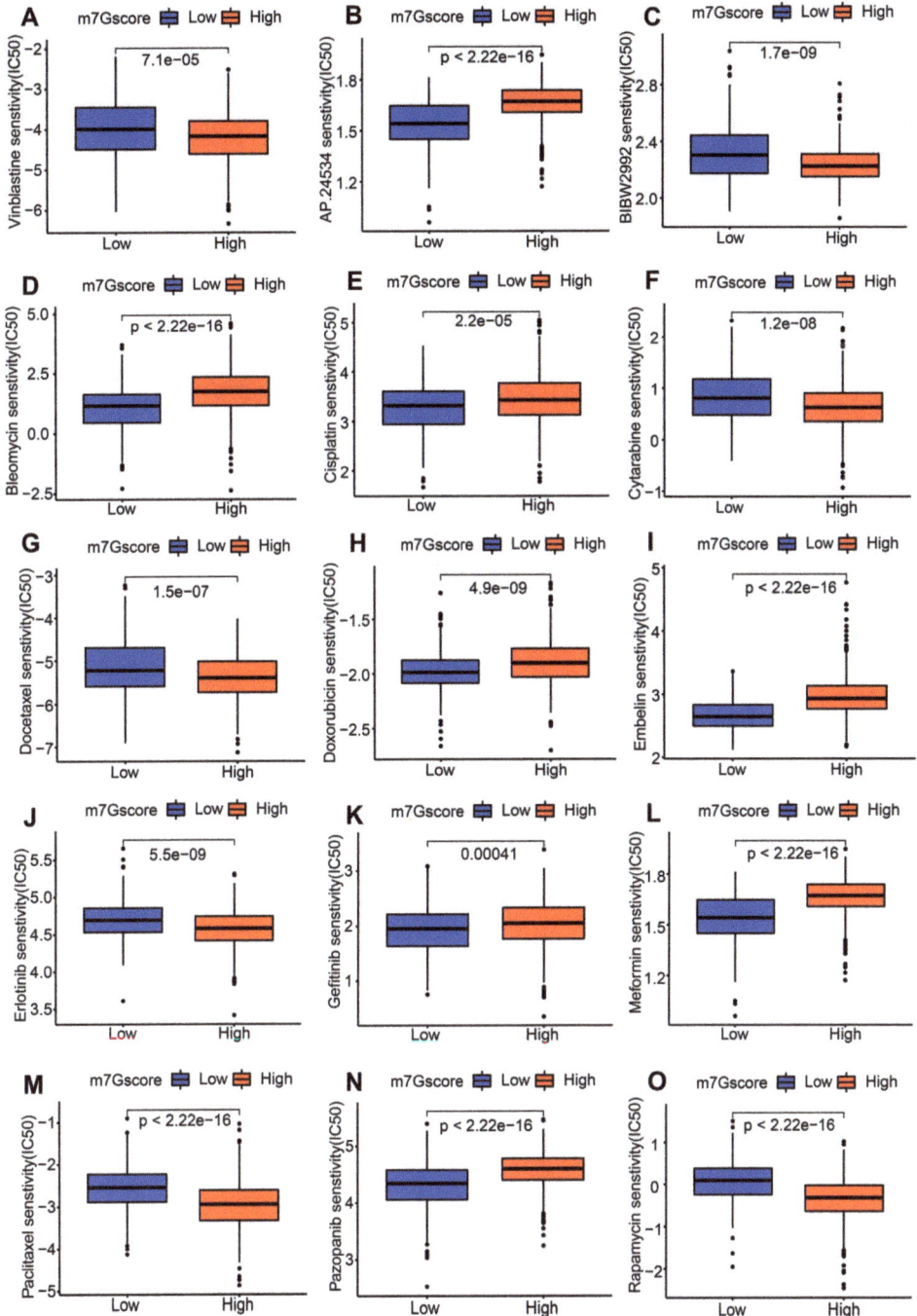

Figure 8. Drug sensitivity in CC patients from different m7G score groups. (**A–O**) Boxplots depicting the IC50 value of Vinblastine (**A**), AP.24534 (**B**), BIBW2992 (**C**), Bleomycin (**D**), Cisplatin (**E**), Cytarabine (**F**), Docetaxel (**G**), Doxorubicin (**H**), Embelin (**I**), Erlotinib (**J**), Gefitinib (**K**), Meformin (**L**), Paclitaxel (**M**), Pazopanib (**N**), and Rapamycin (**O**) in CC patients with different m7G scores.

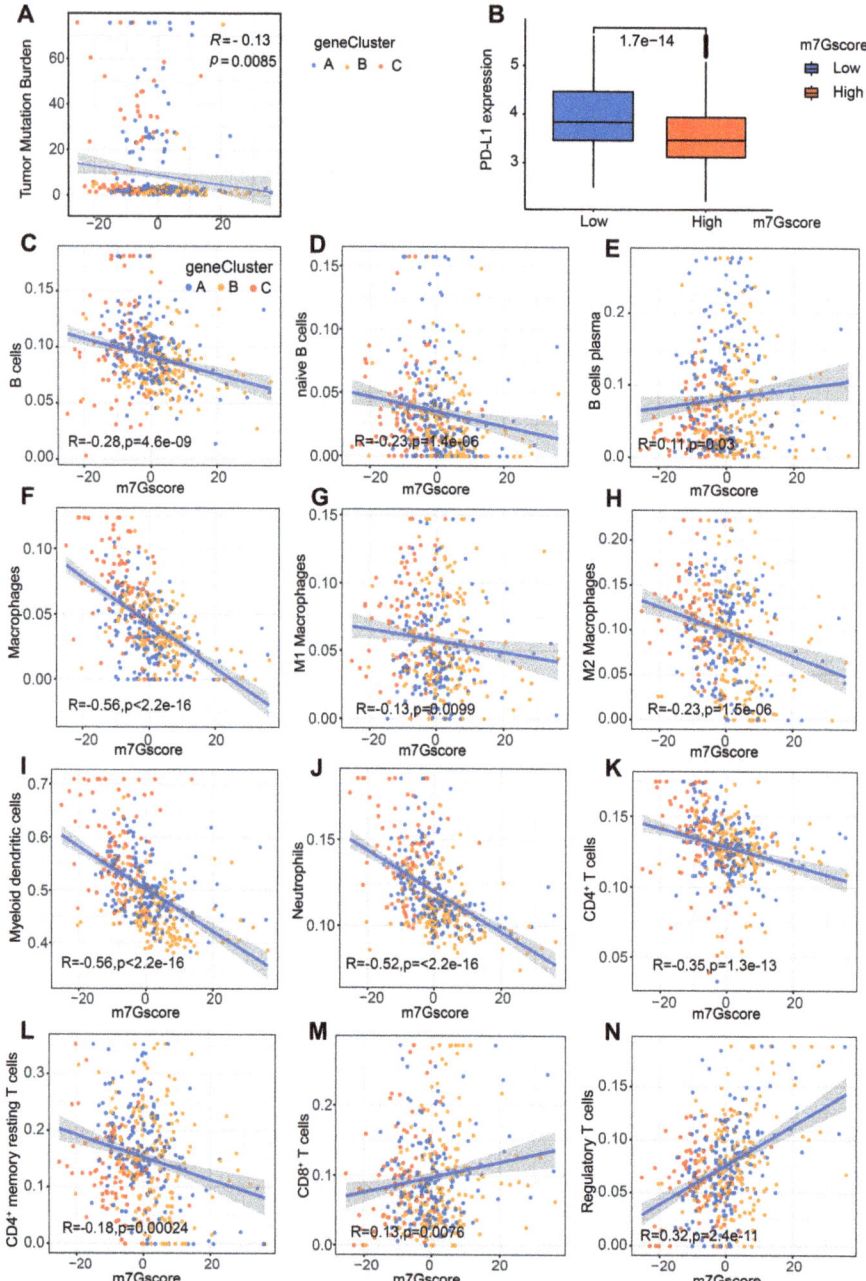

Figure 9. Correlation analysis between m7G score and TMB, as well as tumor immune microenvironment. (**A**) Relevance of TMB and m7G score in CC patients. (**B**) Expression level of immune checkpoint PD-L1 in CC patients from high- and low-m7G score groups. (**C–N**) Correlation analysis between infiltration levels of B cells (**C**), naive B cells (**D**), B cells plasma (**E**), Macrophages (**F**), M1 Macrophages (**G**), M2 Macrophages (**H**), Myeloid dendritic cells (**I**), Neutrophils (**J**), CD4+ T cells (**K**), CD4+ memory resting T cells (**L**), CD8+ T cells (**M**), regulatory T cells (**N**) and m7G score.

4. Discussion

Colon cancer (CC), one of the common malignant tumors worldwide, is a serious challenge to the safeguarding of human health. The current prognostic index is still insufficient to evaluate the prognosis of CC patients in clinical work. Although some research has demonstrated the potential role of m7G genes in the tumorigenesis of several tumors, including acute myeloid leukemia, bladder cancer, and esophageal squamous cell carcinoma, the prognostic value of m7G-related genes is still unclear in CC patients [1,2,21]. Therefore, constructing an effective prognostic model based on m7G genes is of great clinical importance. In this study, the m7G score prognostic model was established via unsupervised clustering and PCA analysis based on data from TCGA-COAD and GSE39582. The GSVA, ssGSEA, GO, KEGG, and KM curve analyses were utilized to identify the biological characteristics of CC patients with different m7G scores. Moreover, the expression levels of 15 prognosis-related m7G genes was further confirmed in human CC cell lines and tissues by qPCR.

Several previous studies have demonstrated the predictive value of m7G-related long noncoding RNAs (lncRNAs) and microRNAs (miRNAs) in different types of cancer. Hong and Du et al. showed that m7G-related miRNA was related to cancer cell migration, tumor immunity, and prognosis [22,23]. Additionally, the predictive value of m7G-related lncRNA has been reported by Ming and Wang, which could be used to assess oncogenesis and treatment response in renal clear cell carcinoma and bladder cancer [24–26]. These studies have inspired us to explore whether m7G-related genes have a similar prognostic prediction effect. The present study constructed the m7G score on the basis of 15 prognostic m7G genes (AGO2, CYFIP1, EIF4E, EIF4E2, EIF4E3, GEMIN5, METTL1, NCBP1, NSUN2, NUDT10, NUDT11, NUDT3, NUDT4, SNUPN, and WDR4) [14,27–30]. In detail, CC patients with higher m7G scores obtained lower PD-L1 expression levels as well as better prognoses.

Tumor mutational burden (TMB) has been reported as an indicator for immunotherapy efficacy in cancer patients, including CC, melanomas, renal cell carcinomas, bladder cancers as well as head and neck squamous cell cancers [27–33]. Usually, cancer patients with high TMB respond better to immunotherapy than those with low TMB [27–32]. Nevertheless, the role of TMB in CC patients remains controversial. Liu et al. illustrated that CC patients with high TMB exhibited a higher OS rate than those with low TMB [27]. In contrast, Zhou et al. demonstrated that CC patients with low TMB had better prognoses than their counterparts in the high TMB group [33]. In accordance with Zhou's findings, our data indicated that CC patients with higher m7G scores obtained lower TMB and higher OS rates. Hence, the correlation between TMB and m7G is worthy of further investigations.

PD-1, located on membrane of T cells, is a well-known immune checkpoint and participates in the immune escape of cancer cells by binding to PD-L1 on the tumor cell surface. Hence, antitumor immunotherapy was developed based on PD-1/PD-L1 blockages or inhibitors, which has achieved tremendous success in cancer patients [34]. Generally, patients with rich but exhausted immunocyte infiltration respond better to PD-1/PD-L1 inhibitors than their counterparts [35–37]. In this study, CC patients in the high-m7G score group exhibited lower expression levels of PD-L1, indicating that m7G-related genes might regulate PD-1/PD-L1 expression and thereby affect the response to anti-PD-1/PD-L1 therapy.

There are some limitations to the present study. To begin with, most data involved in our study were downloaded from public databases, which may inevitably lead to uncertain selection bias. Although we have primarily proven the prognostic value of the m7G score in an external validation cohort and demonstrated differential expression levels of 15 prognostic m7G genes in CC patient samples from our institution, further validation work based on CC cohorts from multiple centers is needed.

5. Conclusions

In summary, our study constructed an m7G score prognostic model for CC patients. The m7G score could play an important role in prognosis prediction and immunotherapy evaluation, which could offer significant benefits in the clinical management of CC patients.

Supplementary Materials: The following supporting information can be downloaded at: https://www.mdpi.com/article/10.3390/cancers14225527/s1, Figure S1: Correlation analysis and construction of m7G clusters; Figure S2: Gene clustering based on prognostic m7G-related DEGs in CC patients; Figure S3: The KM Curves of OS of CC Patients with High and Low m7G Gene Expression; Table S1: List of 29 m7G-related genes; Table S2: List of intersecting genes among different m7G clusters; Table S3: List of 211 prognostic DEGs among different m7G clusters; Table S4: List of 15 prognosis-associated m7G genes; Table S5: Primers of m7G-related genes utilized for qPCR in this study.

Author Contributions: Conceptualization, Z.-Y.X. and T.H.; methodology, T.H.; software, Z.-J.Z.; validation, X.-F.W., Y.-L.C., G.-Z.L. and Y.-W.S.; formal analysis, J.C.; investigation, R.-B.L.; resources, W.-D.P.; data curation, X.-W.H.; writing—original draft preparation, J.C.; writing—review and editing, T.H.; visualization, J.C.; supervision, Z.-Y.X. and T.H.; project administration, Z.-Y.X. and T.H.; funding acquisition, Z.-Y.X. and T.H. All authors have read and agreed to the published version of the manuscript.

Funding: This study was supported by The Starting Funding of Faculty from Sun Yat-sen University (No. 2021276), Science and Technology Planning Project of Guangzhou City (No. 2023A04J1820), National Key Clinical Discipline, and the Discipline Construction Funding for Pancreatic and Hepatobiliary Surgery Department of Sixth Affiliated Hospital of Sun-Yat-Sen University (No. X202102172026091184).

Institutional Review Board Statement: The study was conducted in accordance with the Declaration of Helsinki and approved by the Ethics Committee of the Sixth Affiliated Hospital of Sun Yat-sen University (2016ZSLYEC-056).

Informed Consent Statement: The Ethics Committee of the Sixth Affiliated Hospital of Sun Yat-sen University approved the informed consent waiver.

Data Availability Statement: The processed data that support the findings of this study are available from the corresponding author.

Acknowledgments: We thank Chunbo He and Surendra Shukla (University of Oklahoma Health Sciences Center) for the writing assistance. The authors express our sincere appreciation for the public data obtained from the Gene Expression Omnibus (GEO)and The Cancer Genome Atlas (TCGA).

Conflicts of Interest: The authors declare no conflict of interest.

References

1. Siegel, R.L.; Miller, K.D.; Fuchs, H.E.; Jemal, A. Cancer statistics, 2022. *CA Cancer J Clin.* **2022**, *72*, 7–33. [CrossRef] [PubMed]
2. Sung, H.; Ferlay, J.; Siegel, R.L.; Laversanne, M.; Soerjomataram, I.; Jemal, A.; Bray, F. Global Cancer Statistics 2020: GLOBOCAN Estimates of Incidence and Mortality Worldwide for 36 Cancers in 185 Countries. *CA Cancer J. Clin.* **2021**, *71*, 209–249. [CrossRef] [PubMed]
3. Alexandrov, A.; Martzen, M.R.; Phizicky, E.M. Two Proteins that Form a Complex Are Required for 7-methylguanosine Modification of Yeast tRNA. *RNA* **2002**, *8*, 1253–1266. [CrossRef] [PubMed]
4. Dai, Z.; Liu, H.; Liao, J.; Huang, C.; Ren, X.; Zhu, W.; Zhu, S.; Peng, B.; Li, S.; Lai, J.; et al. N7-Methylguanosine tRNA modification enhances oncogenic mRNA translation and promotes intrahepatic cholangiocarcinoma progression. *Mol. Cell* **2021**, *81*, 3339–3355. [CrossRef]
5. Zhang, W.; Zhang, S.; Wang, Z. Prognostic value of 12 m7G methylation-related miRNA markers and their correlation with immune infiltration in breast cancer. *Front. Oncol.* **2022**, *12*, 929363. [CrossRef]
6. Zhang, C.; Zhou, D.; Wang, Z.; Ju, Z.; He, J.; Zhao, G.; Wang, R. Risk Model and Immune Signature of m7G-Related lncRNA Based on Lung Adenocarcinoma. *Front. Genet.* **2022**, *13*, 907754. [CrossRef]
7. Zhang, M.; Song, J.; Yuan, W.; Zhang, W.; Sun, Z. Roles of RNA Methylation on Tumor Immunity and Clinical Implications. *Front. Immunol.* **2021**, *12*, 641507. [CrossRef]
8. Tomikawa, C. 7-Methylguanosine Modifications in Transfer RNA (tRNA). *Int. J. Mol. Sci.* **2018**, *19*, 4080. [CrossRef]

9. Hong, P.; Du, H.; Tong, M.; Cao, Q.; Hu, D.; Ma, J.; Jin, Y.; Li, Z.; Huang, W.; Tong, G. A Novel M7G-Related MicroRNAs Risk Signature Predicts the Prognosis and Tumor Microenvironment of Kidney Renal Clear Cell Carcinoma. *Front. Genet.* **2022**, *13*, 922358. [CrossRef]
10. Lin, S.; Liu, Q.; Lelyveld, V.S.; Choe, J.; Szostak, J.W.; Gregory, R.I. Mettl1/Wdr4-Mediated m7G tRNA Methylome Is Required for Normal mRNA Translation and Embryonic Stem Cell Self-Renewal and Differentiation. *Mol. Cell* **2018**, *71*, 244–255. [CrossRef]
11. Baradaran Ghavami, S.; Chaleshi, V.; Derakhshani, S.; Aimzadeh, P.; Asadzadeh-Aghdaie, H.; Zali, M.R. Association between TNF-α Rs1799964 and RAF1 Rs1051208 MicroRNA Binding Site SNP and Gastric Cancer Susceptibility in an Iranian Population. *Gastroenterol. Hepatol. Bed Bench* **2017**, *10*, 214–219.
12. Pandolfini, L.; Barbieri, I.; Bannister, A.J.; Hendrick, A.; Andrews, B.; Webster, N.; Murat, P.; Mach, P.; Brandi, R.; Robson, S.C.; et al. METTL1 Promotes Let-7 MicroRNA Processing via m7G Methylation. *Mol. Cell* **2019**, *74*, 1278–1290. [CrossRef] [PubMed]
13. Chen, J.; Li, K.; Chen, J.; Wang, X.; Ling, R.; Cheng, M.; Chen, Z.; Chen, F.; He, Q.; Li, S.; et al. Aberrant Translation Regulated by METTL1/WDR4-mediated tRNA N7-methylguanosine Modification Drives Head and Neck Squamous Cell Carcinoma Progression. *Cancer Commun.* **2022**, *42*, 223–244. [CrossRef] [PubMed]
14. Kiriakidou, M.; Tan, G.S.; Lamprinaki, S.; Planell-Saguer, M.D.; Nelson, P.T.; Mourelatos, Z. An mRNA m7G Cap Binding-like Motif within Human Ago2 Represses Translation. *Cell* **2007**, *129*, 1141–1151. [CrossRef] [PubMed]
15. Osborne, M.J.; Volpon, L.; Memarpoor-Yazdi, M.; Pillay, S.; Thambipillai, A.; Czarnota, S.; Culjkovic-Kraljacic, B.; Trahan, C.; Oeffinger, M.; Cowling, V.H.; et al. Identification and Characterization of the Interaction between the Methyl-7-Guanosine Cap Maturation Enzyme RNMT and the Cap-Binding Protein eIF4E. *J. Mol. Biol.* **2022**, *434*, 167451. [CrossRef] [PubMed]
16. Wang, Z.; Jiao, X.; Carr-Schmid, A.; Kiledjian, M. The hDcp2 Protein Is a Mammalian mRNA Decapping Enzyme. *Proc. Natl. Acad. Sci. USA* **2002**, *99*, 12663–12668. [CrossRef] [PubMed]
17. Wilkerson, M.D.; Hayes, D.N. ConsensusClusterPlus: A Class Discovery Tool with Confidence Assessments and Item Tracking. *Bioinformatics* **2010**, *26*, 1572–1573. [CrossRef] [PubMed]
18. Hänzelmann, S.; Castelo, R.; Guinney, J. GSVA: Gene Set Variation Analysis for Microarray and RNA-Seq Data. *BMC Bioinform.* **2013**, *14*, 7. [CrossRef] [PubMed]
19. Ritchie, M.E.; Phipson, B.; Wu, D.; Hu, Y.; Law, C.W.; Shi, W.; Smyth, G.K. Limma Powers Differential Expression Analyses for RNA-Sequencing and Microarray Studies. *Nucleic Acids Res.* **2015**, *43*, e47. [CrossRef]
20. Becht, E.; Giraldo, N.A.; Lacroix, L.; Buttard, B.; Elarouci, N.; Petitprez, F.; Selves, J.; Laurent-Puig, P.; Sautès-Fridman, C.; Fridman, W.H.; et al. Estimating the Population Abundance of Tissue-Infiltrating Immune and Stromal Cell Populations Using Gene Expression. *Genome Biol.* **2016**, *17*, 218. [CrossRef]
21. Luo, Y.; Yao, Y.; Wu, P.; Zi, X.; Sun, N.; He, J. The potential role of N 7-methylguanosine (m7G) in cancer. *J. Hematol. Oncol.* **2022**, *15*, 63. [CrossRef] [PubMed]
22. Li, L.; Xie, R.; Wei, Q. Network Analysis of miRNA Targeting m6A-Related Genes in Patients with Esophageal Cancer. *PeerJ* **2021**, *9*, e11893. [CrossRef] [PubMed]
23. Miller, K.D.; Nogueira, L.; Devasia, T.; Mariotto, A.B.; Yabroff, K.R.; Jemal, A.; Kramer, J.; Siegel, R.L. Cancer Treatment and Survivorship Statistics, 2022. *CA Cancer J Clin.* **2022**, *72*, 409–436. [CrossRef] [PubMed]
24. Ming, Y.; Wang, C. N7-Methylguanosine-Related lncRNAs: Integrated Analysis Associated with Prognosis and Progression in Clear Cell Renal Cell Carcinoma. *Front. Genet.* **2022**, *13*, 871899. [CrossRef]
25. Ma, T.; Wang, X.; Wang, J.; Liu, X.; Lai, S.; Zhang, W.; Meng, L.; Tian, Z.; Zhang, Y. N6-Methyladenosine-Related Long Non-coding RNA Signature Associated with Prognosis and Immunotherapeutic Efficacy of Clear-Cell Renal Cell Carcinoma. *Front. Genet.* **2021**, *12*, 726369. [CrossRef]
26. Ma, T.; Wang, X.; Meng, L.; Liu, X.; Wang, J.; Zhang, W.; Tian, Z.; Zhang, Y. An Effective N6-Methyladenosine-Related Long Non-coding RNA Prognostic Signature for Predicting the Prognosis of Patients with Bladder Cancer. *BMC Cancer* **2021**, *21*, 1256. [CrossRef]
27. Liu, L.; Bai, X.; Wang, J.; Tang, X.; Wu, D.; Du, S.; Du, X.; Zhang, Y.; Zhu, H.; Fang, Y.; et al. Combination of TMB and CNA Stratifies Prognostic and Predictive Responses to Immunotherapy Across Metastatic Cancer. *Clin. Cancer Res.* **2019**, *25*, 7413–7423. [CrossRef]
28. Ai, L.; Xu, A.; Xu, J. Roles of PD-1/PD-L1 Pathway: Signaling, Cancer, and Beyond. *Adv. Exp. Med. Biol.* **2020**, *248*, 33–59.
29. Luchini, C.; Bibeau, F.; Ligtenberg, M.J.L.; Singh, N.; Nottegar, A.; Bosse, T.; Miller, R.; Riaz, N.; Douillard, J.Y.; Andre, F.; et al. ESMO recommendations on microsatellite instability testing for immunotherapy in cancer, and its relationship with PD-1/PD-L1 expression and tumour mutational burden: A systematic review-based approach. *Ann. Oncol.* **2019**, *30*, 1232–1243. [CrossRef]
30. Samstein, R.M.; Lee, C.H.; Shoushtari, A.N.; Hellmann, M.D.; Shen, R.; Janjigian, Y.Y.; Barron, D.A.; Zehir, A.; Jordan, E.J.; Omuro, A.; et al. Tumor mutational load predicts survival after immunotherapy across multiple cancer types. *Nat. Genet.* **2019**, *51*, 202–206. [CrossRef]
31. Cao, D.; Xu, H.; Xu, X.; Guo, T.; Ge, W. High tumor mutation burden predicts better efficacy of immunotherapy: A pooled analysis of 103078 cancer patients. *Oncoimmunology* **2019**, *8*, e1629258. [CrossRef] [PubMed]
32. Le, D.T.; Uram, J.N.; Wang, H.; Bartlett, B.R.; Kemberling, H.; Eyring, A.D.; Skora, A.D.; Luber, B.S.; Azad, N.S.; Laheru, D.; et al. PD-1 Blockade in Tumors with Mismatch-Repair Deficiency. *N. Engl. J. Med.* **2015**, *372*, 2509–2520. [CrossRef]

33. Zhou, Z.; Xie, X.; Wang, X.; Zhang, X.; Li, W.; Sun, T.; Cai, Y.; Wu, J.; Dang, C.; Zhang, H. Correlations Between Tumor Mutation Burden and Immunocyte Infiltration and Their Prognostic Value in Colon Cancer. *Front. Genet.* **2021**, *12*, 623424. [CrossRef] [PubMed]
34. Gou, Q.; Dong, C.; Xu, H.; Khan, B.; Jin, J.; Liu, Q.; Shi, J.; Hou, Y. PD-L1 degradation pathway and immunotherapy for cancer. *Cell Death Dis.* **2020**, *11*, 955. [CrossRef] [PubMed]
35. Corrò, C.; Dutoit, V.; Koessler, T. Emerging Trends for Radio-Immunotherapy in Rectal Cancer. *Cancers* **2021**, *13*, 1374. [CrossRef]
36. Sun, J.; Zheng, Y.; Mamun, M.; Li, X.; Chen, X.; Gao, Y. Research Progress of PD-1/PD-L1 Immunotherapy in Gastrointestinal Tumors. *Biomed. Pharmacother.* **2020**, *129*, 110504. [CrossRef]
37. Dammeijer, F.; Gulijk, M.V.; Mulder, E.E.; Lukkes, M.; Klaase, L.; Bosch, T.V.D.; Nimwegen, M.V.; Lau, S.P.; Latupeirissa, K.; Schetters, S.; et al. The PD-1/PD-L1-Checkpoint Restrains T cell Immunity in Tumor Draining Lymph Nodes. *Cancer Cell* **2020**, *38*, 685–700. [CrossRef]

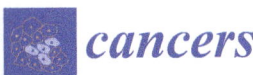

Article

Implementation of an Enhanced Recovery after Surgery Protocol in Advanced and Recurrent Rectal Cancer Patients after beyond Total Mesorectal Excision Surgery: A Feasibility Study

Stefi Nordkamp [1,2,*], Davy M. J. Creemers [1], Sofie Glazemakers [1], Stijn H. J. Ketelaers [1], Harm J. Scholten [3], Silvie van de Calseijde [3], Grard A. P. Nieuwenhuijzen [1], Jip L. Tolenaar [1], Hendi W. Crezee [1], Harm J. T. Rutten [1,2], Jacobus W. A. Burger [1] and Johanne G. Bloemen [1]

1 Department of Surgery, Catharina Hospital, 5623 EJ Eindhoven, The Netherlands; grard.nieuwenhuijzen@catharinaziekenhuis.nl (G.A.P.N.)
2 Department of GROW, School for Oncology and Reproduction, Maastricht University, 6229 ER Maastricht, The Netherlands
3 Department of Anaesthesiology, Catharina Hospital, 5623 EJ Eindhoven, The Netherlands
* Correspondence: stefi.nordkamp@catharinaziekenhuis.nl; Tel.: +31-(0)40-239-8858

Simple Summary: The aim of this study was to evaluate the implementation and outcomes of a tailored ERAS LARRC protocol developed for patients with locally advanced and recurrent rectal cancer who require complex surgical procedures. This study shows that the protocol is feasible with a compliance rate of 73.6% and results in a reduction in postoperative complications. Multimodal anaesthesia could potentially impact the length of stay in a beneficial way, as well as improve the recovery profile.

Abstract: Introduction: The implementation of an Enhanced Recovery After Surgery (ERAS) protocol in patients with locally advanced rectal cancer (LARC) and locally recurrent rectal cancer (LRRC) has been deemed unfeasible until now because of the heterogeneity of this disease and low caseloads. Since evidence and experience with ERAS principles in colorectal cancer care are increasing, a modified ERAS protocol for this specific group has been developed. The aim of this study is to evaluate the implementation of a tailored ERAS protocol for patients with LARC or LRRC, requiring beyond total mesorectal excision (bTME) surgery. Methods: Patients who underwent a bTME for LARC or LRRC between October 2021 and December 2022 were prospectively studied. All patients were treated in accordance with the ERAS LARRC protocol, which consisted of 39 ERAS care elements specifically developed for patients with LARC and LRRC. One of the most important adaptations of this protocol was the anaesthesia procedure, which involved the use of total intravenous anaesthesia with intravenous (iv) lidocaine, iv methadone, and iv ketamine instead of epidural anaesthesia. The outcomes showed compliance with ERAS care elements, complications, length of stay, and functional recovery. A follow-up was performed at 30 and 90 days post-surgery. Results: Seventy-two patients were selected, all of whom underwent bTME for either LARC (54.2%) or LRRC (45.8%). Total compliance with the adjusted ERAS protocol was 73.6%. Major complications were present in 12 patients (16.7%), and the median length of hospital stay was 9 days (IQR 6.0–14.0). Patients who received multimodal anaesthesia (75.0%) stayed in the hospital for a median of 7.0 days (IQR 6.8–15.3). These patients received fewer opioids on the first three postoperative days than patients who received epidural analgesia ($p < 0.001$). Conclusions: The implementation of the ERAS LARRC protocol seemed successful according to its compliance rate of >70%. Its complication rate was substantially reduced in comparison with the literature. Multimodal anaesthesia is feasible in beyond TME surgery with promising effects on recovery after surgery.

Keywords: Enhanced Recovery After Surgery; rectal cancer; locally advanced rectal cancer; locally recurrent rectal cancer; surgery

Citation: Nordkamp, S.; Creemers, D.M.J.; Glazemakers, S.; Ketelaers, S.H.J.; Scholten, H.J.; van de Calseijde, S.; Nieuwenhuijzen, G.A.P.; Tolenaar, J.L.; Crezee, H.W.; Rutten, H.J.T.; et al. Implementation of an Enhanced Recovery after Surgery Protocol in Advanced and Recurrent Rectal Cancer Patients after beyond Total Mesorectal Excision Surgery: A Feasibility Study. *Cancers* **2023**, *15*, 4523. https://doi.org/10.3390/cancers15184523

Academic Editor: Susanne Merkel

Received: 3 August 2023
Revised: 6 September 2023
Accepted: 7 September 2023
Published: 12 September 2023

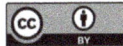

Copyright: © 2023 by the authors. Licensee MDPI, Basel, Switzerland. This article is an open access article distributed under the terms and conditions of the Creative Commons Attribution (CC BY) license (https://creativecommons.org/licenses/by/4.0/).

1. Introduction

The colorectal Enhanced Recovery After Surgery (ERAS) protocol is currently used as the standard mode of care in patients requiring surgical treatment for colorectal cancer [1]. To improve surgical outcomes, a compliance rate of >70% to ERAS care elements has been associated with improved outcomes in minimally invasive colorectal cancer surgery [2]. In patients with locally advanced rectal cancer (LARC) and locally recurrent rectal cancer (LRRC), the implementation of the ERAS protocol has been deemed challenging due to the complexity and heterogeneity of this disease and treatment [3].

Patients with LARC or LRRC require neoadjuvant chemotherapy and radiotherapy, followed by a beyond total mesorectal excision (bTME). This procedure consists of a TME procedure, with an extended resection of the sacral and/or lateral pelvic wall and often multivisceral organ resections [4,5]. As a result, prolonged lengths of hospital stays and higher rates of morbidity and mortality (Clavien–Dindo $\geq$ III of 20–40%) are described in these patients [6–9]. In an earlier study, it was observed that patients with LARC and LRRC are a substantially different group regarding ERAS compliance and postoperative outcomes compared to patients with non-advanced colorectal cancer [10].

Due to the increasing level of experience with ERAS principles in colorectal surgery, it seemed the appropriate time to apply the ERAS principles to advanced rectal cancer surgery. In several high-expertise fields, such as upper gastro-intestinal surgery and cytoreductive surgery with hyperthermal intraperitoneal chemotherapy, ERAS implementation has seemed promising, with good postoperative results [7,11–13]. Therefore, a tailored ERAS protocol for locally advanced and recurrent rectal cancer (LARRC) has been developed by a multidisciplinary team with expertise in advanced rectal cancer [10]. The LARRC protocol was based on the colorectal and pelvic ERAS protocol of Gustafsson [1] and Nygren [12], as well as the pelvic exenteration protocol of Harji et al. [7]. Specific adaptations were made in the anaesthesia protocol, oral intake, postoperative mobilisation, and urological care pathways, as well as strict guidelines for the use of drains and catheters to suit the needs of these patients.

The aim of this study was to evaluate the implementation and outcomes of the tailored ERAS LARRC protocol developed for patients with locally advanced and recurrent rectal cancer who require bTME.

2. Materials and Methods

All consecutive patients with LARC or LRRC who underwent a bTME with curative intent in the Catharina Hospital Eindhoven, a tertiary referral hospital for rectal cancer, were included in this study from October 2021 to December 2022. After the development of the ERAS LARRC protocol in July 2021, a period of 3 months was used for the initiation phase; all involved caretakers (surgeons, anaesthesiologists, intensivists, intensive care nurses, ward nurses, nurse practitioners, stoma care nurses, dieticians, physiotherapists, and surgical residents) were educated to standardise the (digital) system for the care of these patients in the new protocol.

2.1. Patients and Treatment

LARCs were standardly treated with neoadjuvant (chemo)radiotherapy, whereas LRRC patients underwent neoadjuvant chemoradiotherapy or chemo re-irradiation in the case of previous pelvic irradiation [14]. Some patients received induction chemotherapy before chemoradiotherapy [15,16]. After neoadjuvant treatment, a bTME was performed. In this study, a bTME was defined as a total mesorectal excision, with the resection of the sacral and/or lateral pelvic wall and/or multivisceral resections, including partial or total pelvic exenterations. Surgery was often combined with intraoperative radiotherapy (10–12.5 Gy) for the margins considered at risk. Other surgical specialists were consulted if urological, plastic, or vascular reconstructions were required.

2.2. Enhanced Recovery after Surgery Protocol

All patients were treated in accordance with the ERAS LARRC protocol, as shown in Supplementary Material File S1 The ERAS LARRC protocol. It consisted of 39 newly developed ERAS care elements that were analysed for their calculation of compliance and based on colorectal care elements in the EIAS© system [10]. One of the most important adaptations of this protocol was the implementation of a different anaesthesia procedure, which involved the use of total intravenous anaesthesia with intravenous (iv) lidocaine, iv methadone, and iv ketamine, instead of epidural anaesthesia [17–19]. During surgery, continuous wound infusion catheters were applied, which stayed in place for the first two to three postoperative days [20]. As patients commonly suffer from urinary retention after extensive rectal surgery, the use of suprapubic catheters was encouraged. As many of these patients receive urological reconstructions, and postoperative paralytic ileus seems to be associated with radical cystectomies, these patients received postoperative gastric tubes, while all others did not [21–23]. A strict removal procedure followed, and all details about production and removal were registered for analysis. Every patient had a bedside map attached to their bed, along with the information on the protocol (Figure 1).

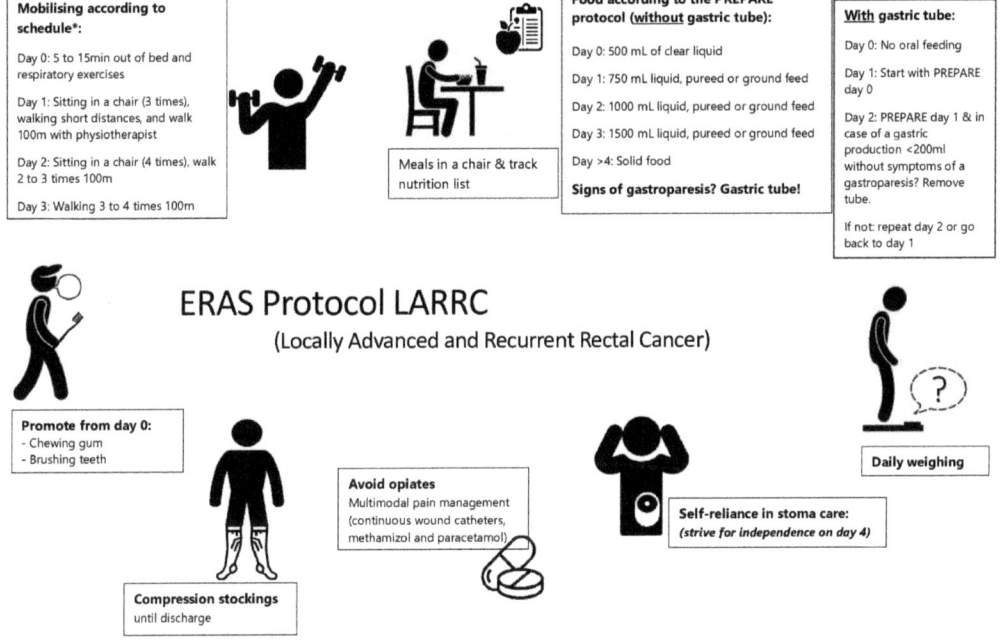

Figure 1. Bed side map of the ERAS LARRC protocol.

2.3. Data Collection and Follow-Up

Patient and tumour characteristics, data on ERAS care elements, complications, and functional recovery (e.g., time until first passage of stool, mobilisation, and length of hospital stay) were prospectively collected from the medical records. Preadmission ERAS elements (e.g., patient education, optimisation of patient's health status), preoperative ERAS elements (e.g., antibiotic and perioperative nausea and vomiting prophylaxis), intraoperative ERAS elements (e.g., anaesthesia, blood loss, duration of procedure and fluid management), and postoperative ERAS elements (e.g., nasogastric tube management, drain management, pain management, and oral intake) were collected. Complications occurring during the first 30 and 90 postoperative days were scored using the Clavien–Dindo classification [24].

2.4. Statistical Analyses

Statistical analyses were performed using SPSS Statistics 29.0 software (IBM, Endicott, NY, USA). The primary endpoints were the percentage of ERAS compliance in comparison to the ERAS LARRC protocol, time to functional recovery, and postoperative complications. Complications were classified using the Clavien–Dindo classification and divided into minor complications (Clavien–Dindo I–IIIa) and major complications (Clavien–Dindo IIIb–IV). Compliance with the protocol was calculated based on the 39 developed ERAS care elements. Secondary endpoints included ERAS-related outcomes per perioperative phase. Demographics were presented for all patients. Sub-analyses were included for the performed anaesthesia and the use of a nasogastric tube because of the diversity of hypotheses in the literature regarding these elements in ERAS care. Continuous data were reported as means with standard deviations or as medians with ranges, depending on parameter distribution. Categorical data were reported as the count with percentages. Group comparisons were performed using the Chi-square test, Fisher's exact test, or the Mann–Whitney U test, as appropriate.

3. Results

A total of 72 patients with rectal cancer underwent bTME surgery between October 2021 and December 2022, of whom 39 (54.2%) were LARC patients and 33 (45.8%) were LRRC patients. Induction chemotherapy was administered in 36 patients (50.0%), while all patients received neoadjuvant radiotherapy. In total, 48 patients (66.7%) received full-course chemoradiotherapy with 50–50.4 Gy, 20 patients (27.8%) received chemoreirradiation with 30–30.6 Gy, and 4 patients (5.5%) received short-course radiotherapy with 25 Gy. Of the bTME surgical procedures, 23 patients (31.9%) underwent pelvic exenteration, 27 patients (37.5%) underwent abdomino-perineal resection (APR), and 18 patients (25.0%) underwent resection with primary (re-)anastomosis. In total, 14 patients (19.4%) underwent additional sacral resection, and 36 patients (50.0%) underwent additional pelvic sidewall resection. The median time of surgery was 306.0 min with a median of 1550.0 mL blood loss. All patient and treatment characteristics are shown in Table 1.

Table 1. Baseline characteristics.

Baseline Characteristics	n = 72 (%)
Age, mean in years (SD)	63.9 (10.7)
Gender	
Male	48 (66.7)
Female	24 (33.3)
ASA class	
I–II	59 (82.0)
III–IV	13 (18.1)
Induction chemotherapy	36 (50.0)
Neoadjuvant radiotherapy	72 (100)
Pathological Tumour stage	
T0–T2	6 (8.3)
T3–T4	37 (51.4)
N.A. *	29 (40.3)
Pathological Nodal stage	
N0	26 (36.1)
N1/2	17 (13.4)
N.A. *	29 (40.3)
Main procedure	
LAR/Re-resection with anastomosis	18 (25.0)
APR	27 (37.5)
Total exenteration	23 (31.9)
Tumour resection n.o.s. **	23 (31.9)

Table 1. *Cont.*

Baseline Characteristics	n = 72 (%)
Intraoperative radiotherapy	58 (80.6)
Bladder resection	24 (33.3)
Urologic reconstruction	34 (47.2)
Partial sacral resection	14 (19.4)
Prostate and/or vesicles resection (male only)	35 (72.9)
Uterus and/or ovaria resection (female only)	13 (54.2)
Vagina resection (female only)	7 (29.2)
Pelvic sidewall resection	36 (50.0)
Lateral lymph node resection	9 (12.5)
Length of operation, median in mL (IQR)	306.0 (219.3–368.8)
Intraoperative blood loss, median in mL (IQR)	1550.0 (762.5–2875.0)
Omentoplasty	51 (70.8)

* N.A. = not applicable in patients with LRRC. ** n.o.s. = not other specified.

3.1. Compliance to the ERAS LARRC Protocol

Total compliance with the ERAS LARRC protocol was 73.6%, in which all 39 items were scored per ERAS care element, as shown in Table 2. The preadmission compliance was 81.9%, the preoperative compliance was 89.4%, the intraoperative compliance was 70.2%, and the postoperative compliance was 62.8% for the total group.

Table 2. Compliance to ERAS LARRC protocol.

	Preadmission Compliance Care Elements	Compliance %
1	Preoperative nutritional status assessed	98.6
2	Preoperative nutritional treatment in case of (risk for) malnutrition	14.3
3	Alcohol (quitted before surgery)	93.1
4	Preadmission patient education	94.4
5	Ostomy introduction	100
6	Patient screened for anaemia preoperatively	94.4
7	Anaemia treatment given when applicable	60
8	Smoker (quitted before surgery)	81.9
9	Prehabilitation (in case of vulnerability)	100
	Preoperative compliance care elements	
10	No oral bowel preparation used unless patients received an LAR	94.4
11	Preoperative oral carbohydrate treatment	91.7
12	No preoperative sedative medication < 65 years	95.8
13	Thrombosis prophylaxis administered until outpatient at 28 days + compression socks	77.8
14	Antibiotic prophylaxis before incision	100
15	PONV prophylaxis administered	100
16	Date of admission = date of surgery (unless they received ureter stents)	81.9
17	SDD administered	73.6
	Intraoperative compliance care elements	
18	No epidural or spinal anaesthesia but use of multimodal anaesthesia	75
19	Nerve blocks or local anaesthesia and continuous wound infusion	75
20	Forced-air heating cover used	100
21	No nasogastric tube placed intraoperatively and used postoperatively unless ileus appeared; it was then removed according to protocol	44.2
22	No resection-site drainage placed according to protocol (pelvic exenteration)	56.9

Table 2. Cont.

	Postoperative compliance care elements	
23	Termination of urinary drainage at end of operation; SPC was used in case of potential retention bladder, Otherwise it was handled according to protocol	84.7
24	Stimulation of gut motility: laxatives and non-medicamental treatment used according to protocol	100
25	Weighted on POD 0	43.1
26	Weighted on POD 1	29.2
27	Weighted on POD 2	65.3
28	Weighted on POD 3	72.2
29	Pain management with CWI, metamizole and paracetamol	72.2
30	PONV prevention	100
31	Energy intake on POD 0 > 500 ml	20.8
32	Energy intake on POD 1 > 750 ml	43.1
33	Energy intake on POD 2 > 1000 mL	37.5
34	Energy intake on POD 3 > 1500 mL	41.7
35	Mobilisation on day of surgery	58.3
36	Mobilisation on POD1 according to protocol	52.8
37	Mobilisation on POD2 according to protocol	69.4
38	Mobilisation on POD3 according to protocol	77.8
39	Follow-up control performed around 30 days postoperatively	100

POD = Postoperative day.

3.2. Comparison of ERAS-Related Outcomes: Anaesthesia and Pain Management

Fifty-four patients (75.0%) received multimodal anaesthesia and postoperative continuous wound infusion (CWI) catheters, while, in 18 patients (25.0%), epidural anaesthesia was used. The use of opioids during the first three postoperative days was significantly lower in the multimodal anaesthesia group ($p < 0.001$) when converted to morphine equivalents. Patients had comparable scores on the numeric pain rating scale (NRS) during the first three postoperative days.

Of the patients with epidural anaesthesia, 17 patients (94.4%) stayed in the ICU compared to 28 patients (51.9%) with multimodal anaesthesia ($p = 0.001$). Of the patients receiving epidural anaesthesia, 14 patients (82.4%) needed hemodynamic support compared to 10 patients (35.7%) in the multimodal anaesthesia group ($p = 0.002$).

Patients with an epidural stayed in the hospital for a median of 10 days (IQR 6.8–15.5) compared to 7.0 days (5.5–14.0) for patients treated with multimodality analgesia ($p = 0.440$) (Table 3).

Table 3. Anaesthesia protocol and postoperative pain management.

Anaesthesia	Multimodal Management	Epidural	
	$n = 54$ (75.0%)	$n = 18$ (25.0%)	p-Value
Postoperative analgesics			
Continuous wound infusion	53 (98.1)	1 (5.6)	<0.001
Patient-controlled analgesia (PCA)	16 (29.6)	8 (44.4)	0.456
Median duration of PCA in days (IQR)	4.0 (3.0–5.0)	3.0 (1.0–4.0)	0.269
Epidural	NA	3.0 (2.0–3.0)	
Postoperative NSAID (Metamizole iv)	49 (90.7)	13 (72.2)	0.063
Median duration of metamizole in days (IQR)	5.0 (3.0–6.0)	5.0 (3.0–6.5)	0.641
Postoperative opioids * POD 0	53 (98.1)	18 (100)	0.750
Postoperative opioids * POD 1	23 (42.6)	18 (100)	<0.001
Postoperative opioids * POD 2	15 (27.8)	18 (100)	<0.001
Postoperative opioids * POD 3	14 (25.9)	17 (94.4)	<0.001
Postoperative opioids * POD 4	13 (24.1)	11 (64.7)	0.002
Postoperative opioids * POD 5	12 (22.2)	7 (41.2)	0.112
Nausea POD 0	10 (18.6)	1 (5.6)	0.380
Nausea POD 1	15 (27.8)	3 (16.7)	0.314

Table 3. Cont.

Anaesthesia	Multimodal Management	Epidural	
	n = 54 (75.0%)	n = 18 (25.0%)	p-Value
Nausea POD 2	16 (45.6)	5 (27.8)	0.987
Nausea POD 3	12 (22.2)	6 (33.3)	0.049
Mobilisation POD 0	33 (61.1)	9 (50.0)	0.554
Mobilisation POD 1	31 (57.4)	7 (38.9)	0.173
Mobilisation POD 2	40 (74.1)	10 (55.6)	0.153
Mobilisation POD 3	45 (83.3)	11 (61.1)	0.050
Complication < 30 days	38 (70.4)	12 (66.7)	0.768
Complication > 30 and <90 days	24 (45.3)	5 (27.8)	0.192
Median time to passage of stool in days (IQR)	3.0 (2.0–4.0)	2.0 (1.0–4.0)	0.411
Median time to tolerating solid food in days (IQR)	4.5 (2.0–6.3)	5.0 (2.8–7.3)	0.987
Median time to recover ADL in days (IQR)	6.0 (4.0–8.0)	6.5 (4.8–9.0)	0.976
Median time to termination of urinary drainage in days (IQR)	5.0 (2.0–10.5)	8.5 (3.8–13.0)	0.798
Median time to functional recovery in days (IQR)	7.0 (5.0–14.0)	10 (7.0–14.3)	0.328
Median length of postoperative ICU stay in days (IQR)	1.0 (0.0–1.0)	2.0 (1.0–2.3)	0.004
Median length of hospital stay in days (IQR)	7.0 (5.5–14.0)	10.0 (6.8–15.5)	0.440

* epidural included, iv or oral opioids.

3.3. Comparison of ERAS-Related Outcomes: Nasogastric Tube Management

A nasogastric tube was placed in 39 patients (54.2%). Among patients requiring a nasogastric tube for a postoperative period longer than 2 days, 13 patients (50.0%) underwent a total pelvic exenteration and a urologic reconstruction, and 23 patients (88.5%) underwent omentoplasty. The median production from the nasogastric tube during the first three postoperative days was 15.0 mL (IQR 0.0–80.0), 50.0 mL (0.0–260.0), 290.0 mL (50.0–800.0), and 300.0 mL (85.0–2025.0), respectively. A nasogastric tube was placed for a median of 3.0 days (IQR 2.0–6.5).

3.4. Comparison of ERAS-Related Outcomes: Urological Management

In 38 patients (52.8%), urethral catheters were placed intraoperatively and used after surgery. These urethral catheters were in place for a median of 6.0 days (IQR 3.0–12.0). In five patients (6.9%), the catheter was replaced due to bladder retention. A total of 10 patients (13.9%) had a urethral catheter at discharge, mostly following psoas hitch reconstruction ($p = 0.040$). A total of 8 patients (11.1%) received a suprapubic catheter, and 4 of these patients were discharged with the catheter. Twenty-three patients (31.9%) had an urostomy because of a total pelvic exenteration.

3.5. Outcomes, Functional Recovery, and Complications

The median hospital stay was 9 days (IQR 6.0–14.0). On the day of surgery, 42 patients (58.3%) were mobilised according to the protocol (out of bed for 5–15 min). On the third postoperative day, 56 patients (77.8%) were mobilised according to the protocol (they were out of bed twice a day for a minimum of one hour and walked around the ward (4–5 times 100 m)).

In total, 51 patients (70.8%) suffered from postoperative complications. Within 30 days after surgery, major complications (Clavien–Dindo > IIIa) were observed in 12 patients (16.7%) and between 31 and 90 days after surgery in 7 patients (9.7%). Most complications were of gastrointestinal origin. Of the total group of patients with complications, 14 patients (19.4%) needed surgical intervention, and 19 patients (26.4%) were readmitted to hospital (Table 4).

Table 4. Functional recovery and complications.

Functional Outcomes and Complications	n = 72 (%)
Median time to oral pain control in days (IQR)	4.0 (3.0–4.0)
Median time to passage of stool in days (IQR)	3.0 (2.0–4.0)
Median time to tolerating solid food in days (IQR)	5.0 (2.0–7.0)

Table 4. Cont.

Functional Outcomes and Complications	n = 72 (%)
Median time to recover ADL in days (IQR)	6.0 (4.0–8.0)
Median time to termination of urinary drainage in days (IQR)	6.0 (3.0–12.0)
Median time to termination of resection-site drain in days (IQR)	3.0 (2.0–4.0)
Median time to termination of nasogastric tube in days (IQR)	3.0 (2.0–6.5)
Mobilisation according to protocol	47 (65.3)
Median length of hospital stay in days (IQR)	9.0 (6.0–14.0)
Complications	51 (70.8)
Complications < 30 days	44 (61.1)
Most severe complication < 30 days (Clavien–Dindo)	
None	21 (29.2)
I–IIIa	39 (54.2)
IIIb–IV	12 (16.7)
Complications > 30 days <90 days	29 (40.3)
Gastro-intestinal complications	
Gastroparesis/paralytic ileus	18 (25.0)
Intra-abdominal abscess	8 (11.1)
Leakage anastomosis	6 (8.3)
Wound infection/dehiscence	12 (16.7)
Mechanical ileus	4 (5.6)
Urological complications	
Bladder retention	5 (6.9)
Urinary tract infection	9 (12.5)
Other	6 (8.3)
Neurological complications	9 (12.5)
Cardio-pulmonary complications	10 (13.9)
Vascular complications	3 (4.2)
Reoperations	14 (19.4)
Readmissions	19 (26.4)

4. Discussion

This study demonstrates the feasibility of implementing an ERAS protocol specifically designed for patients undergoing bTME for LARC or LRRC with a compliance rate of 73.6%. Patients treated within the ERAS LARRC protocol had lower rates of postoperative complications in comparison to the literature [6–9]. The use of multimodal analgesia, instead of epidural analgesia, was effective in postoperative pain management, with potentially beneficial effects on functional recovery and length of stay.

In the literature, evidence for the beneficial effects of an ERAS protocol for patients with LARC or LRRC undergoing bTME is lacking, as this heterogeneous and complex patient group is commonly excluded from ERAS-related studies [25]. The potential benefit of an ERAS protocol in these patients could be extensive as they suffer from poor postoperative outcomes due to a long period of functional recovery and a high complication rate. However, to expect an improvement in postoperative outcomes and time to functional recovery via ERAS implementation, compliance rates of at least 70% appear necessary [26,27].

The development and implementation of a new ERAS protocol is challenging. The implementation of the ERAS LARRC protocol in this centre was facilitated due to the prior implementation of an ERAS protocol for non-advanced colorectal surgical care. Certain elements could be implemented directly, such as proactive education and nursing pathways, careful fluid management, and attention to nausea and vomiting, as these elements have a significant effect on functional recovery after any gastrointestinal surgical procedure [5]. Other elements could not be implemented directly or had to be altered, taking into account the extensive surgical procedure and the increased likelihood of postoperative morbidity in LARRC patients. In the minimally invasive colorectal ERAS protocol, epidural analgesia is obsolete, but in beyond TME surgery for LARC or LRCC, it is considered necessary for adequate postoperative pain management [7]. In our multidisciplinary team, a novel multimodal approach with the use of methadone, lidocaine, and ketamine was proposed instead of using epidural analgesia. The use of multimodal analgesia was implemented gradually during the study period with promising results.

Epidural analgesia is not easily changed to a multimodal approach, as it remains the golden standard in treating postoperative pain. At the beginning of the studied period, all patients with sacral resections received epidural analgesia, while during implementation, more patients received multimodal analgesia with increasingly promising results. This resulted in more affinity with the multimodal approach and a reduction in used epidural analgesia. However, selection bias was not prevented and should be investigated in future research.

Even so, the implementation of the adjusted ERAS protocol seems feasible, and the postoperative results are also encouraging. Comparing the outcomes of this study to other examples in the literature in terms of ERAS care elements is challenging, and, to our knowledge, ERAS has not yet been implemented in patients with LARC or LRRC. One ERAS implementation study conducted by Harji et al. investigated the implementation of an ERAS protocol adjusted specifically for patients with pelvic malignancies undergoing pelvic exenteration [7]. A few other studies have presented postoperative outcomes after bTME in rectal cancer, investigating outcomes after pelvic exenteration for pelvic malignancies of any kind without the implementation of a specific ERAS protocol [6,28–32]. In these studies, patient characteristics and procedures were comparable to this study, such as operating time and blood loss. The length of stay in these studies varied between 9 and 19 days, while in this study, the median hospital stay was 9 days. Stays in the intensive care unit were reduced, as patients remained there for 1 to 2 days, compared to 3 to 4 days in other studies. In the literature, the major complication rate (Clavien–Dindo > IIIa) showed a median of 22.6% to 61.3%, compared to a median major complication rate of 16.7% in this cohort. In conclusion, the results of this study seem rather promising.

Based on the results of this study, the presented ERAS LARRC protocol is implementable and valuable and can be applied in clinical practise. However, the current protocol still should be tailored to some care elements. The heterogeneity of this disease and type of surgical procedure complicates implementation, and some exceptions or deviations from protocol are inevitable. The quality of the protocol lies within the combination of all individual ERAS care elements, and successful implementation requires continuous effort, feedback, and further development. As with all new protocol implementations, compliance increases over time by gaining more affinity and experience with the protocol. In our centre, caretakers were already familiar with ERAS, which facilitated the implementation. Even so, as compliance was already >70%, it should increase even further over time due to the increased affinity of caretakers with it, as well as the continuous evolution of the protocol.

It is essential to identify factors that are associated with compliance and functional recovery in patients with LARC and LRRC. Postoperative care elements have the greatest impact on overall recovery, yet they are also the most difficult to comply with [7]. This was reflected in this study. Even though the overall compliance rate was >70%, postoperative compliance was only 62.8%. This was mainly due to an inability to attain a sufficient amount of oral intake and the inability to weigh patients postoperatively in order to manage the fluid balance. As 54.2% of patients had a nasogastric tube postoperatively, the appropriate intake could not be accomplished in these patients. As most patients seemed to develop gastroparesis and/or paralytic ileus on the second postoperative day, it appears possible to abstain from using a nasogastric tube for the first two postoperative days in most patients. A potential additional benefit of omitting a nasogastric tube may be that patients are less constrained in postoperative mobilisation. As oral intake is increased gradually within the ERAS LARRC protocol, a nasogastric tube could still be inserted in case of gastroparesis and/or paralytic ileus. Another future adjustment is the promotion of suprapubic catheters as an alternative to urethral catheters in case of expected bladder retention after surgery. However, a patient cohort that might benefit from a suprapubic catheter cannot be defined based on the current study. In upcoming years, implementation in other centres is needed to investigate all specific care elements and guarantee an effective ERAS LARRC protocol as the new standard of care.

5. Conclusions

This study shows that an ERAS protocol developed for patients undergoing bTME for LARC or LRRC is feasible. In comparison to prior studies in the literature, the current ERAS LARRC protocol results in a reduction in complications. Multimodal anaesthesia could potentially impact the length of stay in a beneficial way, as well as improve the recovery profile. Despite the fact that the presented cohort study is a work in progress, it shows that even in this heterogenic group, standardisation in perioperative care is achievable and may yield promising results.

Supplementary Materials: The following supporting information can be downloaded at: https://www.mdpi.com/article/10.3390/cancers15184523/s1, References [1,12,33–49] are cited in the supplementary materials. File S1: The ERAS LARRC protocol.

Author Contributions: Conceptualization, S.N., H.J.S., S.v.d.C., G.A.P.N., J.L.T., H.W.C., H.J.T.R., J.W.A.B. and J.G.B.; Methodology, S.N.; Formal analysis, S.N.; Investigation, S.N., D.M.J.C., S.G., S.H.J.K., H.J.S., S.v.d.C., G.A.P.N., J.L.T., H.W.C., H.J.T.R., J.W.A.B. and J.G.B.; Writing—original draft, S.N.; Writing—review & editing, S.N., D.M.J.C., S.G., S.H.J.K., H.J.S., H.J.T.R. and J.G.B.; Visualization, S.N.; Supervision, H.J.T.R., J.W.A.B. and J.G.B. All authors have read and agreed to the published version of the manuscript.

Funding: This research received no external funding.

Institutional Review Board Statement: This study was reviewed and approved by the Medical Research Ethics Committees United–Nieuwegein (registration number W22.021). The study was not subject to the Medical Research Involving Human Subjects Act.

Informed Consent Statement: Written informed consent for participation was waived for this study since this study evaluated standard of care, in accordance with the national legislation and the institutional requirements.

Data Availability Statement: Data is available upon request to the corresponding author with specification of the purpose of the request.

Conflicts of Interest: The authors declare no conflict of interest.

References

1. Gustafsson, U.O.; Scott, M.J.; Hubner, M.; Nygren, J.; Demartines, N.; Francis, N.; Rockall, T.A.; Young-Fadok, T.M.; Hill, A.G.; Soop, M.; et al. Guidelines for Perioperative Care in Elective Colorectal Surgery: Enhanced Recovery After Surgery (ERAS®) Society Recommendations: 2018. *World J. Surg.* **2019**, *43*, 659–695. [CrossRef] [PubMed]
2. Gustafsson, U.O.; Hausel, J.; Thorell, A.; Ljungqvist, O.; Soop, M.; Nygren, J.; Group, E.R.A.S.S. Adherence to the Enhanced Recovery After Surgery Protocol and Outcomes After Colorectal Cancer Surgery. *Arch. Surg.* **2011**, *146*, 571–577. [CrossRef] [PubMed]
3. Collaborative, P. Perioperative management and anaesthetic considerations in pelvic exenterations using Delphi methodology: Results from the PelvEx Collaborative. *BJS Open* **2021**, *5*, zraa055. [CrossRef] [PubMed]
4. Denost, Q.; Rullier, E.; Maillou-Martinaud, H.; Tuech, J.-J.; Ghouti, L.; Cotte, E.; Panis, Y.; Lelong, B.; Rouanet, P.; Broc, G.; et al. International variation in managing locally advanced or recurrent rectal cancer: Prospective benchmark analysis. *Br. J. Surg.* **2020**, *107*, 1846–1854. [CrossRef]
5. Tekkis, P.; Road, F. Consensus statement on the multidisciplinary management of patients with recurrent and primary rectal cancer beyond total mesorectal excision planes. *Br. J. Surg.* **2013**, *100*, 1009–1014. [CrossRef]
6. Mariathasan, A.B.; Boye, K.; Giercksky, K.E.; Brennhovd, B.; Gullestad, H.P.; Emblemsvåg, H.L.; Grøholt, K.K.; Dueland, S.; Flatmark, K.; Larsen, S.G. Beyond total mesorectal excision in locally advanced rectal cancer with organ or pelvic side-wall involvement. *Eur. J. Surg. Oncol.* **2018**, *44*, 1226–1232. [CrossRef] [PubMed]
7. Harji, D.; Mauriac, P.; Bouyer, B.; Berard, X.; Gille, O.; Salut, C.; Rullier, E.; Celerier, B.; Robert, G.; Denost, Q. The feasibility of implementing an enhanced recovery programme in patients undergoing pelvic exenteration. *Eur. J. Surg. Oncol.* **2021**, *47*, 3194–3201. [CrossRef]

8. Ketelaers, S.H.J.; Voogt, E.L.K.; Simkens, G.A.; Bloemen, J.G.; Nieuwenhuijzen, G.A.P.; de Hingh, I.H.J.; Rutten, H.J.T.; Burger, J.W.A.; Orsini, R.G. Age-related differences in morbidity and mortality after surgery for primary clinical T4 and locally recurrent rectal cancer. *Color. Dis.* **2021**, *23*, 1141–1152. [CrossRef]
9. Toh, J.W.T.; Cecire, J.; Hitos, K.; Shedden, K.; Gavegan, F.; Pathmanathan, N.; El Khoury, T.; Di Re, A.; Cocco, A.; Limmer, A.; et al. The impact of variations in care and complications within a colorectal enhanced recovery after surgery (ERAS) program on length of stay. *Ann. Coloproctol.* **2021**, *38*, 36–46. [CrossRef]
10. Nordkamp, S.; Ketelaers, S.H.J.; Piqeur, F.; Scholten, H.J.; van de Calseijde, S.; Tolenaar, J.; Nieuwenhuijzen, G.A.P.; Rutten, H.J.T.; Burger, J.W.A.; Bloemen, J.G. Current perioperative care in patients undergoing bTME for rectal cancer: What are the differences with the colorectal Enhanced Recovery After Surgery protocol? *Color. Dis.*. under review.
11. Robella, M.; Tonello, M.; Berchialla, P.; Sciannameo, V.; Ilari Civit, A.M.; Sommariva, A.; Sassaroli, C.; Di Giorgio, A.; Gelmini, R.; Ghirardi, V.; et al. Enhanced Recovery after Surgery (ERAS) Program for Patients with Peritoneal Surface Malignancies Undergoing Cytoreductive Surgery with or without HIPEC: A Systematic Review and a Meta-Analysis. *Cancers* **2023**, *15*, 570. [CrossRef] [PubMed]
12. Nygren, J.; Thacker, J.; Carli, F.; Fearon, K.C.H.; Norderval, S.; Lobo, D.N.; Ljungqvist, O.; Soop, M.; Ramirez, J. Guidelines for perioperative care in elective rectal/pelvic surgery: Enhanced Recovery After Surgery (ERAS®) Society recommendations. *World J. Surg.* **2013**, *37*, 285–305. [CrossRef] [PubMed]
13. Cerantola, Y.; Valerio, M.; Persson, B.; Jichlinski, P.; Ljungqvist, O.; Hubner, M.; Kassouf, W.; Muller, S.; Baldini, G.; Carli, F.; et al. Guidelines for perioperative care after radical cystectomy for bladder cancer: Enhanced Recovery After Surgery (ERAS®) society recommendations. *Clin. Nutr.* **2013**, *32*, 879–887. [CrossRef]
14. Federation of Medical Specialists. Dutch National Guidelines Colorectal Cancer. 2020. Available online: https://richtlijnendatabase.nl/richtlijn/colorectaal_carcinoom_crc/startpagina_-_crc.html (accessed on 6 September 2023).
15. Voogt, E.L.K.; Nordkamp, S.; Rutten, H.J.T.; Burger, J.W.A.; Collaborative, P. Induction chemotherapy followed by chemoradiotherapy versus chemoradiotherapy alone as neoadjuvant treatment for locally recurrent rectal cancer: The PelvEx II study. *Eur. J. Surg. Oncol.* **2021**, *47*, e22–e23. [CrossRef]
16. Van den Berg, K.; Schaap, D.P.; Voogt, E.L.K.; Buffart, T.E.; Verheul, H.M.W.; de Groot, J.W.B.; Verhoef, C.; Melenhorst, J.; Roodhart, J.M.L.; de Wilt, J.H.W.; et al. Neoadjuvant FOLFOXIRI prior to chemoradiotherapy for high-risk ("ugly") locally advanced rectal cancer: Study protocol of a single-arm, multicentre, open-label, phase II trial (MEND-IT). *BMC Cancer* **2022**, *22*, 957. [CrossRef]
17. Kendall, M.C.; Alves, L.J.; Pence, K.; Mukhdomi, T.; Croxford, D.; De Oliveira, G.S. The Effect of Intraoperative Methadone Compared to Morphine on Postsurgical Pain: A Meta-Analysis of Randomized Controlled Trials. *Anesthesiol. Res. Pract.* **2020**, *2020*, 6974321. [CrossRef]
18. Murphy, G.S.; Szokol, J.W.; Avram, M.J.; Greenberg, S.B.; Marymont, J.H.; Shear, T.; Parikh, K.N.; Patel, S.S.; Gupta, D.K. Intraoperative Methadone for the Prevention of Postoperative Pain: A Randomized, Double-blinded Clinical Trial in Cardiac Surgical Patients. *Anesthesiology* **2015**, *122*, 1112–1122. [CrossRef]
19. Richlin, D.M.; Reuben, S.S. Postoperative pain control with methadone following lower abdominal surgery. *J. Clin. Anesth.* **1991**, *3*, 112–116. [CrossRef]
20. Ketelaers, S.H.J.; Dhondt, L.; van Ham, N.; Harms, A.S.; Scholten, H.J.; Nieuwenhuijzen, G.A.P.; Rutten, H.J.T.; Burger, J.W.A.; Bloemen, J.G.; Vogelaar, F.J. A prospective cohort study to evaluate continuous wound infusion with local analgesics within an enhanced recovery protocol after colorectal cancer surgery. *Color. Dis.* **2022**, *24*, 1172–1183. [CrossRef]
21. Ramirez, J.A.; McIntosh, A.G.; Strehlow, R.; Lawrence, V.A.; Parekh, D.J.; Svatek, R.S. Definition, incidence, risk factors, and prevention of paralytic ileus following radical cystectomy: A systematic review. *Eur. Urol.* **2013**, *64*, 588–597. [CrossRef]
22. Marcq, G.; Kassouf, W. Postoperative ileus: A systematic pathway for radical cystectomy candidates? *Can. Urol. Assoc. J.* **2021**, *15*, 40–41. [CrossRef] [PubMed]
23. Raynor, M.C.; Pruthi, R.S. Postoperative Ileus After Radical Cystectomy: Looking for Answers to an Age-old Problem. *Eur. Urol.* **2014**, *66*, 273–274. [CrossRef] [PubMed]
24. Dindo, D.; Demartines, N.; Clavien, P.-A. Classification of surgical complications: A new proposal with evaluation in a cohort of 6336 patients and results of a survey. *Ann. Surg.* **2004**, *240*, 205–213.
25. Bellato, V.; An, Y.; Cerbo, D.; Campanelli, M.; Franceschilli, M.; Khanna, K.; Sensi, B.; Siragusa, L.; Rossi, P.; Sica, G.S. Feasibility and outcomes of ERAS protocol in elective cT4 colorectal cancer patients: Results from a single-center retrospective cohort study. *World J. Surg. Oncol.* **2021**, *19*, 196. [CrossRef]
26. Sánchez-Iglesias, J.L.; Gómez-Hidalgo, N.R.; Pérez-Benavente, A.; Carbonell-Socias, M.; Manrique-Muñoz, S.; Serrano, M.P.; Gutiérrez-Barceló, P.; Bradbury, M.; Nelson, G.; Gil-Moreno, A. Importance of Enhanced Recovery After Surgery (ERAS) Protocol Compliance for Length of Stay in Ovarian Cancer Surgery. *Ann. Surg. Oncol.* **2021**, *28*, 8979–8986. [CrossRef] [PubMed]
27. Tejedor, P.; González Ayora, S.; Ortega López, M.; León Arellano, M.; Guadalajara, H.; García-Olmo, D.; Pastor, C. Implementation barriers for Enhanced Recovery After Surgery (ERAS) in rectal cancer surgery: A comparative analysis of compliance with colon cancer surgeries. *Updates Surg.* **2021**, *73*, 2161–2168. [CrossRef]
28. Rahbari, N.N.; Ulrich, A.B.; Bruckner, T.; Münter, M.; Nickles, A.; Contin, P.; Löffler, T.; Reissfelder, C.; Koch, M.; Büchler, M.W.; et al. Surgery for locally recurrent rectal cancer in the era of total mesorectal excision: Is there still a chance for cure? *Ann. Surg.* **2011**, *253*, 522–533. [CrossRef]

29. Factors affecting outcomes following pelvic exenteration for locally recurrent rectal cancer. *Br. J. Surg.* **2018**, *105*, 650–657. [CrossRef]
30. Liccardo, F.; Baird, D.L.H.; Pellino, G.; Rasheed, S.; Kontovounisios, C.; Tekkis, P.P. Predictors of short-term readmission after beyond total mesorectal excision for primary locally advanced and recurrent rectal cancer. *Updates Surg.* **2019**, *71*, 477–484. [CrossRef]
31. Steffens, D.; Solomon, M.J.; Lee, P.; Austin, K.; Koh, C.; Byrne, C.; Karunaratne, S.; Hatcher, S.; Taylor, K.; McBride, K. Surgical, survival and quality of life outcomes in over 1000 pelvic exenterations: Lessons learned from a large Australian case series. *ANZ J. Surg.* **2023**, *93*, 1232–1241. [CrossRef]
32. Assi, H.; Persson, A.; Palmquist, I.; Öberg, M.; Buchwald, P.; Lydrup, M.-L. Short-term outcomes following beyond total mesorectal excision and reconstruction using myocutaneous flaps: A retrospective cohort study. *Eur. J. Surg. Oncol.* **2022**, *48*, 1161–1166. [CrossRef] [PubMed]
33. Han, C.Y.; Sharma, Y.; Yaxley, A.; Baldwin, C.; Miller, M. Use of the Patient-Generated Subjective Global Assessment to Identify Pre-Frailty and Frailty in Hospitalized Older Adults. *J. Nutr. Health Aging* **2021**, *25*, 1229–1234. [PubMed]
34. Van Rooijen, S.; Carli, F.; Dalton, S.; Thomas, G.; Bojesen, R.; Le Guen, M.; Barizien, N.; Awasthi, R.; Minnella, E.; Beijer, S.; et al. Multimodal prehabilitation in colorectal cancer patients to improve functional capacity and reduce postoperative complications: The first international randomized controlled trial for multimodal prehabilitation. *BMC Cancer* **2019**, *19*, 98.
35. Ghignone, F.; Hernandez, P.; Mahmoud, M.N.; Ugolini, G. Functional recovery in senior adults undergoing surgery for colorectal cancer: Assessment tools and strategies to preserve functional status. *Eur. J. Surg. Oncol. J. Eur. Soc. Surg. Oncol. Br. Assoc. Surg. Oncol.* **2020**, *46*, 387–393.
36. Brady, M.; Kinn, S.; Stuart, P. Preoperative fasting for adults to prevent perioperative complications. *Cochrane Database Syst. Rev.* **2003**, CD004423. [CrossRef]
37. Smith, M.D.; McCall, J.; Plank, L.; Herbison, G.P.; Soop, M.; Nygren, J. Preoperative carbohydrate treatment for enhancing recovery after elective surgery. *Cochrane Database Syst. Rev.* **2014**, CD009161. [CrossRef]
38. Carli, F. Physiologic considerations of Enhanced Recovery After Surgery (ERAS) programs: Implications of the stress response. *Can. J. Anaesth.* **2015**, *62*, 110–119. [CrossRef]
39. Abis, G.S.A.; Stockmann, H.B.A.C.; van Egmond, M.; Bonjer, H.J.; Vandenbroucke-Grauls, C.M.J.E.; Oosterling, S.J. Selective decontamination of the digestive tract in gastrointestinal surgery: Useful in infection prevention? A systematic review. *J. Gastrointest. Surg. Off. J. Soc. Surg. Aliment. Tract.* **2013**, *17*, 2172–2178.
40. Abis, G.S.A.; Stockmann, H.B.A.C.; Bonjer, H.J.; van Veenendaal, N.; van Doorn-Schepens, M.L.M.; Budding, A.E.; Wilschut, J.A.; van Egmond, M.; Oosterling, S.J.; de Lange, E.S.M.; et al. Randomized clinical trial of selective decontamination of the digestive tract in elective colorectal cancer surgery (SELECT trial). *Br. J. Surg.* **2019**, *106*, 355–363.
41. Kwon, S.; Thompson, R.; Dellinger, P.; Yanez, D.; Farrohki, E.; Flum, D. Importance of perioperative glycemic control in general surgery: A report from the Surgical Care and Outcomes Assessment Program. *Ann. Surg.* **2013**, *257*, 8–14. [CrossRef]
42. Weibel, S.; Rücker, G.; Eberhart, L.H.; Pace, N.L.; Hartl, H.M.; Jordan, O.L.; Mayer, D.; Riemer, M.; Schaefer, M.S.; Raj, D.; et al. Drugs for preventing postoperative nausea and vomiting in adults after general anaesthesia: A network meta-analysis. *Cochrane Database Syst. Rev.* **2020**, *10*, CD012859. [PubMed]
43. Watanabe, J.; Miki, A.; Koizumi, M.; Kotani, K.; Sata, N. Effect of Postoperative Coffee Consumption on Postoperative Ileus after Abdominal Surgery: An Updated Systematic Review and Meta-Analysis. *Nutrients* **2021**, *13*, 4394. [CrossRef] [PubMed]
44. Short, V.; Herbert, G.; Perry, R.; Atkinson, C.; Ness, A.R.; Penfold, C.; Thomas, S.; Andersen, H.K.; Lewis, S.J. Chewing gum for postoperative recovery of gastrointestinal function. *Cochrane Database Syst. Rev.* **2015**, CD006506. [CrossRef]
45. Felder, S.; Rasmussen, M.S.; King, R.; Sklow, B.; Kwaan, M.; Madoff, R.; Jensen, C. Prolonged thromboprophylaxis with low molecular weight heparin for abdominal or pelvic surgery. *Cochrane Database Syst. Rev.* **2019**, *3*, CD004318.
46. Sachdeva, A.; Dalton, M.; Amaragiri, S.V.; Lees, T. Elastic compression stockings for prevention of deep vein thrombosis. *Cochrane Database Syst. Rev.* **2010**, CD001484. [CrossRef]
47. Changchien, C.R.; Yeh, C.Y.; Huang, S.T.; Hsieh, M.-L.; Chen, J.-S.; Tang, R. Postoperative urinary retention after primary colorectal cancer resection via laparotomy: A prospective study of 2355 consecutive patients. *Dis. Colon Rectum* **2007**, *50*, 1688–1696. [CrossRef] [PubMed]
48. Buckley, B.S.; Lapitan, M.C.M. Drugs for treatment of urinary retention after surgery in adults. *Cochrane Database Syst. Rev.* **2010**, CD008023. [CrossRef] [PubMed]
49. McPhail, M.J.W.; Abu-Hilal, M.; Johnson, C.D. A meta-analysis comparing suprapubic and transurethral catheterization for bladder drainage after abdominal surgery. *Br. J. Surg.* **2006**, *93*, 1038–1044. [CrossRef] [PubMed]

Disclaimer/Publisher's Note: The statements, opinions and data contained in all publications are solely those of the individual author(s) and contributor(s) and not of MDPI and/or the editor(s). MDPI and/or the editor(s) disclaim responsibility for any injury to people or property resulting from any ideas, methods, instructions or products referred to in the content.

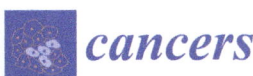

Article

Treatment of Colorectal Cancer in Certified Centers: Results of a Large German Registry Study Focusing on Long-Term Survival

Vinzenz Völkel [1,*], Michael Gerken [1,2], Kees Kleihues-van Tol [3], Olaf Schoffer [4], Veronika Bierbaum [4], Christoph Bobeth [4], Martin Roessler [4], Christoph Reissfelder [5], Alois Fürst [6], Stefan Benz [3,7], Bettina M. Rau [8], Pompiliu Piso [9], Marius Distler [10], Christian Günster [11], Judith Hansinger [1], Jochen Schmitt [4] and Monika Klinkhammer-Schalke [1,3]

[1] Tumor Center Regensburg, Center of Quality Management and Health Services Research, University of Regensburg, 93053 Regensburg, Germany; monika.klinkhammer-schalke@klinik.uni-regensburg.de (M.K.-S.)
[2] Bavarian Cancer Registry, Regional Center Regensburg, Bavarian Health and Food Safety Authority, 93053 Regensburg, Germany
[3] Arbeitsgemeinschaft Deutscher Tumorzentren e.V. (ADT), 14057 Berlin, Germany
[4] Center for Evidence-Based Healthcare (ZEGV), Faculty of Medicine, University Hospital Carl Gustav Carus and Carl Gustav Carus, Dresden University of Technology (TU Dresden), 01307 Dresden, Germany; olaf.schoffer@ukdd.de (O.S.); jochen.schmitt@ukdd.de (J.S.)
[5] Department of Surgery, Universitätsmedizin Mannheim, Medical Faculty Mannheim, Heidelberg University, 68167 Mannheim, Germany
[6] Klinik für Allgemein-, Viszeral-, Thoraxchirurgie und Adipositasmedizin, Caritas Krankenhaus St., 93053 Regensburg, Germany
[7] Klinik für Allgemein-, Viszeral-, Thorax- und Kinderchirurgie, 71032 Böblingen, Germany
[8] Department of General, Visceral and Thoracic Surgery, Hospital of Neumarkt, 92318 Neumarkt in der Oberpfalz, Germany
[9] Klinik für Allgemein- und Viszeralchirurgie, Krankenhaus der Barmherzigen Brüder, 93049 Regensburg, Germany
[10] Department of Visceral, Thoracic and Vascular Surgery, University Hospital Carl Gustav Carus Dresden, Faculty of Medicine Carl Gustav Carus, Dresden University of Technology (TU Dresden), 01307 Dresden, Germany
[11] WIdO—AOK Research Institute, 10178 Berlin, Germany
* Correspondence: vinzenz.voelkel@ur.de

Citation: Völkel, V.; Gerken, M.; Kleihues-van Tol, K.; Schoffer, O.; Bierbaum, V.; Bobeth, C.; Roessler, M.; Reissfelder, C.; Fürst, A.; Benz, S.; et al. Treatment of Colorectal Cancer in Certified Centers: Results of a Large German Registry Study Focusing on Long-Term Survival. *Cancers* **2023**, *15*, 4568. https://doi.org/10.3390/cancers15184568

Academic Editor: Susanne Merkel

Received: 17 August 2023
Revised: 8 September 2023
Accepted: 13 September 2023
Published: 15 September 2023

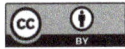

Copyright: © 2023 by the authors. Licensee MDPI, Basel, Switzerland. This article is an open access article distributed under the terms and conditions of the Creative Commons Attribution (CC BY) license (https://creativecommons.org/licenses/by/4.0/).

Simple Summary: Certification in oncology aims to establish structural and procedural standards according to evidence-based guidelines. The WiZen study is the largest study so far to analyze the effect of the certification of designated cancer centers on survival in Germany. Based on clinical cancer registry data of 47.440 colorectal cancer patients treated between 2009 and 2017, the present study shows that treatment at colorectal cancer centers has been associated with significantly better outcomes. Patients treated at certified facilities had an eleven percent (colon)/nine percent (rectum) lower risk of dying within the first five years after diagnosis. These findings support the shift towards a more structured cancer care system.

Abstract: (1) Background: The WiZen study is the largest study so far to analyze the effect of the certification of designated cancer centers on survival in Germany. This certification program is provided by the German Cancer Society (GCS) and represents one of the largest oncologic certification programs worldwide. Currently, about 50% of colorectal cancer patients in Germany are treated in certified centers. (2) Methods: All analyses are based on population-based clinical cancer registry data of 47.440 colorectal cancer (ICD-10-GM C18/C20) patients treated between 2009 and 2017. The primary outcome was 5-year overall survival (OAS) after treatment at certified cancer centers compared to treatment at other hospitals; the secondary endpoint was recurrence-free survival. Statistical methods included Kaplan–Meier analysis and multivariable Cox regression. (3) Results: Treatment at certified hospitals was associated with significant advantages concerning 5-year overall survival (HR 0.92, 95% CI 0.89, 0.96, adjusted for a broad range of confounders) for colon cancer patients. Concentrating on UICC stage I–III patients, for whom curative treatment is possible, the survival benefit was even larger (colon cancer: HR 0.89, 95% CI 0.84, 0.94; rectum cancer:

HR 0.91, 95% CI 0.84, 0.97). (4) Conclusions: These results encourage future efforts for further implementation of the certification program. Patients with colorectal cancer should preferably be directed to certified centers.

Keywords: certified cancer center; colon cancer; rectal cancer; cohort study; registries; survival; quality of cancer care; evidence-based medicine; WiZen; German Cancer Society

1. Introduction

Colorectal cancer is one of the most common malignancies worldwide [1,2]. In Germany, 5.3% of women and 6.7% of men will be diagnosed with colorectal cancer in the course of their life; this corresponds to a national incidence of approximately 60,000 diagnoses per year [3]. With these figures, colorectal cancer belongs to the three most frequent tumor diseases in Germany. The observed survival rate after five years for all stages has been constantly improving over the past decades and amounts to 54% among female and 52% among male patients [3]. Depending on the tumor location, Union for International Cancer Control (UICC) stage, and therapy intention, the treatment of colorectal cancer relies on surgical resection in locally advanced and metastatic cases combined with pre- or postoperative chemo-, radio-, or targeted therapy [4].

Health care systems worldwide aim to improve cancer care quality by means of the accreditation or certification of specialized hospitals [5–8]. To promote optimal, guideline-based therapy pathways, a certification program for treating facilities has been established in Germany. Since 2003, the German Cancer Society (GCS; German: Deutsche Krebsgesellschaft, DKG) has offered organ-specific certification programs [9–11]. As of today, there exist 18 different GCS certification programs and 1402 GCS-certified centers [12]. Of those, 314 are specialized in colorectal cancer [13]. To obtain GCS certification, a hospital has to fulfill a broad variety of requirements. They include structural measures concerning, e.g., regular interdisciplinary communication and consensus decision making in structured tumor boards, or the maintenance of multi-professional outreach networks. Moreover, they have to report about 30 performance indicators reflecting process and outcome quality in compliance with official treatment guidelines (e.g., minimal annual caseloads of 30 colon and 20 rectum cancer resections per certified center and year, share of therapy pathways deviating from tumor board decisions) [14]. Certified colorectal cancer centers must undergo regular external audits and their performance indicators are included in publicly available annual quality reports published by the GCS [15].

In 2018, a registry-based health service analysis showed that treatment at GCS-certified colorectal cancer facilities might be associated with significant survival benefits [16]. However, this study and a few other analyses for different tumor entities from other countries [17–21] were subject to some limitations (e.g., concerning the coverage area, transferability from other health care systems to Germany), leaving room for discussion. The WiZen study (German Innovation Fund, grant number 01VSF17020) currently represents the largest study on the topic. The present publication aims to provide an in-depth overview of the study's specific results regarding colorectal cancer with a special focus on clinical cancer registry-based analyses (the statutory health insurance-based analyses will be published elsewhere).

2. Materials and Methods

2.1. Aim

The WiZen study has been jointly conducted by four different institutions with expertise in clinical epidemiology and evidence-based medicine: Zentrum für Evidenzbasierte Gesundheitsversorgung (ZEGV)/Hochschulmedizin Dresden, Germany, Tumorzentrum Regensburg (TZR), Germany, Arbeitsgemeinschaft Deutscher Tumorzentren e. V. (ADT), Berlin, Germany and Wissenschaftliches Institut der AOK (WIdO), Berlin, Germany. Cooperation partners who provided relevant data from cancer registries and the certification program were GCS, Berlin, Germany. Klinisches Krebsregister Dresden (KKRD), Germany, Klinisches Krebsregister Erfurt (KKRE), Germany, and Klinisches Krebsregister für Brandenburg und Berlin (KKRBB), Germany.

The WiZen study has been designed as a set of retrospective cohort studies aiming to evaluate whether treatment in a GCS-certified cancer center is associated with better overall survival. Besides colorectal cancer, it focuses on seven other tumor entities (breast cancer, gynecological cancer, head and neck cancer, lung cancer, neurooncological tumors, pancreatic cancer, and prostate cancer; a general report of the project results is available online [22]).

2.2. Data Source

The findings reported in this publication are based on a comprehensive dataset provided by four large clinical cancer registries (TZR, KKRD, KKRE, KKRBB). These cancer registries fulfill an official mandate and collect data on all cancer patients registered in their catchment area. The dataset contained demographic characteristics (age, sex, date of death), detailed tumor characteristics (date of diagnosis, histological subtype, tumor stage according to the International Union against Cancer, UICC, tumor grade, lymphatic and venous invasion), as well as information about treatment procedures. It covered an observation period from 2006 to 2017.

2.3. Inclusion and Exclusion Criteria

The following criteria were used to define the population for the analyses shown in this paper:

(a) Diagnosis of colorectal cancer according to the ICD-10-GM codes C18 (malignant neoplasm of the colon) or C20 (malignant neoplasm of the rectum).
(b) Age of at least 18 years at the time of diagnosis.
(c) No previous diagnoses of colorectal cancer (a patient was only considered as incident between 2009 and 2017 if there were no earlier diagnoses of colorectal cancer recorded; to avoid issues with missing information concerning earlier tumor diagnoses, patients with a cancer diagnosis between 2006 and 2008 were excluded a priori following the guideline "good practice of secondary data analysis" [23] since it would not have been possible to assess a case's compliance to this inclusion criterion). Previous diagnoses of other, non-colorectal cancer were no exclusion criterion.
(d) Sufficient information concerning the certification status of the treating hospital (in this context, treatment at a non-certified institution that belongs to an association containing a GCS-certified colorectal cancer center was also considered a certified center treatment).
(e) Consistent histological subtype (only adenocarcinoma, exclusion of, e.g., lymphoma or sarcoma).

2.4. Statistical Analysis

The primary outcome was overall survival up to five years after diagnosis, and the secondary outcome was 5-year recurrence-free survival. Each included patient was considered to be at risk of death or tumor recurrence from the date of diagnosis onwards. The follow-up period ended at the date of death or tumor recurrence, or on 31 December 2017, in the absence of an event. To compare the unadjusted survival rates between GCS-certified colorectal cancer centers and non-certified hospitals, the Kaplan–Meier method was employed. To adjust for a variety of important confounders (age, sex, year of diagnosis, UICC stage, grade, lymphatic and venous invasion), multivariable Cox regression models were developed. All significance tests were two-sided with a significance level of 0.05. All reported results are presented together with the corresponding p-value and/or the upper and the lower border of the 95% confidence interval. The analyses were performed with IBM SPSS 25 (IBM SPSS Statistics for Windows, Version 25.0. Armonk, NY, USA: IBM Corp.).

2.5. Data Protection and Ethics

The data were pseudonymized at the participating cancer registries. The pseudonymized data were analyzed at TZR. The WiZen study was approved by the ethics committee of the TU Dresden (approval number: EK95022019). The study was registered at ClinicalTrials.gov (identifier: NCT04334239). The data processing and analyses were conducted in line with the Declaration of Helsinki and the General Data Protection Regulation of the European Union.

3. Results

3.1. Inclusion Process

Between 2009 and 2017, the dataset contained 30,742 patients with colon (ICD-10-GM C18) and 17,040 with rectum cancer (ICD-10-GM C20). After the application of all inclusion criteria, 30,497 (99.2%), and 16,943 (99.4%) patients, respectively, were used for the projected analyses.

3.2. Share of Patients Treated in GCS-Certified Colorectal Cancer Centers

The share of patients treated in GCS-certified colorectal cancer centers was 27.9% (colon; rectum: 31.7%) at the beginning of the observation period in 2009 and increased to 51.9% (colon; rectum: 49.4%) in 2016; thereafter, it slightly dropped (Figure 1).

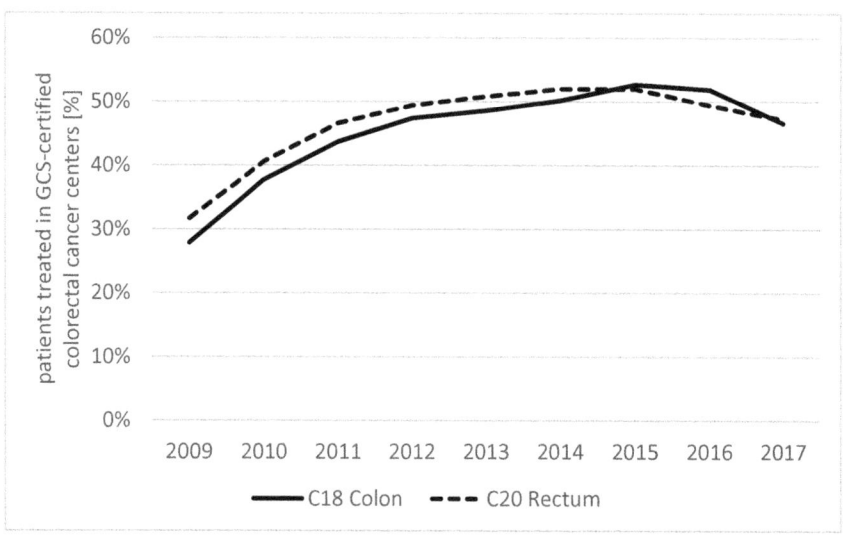

Figure 1. Share of patients treated in GCS-certified colorectal cancer centers according to diagnosis.

3.3. Description of Collectives

The colon cancer patients treated in GCS-certified centers showed a similar sex distribution to the patients from non-certified hospitals. Among the rectum cancer patients, the share of male patients was only slightly higher in non-certified hospitals (66.5% vs. 62.9%). Concerning the age distribution, no relevant differences between centers and other hospitals were seen, either. The colon and rectum cancer patients treated at certified centers suffered from advanced UICC stages (III and IV) more often; moreover, an unknown tumor stage was seen less frequently in center patients (colon: 6.7% vs. 17.5%; rectum: 6.9% vs. 16.2%). More details can be found in Tables 1 and 2.

Table 1. Patient characteristics according to diagnosis and treatment status.

	C18 Colon				C20 Rectum			
Treatment in GCS-Certified Centers	Yes		No		Yes		No	
	n	%	n	%	n	%	n	%
Sex								
Female	6043	43.9	7515	44.9	2650	33.5	3353	37.1
Male	7717	56.1	9222	55.1	5254	66.5	5686	62.9
Age								
18–49	915	6.6	765	4.6	574	7.3	481	5.3
50–59	1801	13.1	1918	11.5	1553	19.6	1611	17.8
60–69	3086	22.4	3569	21.3	2136	27.0	2333	25.8
70–79	4860	35.3	6353	38.0	2480	31.4	3047	33.7
80+	3098	22.5	4132	24.7	1161	14.7	1567	17.3
Year of diagnosis								
2009–2011	3725	27.1	6504	38.9	2246	28.4	3409	37.7
2012–2014	4883	35.5	5136	30.7	2878	36.4	2793	30.9
2015–2017	5152	37.4	5097	30.5	2780	35.2	2837	31.4
Total	13,760	100.0	16,737	100.0	7904	100.0	9039	100.0

Table 2. Tumor characteristics according to diagnosis and treatment status.

	C18 Colon				C20 Rectum			
Treatment in GCS-Certified Centers	Yes		No		Yes		No	
	n	%	n	%	n	%	n	%
UICC stage								
I	2622	19.1	2915	17.4	1348	17.1	1511	16.7
II	3694	26.8	4190	25.0	1348	17.1	1577	17.4
III	2892	21.0	3352	20.0	2913	36.9	2770	30.6
IV	3634	26.4	3344	20.0	1747	22.1	1718	19.0
X	918	6.7	2936	17.5	548	6.9	1463	16.2
Grade								
G1	742	5.4	1232	7.4	400	5.1	683	7.6
G2	8913	64.8	10,286	61.5	5431	68.7	5704	63.1
G3/4	3059	22.2	3932	23.5	1127	14.3	1650	18.3
GX	1046	7.6	1287	7.7	946	12.0	1002	11.1
Lymphatic invasion								
L0	6783	49.3	7726	46.2	4297	54.4	3999	44.2
L1	4711	34.2	5905	35.3	1705	21.6	2304	25.5
LX	2266	16.5	3106	18.6	1902	24.1	2736	30.3
Vein invasion								
V0	9405	68.4	11,075	66.2	5157	65.2	5251	58.1
V1/2	1905	13.8	2401	14.3	779	9.9	1000	11.1
VX	2450	17.8	3261	19.5	1968	24.9	2788	30.8
Total	13,760	100.0	16,737	100.0	7904	100.0	9039	100.0

3.4. Survival Analyses

The mean follow-up—estimated by means of the reverse Kaplan–Meier method—was 3.39 years in the complete cohort (95% CI 3.36–3.42) and the median follow-up was 3.20

(95% CI 3.14–3.25). In patients treated at certified centers, the mean follow-up was 3.57 years (95% CI 3.53–3.61; median 3.51, 95% CI 3.44–3.58) and in patients treated at non-certified hospitals was 3.23 years (95% CI 3.18–3.28; median 2.84, 95% CI 2.75–2.93), respectively.

3.4.1. Overall Survival

For colon cancer patients of GCS-certified centers, the 5-year Kaplan–Meier survival rate over all stages was 45% compared to 39% for patients from other non-certified hospitals (Figure 2a). The difference between the two survival curves was highly significant ($p < 0.001$). Moreover, 48% of the rectum cancer patients treated in GCS-certified centers were still alive after five years; among patients of other hospitals, this estimated rate was 41%. Again, the difference between the two Kaplan–Meier survival curves was highly significant ($p < 0.001$, Figure 2b).

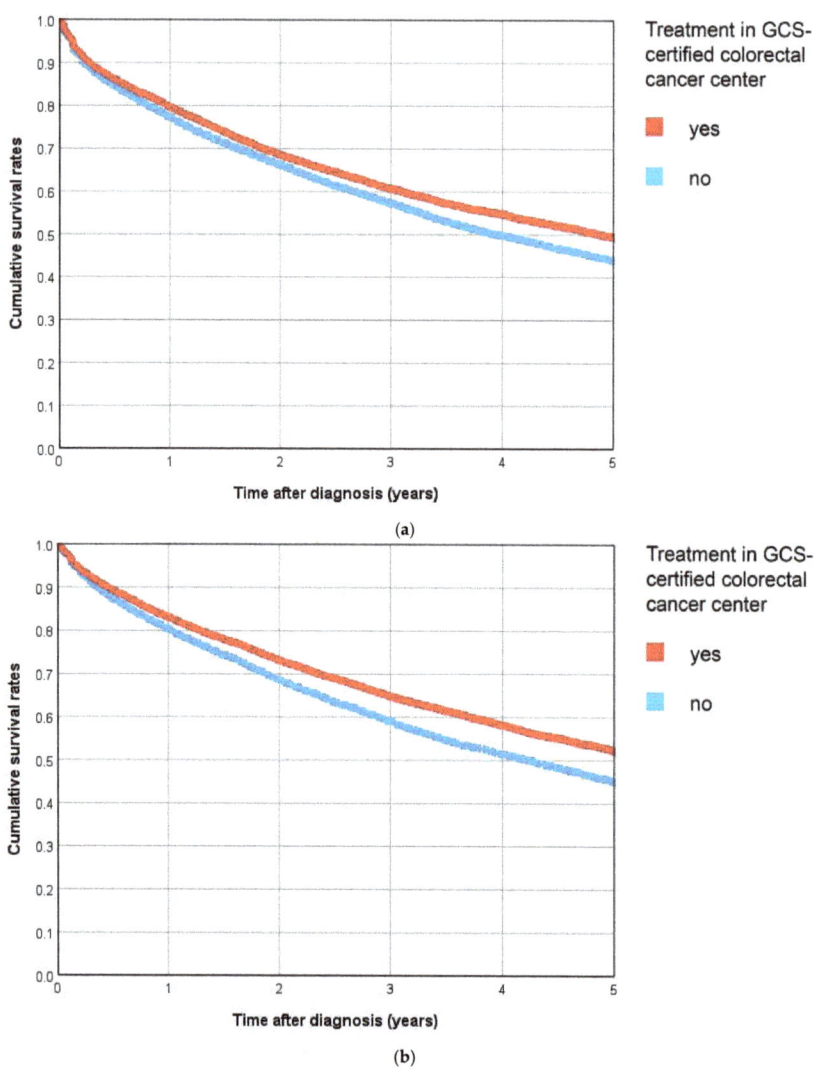

Figure 2. (**a**) C18 Colon, (**b**) C20 Rectum. Kaplan–Meier curves for overall survival according to diagnosis and treatment status.

For colon cancer patients, the unadjusted hazard ratio over all patients for all-cause mortality was 0.868 (95% CI 0.837, 0.900) for treatment in a GCS-certified cancer center compared to other hospitals. Adjusting for age, sex, year of diagnosis, UICC stage, grade, and lymphatic and venous invasion, it changed to 0.921 (95% CI 0.887, 0.956, Figure 3). The results for all covariates contained in the adjusted Cox regression model can be found in Supplementary Table S1. For rectal cancer patients, the corresponding hazard ratios were 0.820 (unadjusted, 95% CI 0.780, 0.862) and 0.978 (adjusted, 95% CI 0.929, 1.029), respectively. For colon cancer, this indicates a moderate, yet significant superiority concerning overall survival for treatment in a GCS-certified colorectal cancer center ($p < 0.001$), while no significant difference was seen for rectum cancer patients of all stages combined.

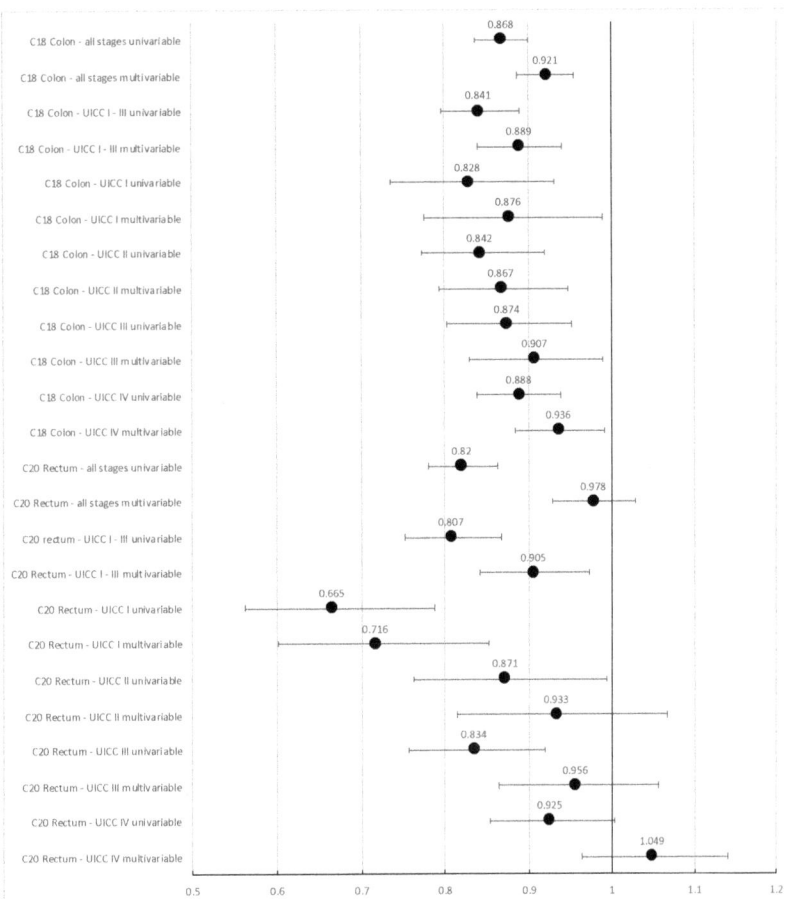

Figure 3. Unadjusted and adjusted (adjusted for age, sex, year of diagnosis, UICC stage—if not stratified for, grade, and lymphatic and venous invasion) hazard ratios with 95% CI for all-cause mortality following treatment in GCS-certified colorectal cancer centers compared to treatment in non-certified hospitals, stratified for location and UICC stage.

Excluding patients with unknown UICC stage, the adjusted hazard ratio for all-cause mortality changed to 0.908 (colon cancer, 95% CI 0.873, 0.945) and 0.961 (rectum cancer, 95% CI 0.909, 1.014) in favor of treatment in GCS-certified cancer centers (Supplementary Table S2). Analyzing UICC stage I to III patients only, the effect of treatment in a GCS-certified center increased (colon cancer: HR 0.889; 95% CI 0.840, 0.940) and became significant for rectum cancer, too (HR 0.905, 95% CI 0.841, 0.973, Figure 3).

For both tumor locations, the effect of center treatment was stronger at lower (colon cancer: UICC I: HR 0.876, UICC II: HR 0.867; rectum cancer: UICC I: HR 0.716, UICC II: HR 0.933, Figure 3) than in higher stages (colon cancer: UICC III: HR 0.907, UICC IV: HR 0.936; rectum cancer: UICC III: HR 0.956, UICC IV: HR 1.049, Figure 3).

3.4.2. Recurrence-Free Survival

For R0-resected UICC stage I–III patients, it was also possible to analyze recurrence-free survival. For colon cancer patients treated at GCS-certified centers, the 5-year recurrence-free survival rate was 61% compared to 55% for patients from non-certified hospitals ($p < 0.001$, Figure 4a). For rectal cancer patients, the 5-year recurrence-free survival rates were 62% and 54%, respectively ($p < 0.001$, Figure 4b).

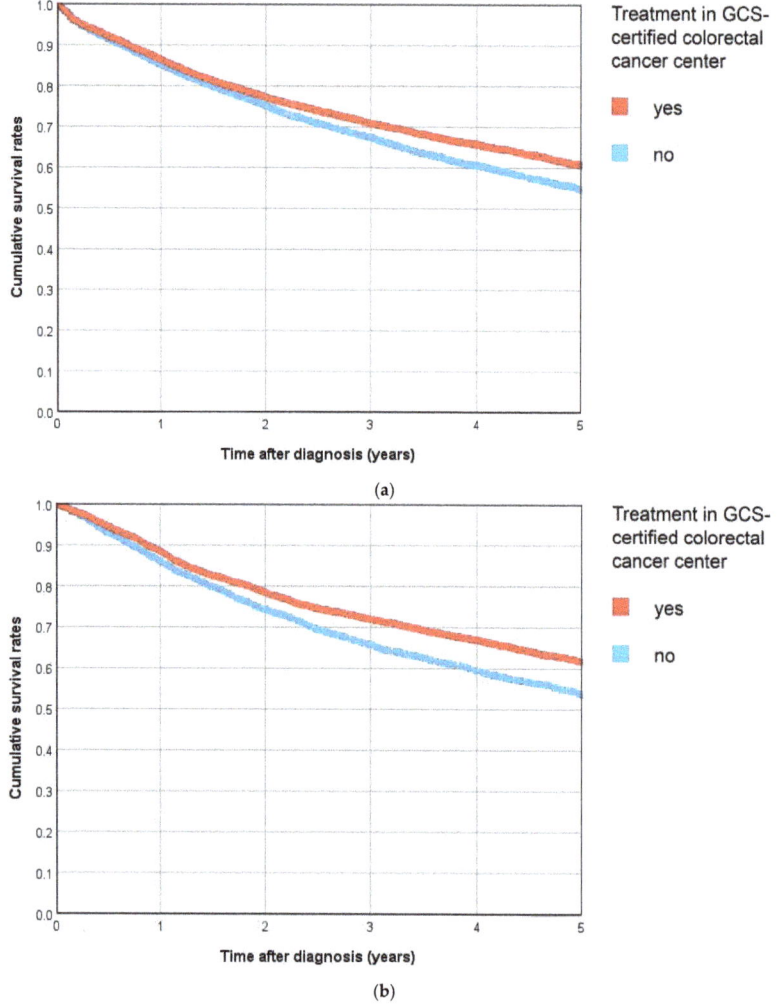

Figure 4. (**a**) C18 Colon, (**b**) C20 Rectum. Kaplan–Meier curves for recurrence-free survival in R0-resected patients with UICC stage I–III according to diagnosis and treatment status.

The adjusted hazard ratio for death or tumor recurrence was 0.878 (colon cancer, 95% CI 0.832, 0.927) and 0.856 (rectum cancer, 95% CI 0.796, 0.921, Table 3), indicating the significant superiority of center treatment.

Table 3. Adjusted hazard ratios with 95% CI for recurrence-free survival (CCR data, UICC stage I–III, R0 only) following treatment in GCS-certified colorectal cancer centers, ref.: treatment in non-certified hospitals.

	HR	Lower 95% CI	Upper 95% CI
C18 Colon all stages univariable	0.845	0.802	0.891
C18 Colon all stages multivariable *	0.878	0.832	0.927
C20 Rectum all stages univariable	0.786	0.732	0.844
C20 Rectum all stages multivariable *	0.856	0.796	0.921

* adjusted for age, sex, year of diagnosis, UICC stage, grade, and lymphatic and venous invasion.

4. Discussion

4.1. Summary

Since 2003, the German Cancer Society has certified hospitals specializing in the treatment of cancer and fulfilling certain quality standards. Currently, there exist 314 designated colorectal cancer centers in Germany [13], but evidence as to whether treatment at certified facilities is associated with better survival is scarce. With 47,440 included patients, the analyses presented in this publication represent the largest registry-based study on the topic.

After adjustment for important covariates like age, tumor stage, and the year of index treatment, the hazard of death was significantly lower by 7.9 percent in colon cancer patients treated in certified centers (HR 0.921), whereas only a small and non-significant hazard reduction was seen in rectum cancer patients (HR 0.978). If only patients in non-metastatic stages (UICC I–III) were analyzed, the hazard ratio for center treatment decreased to 0.889 in colon and 0.905 in rectum cancer patients, indicating a substantial and significant survival benefit for both tumor entities.

4.2. Effect of Certification

In oncology, great efforts are taken to achieve rather modest improvements of prognosis. In comparison to this, a broader implementation of certification programs and concentration of cancer treatment in certified institutions is associated with larger survival benefits and lower costs for the health care system. Slightly longer traveling distances to the next certified colorectal cancer center (in over 50% of the cases, 20 min or less [24]) seem a rather modest price for an overall survival benefit of up to 28 percent, depending on the UICC stage. Moreover, previous studies show that treatment at GCS-certified colorectal cancer centers is associated with significantly lower treatment costs, even if additional expenses induced by certification requirements are taken into account [25].

The findings presented in this paper are in concordance with other analyses of the WiZen study based on statutory health insurance data [22]. For colon cancer, the adjusted hazard ratio for treatment in certified centers was identical, underlining the high external validity of the presented results. Moreover, the results of the present study support the findings of earlier studies on the topic, which were limited by smaller sample sizes and locally restricted study cohorts. Using clinical cancer registry data from a southern German region with 1.1 million inhabitants from 2004 to 2013, Völkel et al. [16] observed a significant overall survival benefit (HR 0.81) for center treatment. Trautmann et al. analyzed statutory health insurance data from 2005 to 2015 from Saxony, Germany, and also reported a significant survival benefit for patients treated in certified hospitals (OAS: HR 0.90, [26]). Similar results can be found in the international literature, although a comparison to differently structured health care systems and specific interventions within these systems is always difficult. In 2008, Paulson et al. [27] retrospectively analyzed more than 40,000 patients from the US having received surgery for colon and rectum carcinoma. The postoperative mortality in National Cancer Institute (NCI)-designated centers was lower (3.2% vs. 6.7%); additionally, they observed a significant long-term survival benefit for colon (HR 0.84) and rectum cancer patients (HR 0.85), which is comparable to the results presented in this study. In 2021, Okawa et al. [28] published a registry-based observational study about the health care system in Japan, where accredited, high-capacity, highly experienced cancer care hospitals also exist; the findings showed that treatment in these intuitions is associated with higher adjusted all-site 3-year survival rates (86.6%) compared to non-designated hospitals (78.8%).

The fact that the survival benefits observed in the present study were particularly high in UICC stage I–III patients is hardly surprising; for these patients, clear guideline recommendations and quality standards for surgery and (neo-)adjuvant procedures [4] are provided and implemented. Correspondingly, GCS certification strongly focuses on guideline-adherent therapy pathways and is more than a simple volume-based centralization process. Concerning the predominantly palliative UICC stage IV patients, it has to be acknowledged that prolongation of survival is not always the primary treatment aim [29,30]. Future studies on this topic for this specific patient group should implement additional outcome variables reflecting aspects like quality of life and the patients' perspective.

4.3. Strengths and Limitations

For ethical and practical reasons, it is impossible to conduct a randomized controlled trial to analyze the effectiveness of center-based cancer treatment [31–33]. Patients are free to present to their hospital of choice. Usually, their decision incorporates factors like regional accessibility, patient mobility, referral by other health professionals, advice from other patients, and many more [34]. Subjecting cancer patients to a random allocation process would impair their right of self-determination. Consequently, an observational study design with independent standardized controlled prospective data collection represents the most adequate methodology. Using population-based clinical cancer registry data of four large German cancer registries covering different regions, the results of this study are highly reliable and representative. Every patient with colorectal cancer registered within the catchment area of these cancer registries is part of the truly population-based study collective. No patient was excluded due to unfavorable characteristics like high age or advanced tumor stages [35,36].

With observational data and non-randomized group allocation, adjustment for potential confounders is crucial. Making use of a comprehensive dataset, it was possible to include a broad range of demographic and disease-specific items in the multivariable regression analyses. For certain variables like, e.g., tumor stage, information was partially missing—this was more often the case in patients from non-certified hospitals, which might be a consequence of lower documentation standards in these hospitals. However, sensitivity analyses with the inclusion and exclusion of patients with incomplete information were performed and the results remained stable.

The strength of the cancer registry-based part of the WiZen analyses presented in our manuscript consists of the detailed information about tumor characteristics. Nevertheless, it would have been desirable to include additional confounders like teaching status or hospital volume. However, for some of the cases, no documentation about the specific institution a case was treated in was available. For these cases, certification status was retrieved from a generic variable "center treatment yes/no". Notwithstanding this, it was possible to adjust for these factors in separate analyses of the WiZen project, which were based on statutory health insurance data and that will be published elsewhere. In these analyses, one can see that hospital size and teaching status are seen more often among certified centers; these factors did indeed have a significant influence on survival, but even after adjustment for these factors, certification as colorectal cancer center was associated with a substantial and significant survival benefit.

Also, there was no information available on whether a resection was performed as an emergency procedure. This might be a limitation of our analyses, since an earlier study on the topic from Germany using comprehensive hospital billing data [37] found lower rates of emergency procedures in hospitals with larger caseloads. Given the association of larger hospital size and certification status, this finding might be partly transferable to our study setting. However, the share of emergency procedures in the earlier study ranged between 30.7% for very low-volume and 28.1% for very high-volume hospitals, indicating a rather moderate difference. Moreover, it is known that reasons for surgery performed as emergency procedure are, e.g., more advanced tumor stages, lymphatic invasion, venous invasion, and higher age [38]. By adjusting for all of these factors, we are confident that we at least partially adjusted for the adverse effect of emergency procedures.

Therapy modalities like, e.g., the TME technique or the application of postoperative chemo protocols were deliberately excluded in the multivariable regression models, since the realization of guideline-adherent therapy might be a characteristic of certified centers and, thus, a reason for better survival after treatment at these institutions. However, delving deeper into the differences between therapy pathways of center- and non-center patients would definitely be an interesting topic for future research. To achieve reliable and valid results, the WiZen study followed a conservative approach, which might have led to an underestimation of the center effect. Patients treated in a hospital that forms part of an association with a GCS-certified cancer center were regarded as center patients, although their treatment might still not have met center standards. Furthermore, patients treated in hospitals that later became certified were allocated to the group treated in non-certified hospitals.

5. Conclusions

The results of the WiZen study contribute to a continuously growing international evidence base pointing towards the additional value of cancer treatment in designated centers that are defined not only by their caseload, but also by other quality indicators like guideline adherence. It represents the largest study to date on the efficacy of certification programs in the German health care system. The presented results show that treatment at certified colorectal cancer centers is associated with significant and substantial long-term benefits concerning overall and recurrence-free survival. In early-stage colon cancer, treatment at a certified institution contributes to lowering the overall mortality risk by more than 25%. This important information should be widely distributed to patients, referring outpatient physicians, and decision makers.

Supplementary Materials: The following supporting information can be downloaded at: https://www.mdpi.com/article/10.3390/cancers15184568/s1: Table S1. Full results of multivariable Cox regression for all-cause mortality according to diagnosis. Table S2. Sensitivity analyses: Unadjusted and adjusted* hazard ratios with 95% CI for all-cause mortality following treatment in GCS-certified colorectal cancer centers compared to treatment in non-certified hospitals.

Author Contributions: Conceptualization: O.S., C.R., A.F., S.B., B.M.R., P.P., M.D., J.S. and M.K.-S.; data curation: M.G. and K.K.-v.T.; formal analysis: V.V., M.G. and J.H.; funding acquisition: J.S. and M.K.-S.; investigation: V.V., M.G., K.K.-v.T., O.S., V.B., C.B. and M.R.; methodology: M.G., K.K.-v.T. and O.S.; project administration: O.S., J.S. and M.K.-S.; resources: O.S. and M.K.-S.; software: M.G. and K.K.-v.T.; supervision: J.S. and M.K.-S.; validation: V.V., M.G., K.K.-v.T., O.S., V.B., C.B., M.R., C.R., A.F., S.B., B.M.R., P.P., M.D., C.G., J.H., J.S. and M.K.-S.; visualization: V.V. and M.G.; writing—original draft: V.V. and M.G., Writing—review and editing: K.K.-v.T., O.S., V.B., C.B., M.R., C.R., A.F., S.B., B.M.R., P.P., M.D., C.G., J.H., J.S. and M.K.-S. All authors have read and agreed to the published version of the manuscript.

Funding: This research was funded by the German Federal Joint Committee as part of the Innovationsfonds (funding number 01VSF17020).

Institutional Review Board Statement: The WiZen study was approved by the ethics committee of the TU Dresden (date of approval: 14 Februray 2019; approval number: EK95022019, IRB 00001473, OHRP IORG0001076). Data processing and analyses were conducted in line with the Declaration of Helsinki and the General Data Protection Regulation of the European Union.

Informed Consent Statement: Since the analysis relies on pseudonymized, secondary data, individual consent to participate has not been required as confirmed by the ethics committee of the TU Dresden (reference number: EK95022019).

Data Availability Statement: The authors confirm that the data utilized in this study cannot be made available in the manuscript, the supplemental files, or in a public repository due to German data protection laws ('Bundesdatenschutzgesetz', BDSG).

Acknowledgments: The authors thank the clinical cancer registries Tumorzentrum Regensburg (TZR), Klinisches Krebsregister Dresden (KKRD), Klinisches Krebsregister Erfurt (KKRE), and Klinisches Krebsregister für Brandenburg und Berlin (KKRBB) for providing the data to conduct the presented analyses.

Conflicts of Interest: A.F., B.M.R., C.R., J.S., M.D., O.S., P.P. and S.B. work at institutions with certified cancer centers; M.R., C.B., V.B. and V.V. worked at institutions with certified cancer centers in the past. Unrelated to this study, J.S. reports institutional grants for investigator-initiated research from the German GBA, the BMG, BMBF, EU, Federal State of Saxony, Novartis, Sanofi, ALK, and Pfizer. He also participated in advisory board meetings as a paid consultant for Sanofi, Lilly, and ALK. J.S. serves the German Ministry of Health as a member of the Sachverständigenrat Gesundheit und Pflege. O.S. is a member of the certification commission "Skin Cancer Centers" of the German Cancer Society and a member of the expert panel in the project "Development of Criteria for the Evaluation of Certificates and Quality Seals in Accordance with Section 137a (3) Sentence 2 Number 7 SGB V" for the Institute for Quality Assurance and Transparency in Health Care (IQTIG). Unrelated to this study, O.S. worked as a paid consultant for Novartis.

References

1. World Health Organization. *World Cancer Report: Cancer Research for Cancer Prevention*; World Cancer Reports; Wild, C.P., Weiderpass, E., Stewart, B.W., Eds.; World Health Organization: Geneva, Switzerland, 2020.
2. Siegel, R.L.; Miller, K.D.; Goding Sauer, A.; Fedewa, S.A.; Butterly, L.F.; Anderson, J.C.; Cercek, A.; Smith, R.A.; Jemal, A. Colorectal cancer statistics, 2020. *CA Cancer J. Clin.* **2020**, *70*, 145–164. [CrossRef]
3. *Krebs in Deutschland für 2017/2018*, 13th ed.; Robert Koch-Institut; Gesellschaft der Epidemiologischen Krebsregister in Deutschland e.V. (Eds.) Zentrum für Krebsregisterdaten: Berlin, Germany, 2021; ISBN 978-3-89606-309-0. [CrossRef]
4. Leitlinienprogramm Onkologie (Deutsche Krebsgesellschaft, Deutsche Krebshilfe, AWMF): S3-Leitlinie Kolorektales Karzinom, Langversion 2.1, 2019, AWMF Registrierungsnummer: 021/007OL. Available online: https://www.leitlinienprogramm-onkologie.de/leitlinien/kolorektales-karzinom/ (accessed on 21 June 2023).
5. Griesshammer, E.; Adam, H.; Sibert, N.T.; Wesselmann, S. Implementing quality metrics in European Cancer Centers (ECCs). *World J. Urol.* **2021**, *39*, 49–56. [CrossRef]
6. Wind, A.; Rajan, A.; van Harten, W.H. Quality assessments for cancer centers in the European Union. *BMC Health Serv. Res.* **2016**, *16*, 474. [CrossRef]
7. Available online: https://www.cancer.gov/research/infrastructure/cancer-centers (accessed on 15 January 2023).
8. Kato, M. Designated cancer hospitals and cancer control in Japan. *J. Natl. Inst. Public Health* **2012**, *61*, 549–555.
9. Bundesministerium für Gesundheit. Nationaler Krebsplan. Available online: https://www.bundesgesundheitsministerium.de/themen/praevention/nationaler-krebsplan.html (accessed on 15 January 2023).
10. Brucker, S.Y.; Schumacher, C.; Sohn, C.; Rezai, M.; Bamberg, M.; Wallwiener, D. Benchmarking the quality of breast cancer care in a nationwide voluntary system: The first five-year results (2003–2007) from Germany as a proof of concept. *BMC Cancer* **2008**, *8*, 358. [CrossRef]
11. Kowalski, C.; Graeven, U.; von Kalle, C.; Lang, H.; Beckmann, M.W.; Blohmer, J.-U.; Burchardt, M.; Ehrenfeld, M.; Fichtner, J.; Grabbe, S.; et al. Shifting cancer care towards Multidisciplinarity: The cancer center certification program of the German cancer society. *BMC Cancer* **2017**, *17*, 850. [CrossRef]
12. GCS-Certification, Center Search. Available online: https://www.krebsgesellschaft.de/deutsche-krebsgesellschaft/zertifizierung/zentrumssuche.html (accessed on 15 January 2023).
13. oncoMAP. Available online: https://www.oncomap.de/centers?selectedOrgans=[Darm]&showMap=1 (accessed on 5 July 2023).
14. GCS-Certification Documents. Available online: https://www.krebsgesellschaft.de/zertdokumente.html (accessed on 5 July 2023). (In German).
15. GCS-Certification, Annual Reports. Available online: https://www.krebsgesellschaft.de/jahresberichte.html (accessed on 8 September 2023).
16. Völkel, V.; Draeger, T.; Gerken, M.; Fürst, A.; Klinkhammer-Schalke, M. Long-Term Survival of Patients with Colon and Rectum Carcinomas: Is There a Difference between Cancer Centers and Non-Certified Hospitals? *Gesundheitswesen* **2019**, *81*, 801–807. [CrossRef]
17. Birkmeyer, N.J.O.; Goodney, P.P.; Stukel, T.A.; Hillner, B.E.; Birkmeyer, J.D. Do cancer centers designated by the National Cancer Institute have better surgical outcomes? *Cancer* **2005**, *103*, 435–441. [CrossRef]
18. Mehta, R.; Ejaz, A.; Hyer, J.M.; Tsilimigras, D.I.; White, S.; Merath, K.; Sahara, K.; Bagante, F.; Paredes, A.Z.; Cloyd, J.M.; et al. The Impact of Dedicated Cancer Centers on Outcomes among Medicare Beneficiaries Undergoing Liver and Pancreatic Cancer Surgery. *Ann. Surg. Oncol.* **2019**, *26*, 4083–4090. [CrossRef]

19. Butea-Bocu, M.C.; Müller, G.; Pucheril, D.; Kröger, E.; Otto, U. Is there a clinical benefit from prostate cancer center certification? An evaluation of functional and oncologic outcomes from 22,649 radical prostatectomy patients. *World J. Urol.* **2021**, *39*, 5–10. [CrossRef]
20. Richter, M.; Sonnow, L.; Mehdizadeh-Shrifi, A.; Richter, A.; Koch, R.; Zipprich, A. German oncology certification system for colorectal cancer—Relative survival rates of a single certified centre vs. national and international registry data. *Innov. Surg. Sci.* **2021**, *6*, 67–73. [CrossRef] [PubMed]
21. Kranz, J.; Grundmann, R.; Steffens, J. Does structural and process quality of certified prostate cancer centers result in better medical care? *Urol. A* **2021**, *60*, 59–66. [CrossRef]
22. Available online: https://innovationsfonds.g-ba.de/downloads/beschluss-dokumente/268/2022-10-17_WiZen_Ergebnisbericht.pdf (accessed on 28 July 2023).
23. Arbeitsgruppe Erhebung und Nutzung von Sekundärdaten der Deutschen Gesellschaft fur Sozialmedizin und Prävention. Arbeitsgruppe Epidemiologische Methoden der Deutschen Gesellschaft für Epidemiologie. Deutsche Gesellschaft für Medizinische Informatik Biometrie und Epidemiologie, Deutsche Gesellschaft für Sozialmedizin und Prävention. Good practice of secondary data analysis, first revision. *Gesundheitswesen* **2008**, *70*, 54–60.
24. Fünfte Stellungnahme der Regierungskommission für eine Moderne und bedarfsgerechte Krankenhausversorgung: Verbesserung von Qualität und Sicherheit der Gesundheitsversorgung Potenzialanalyse Anhand exemplarischer Erkrankungen. Available online: https://www.bundesgesundheitsministerium.de/fileadmin/Dateien/3_Downloads/K/Krankenhausreform/5_Stellungnahme_Potenzialanalyse_bf_Version_1.1.pdf (accessed on 11 August 2023).
25. Cheng, C.; Datzmann, T.; Hernandez, D.; Schmitt, J.; Schlander, M. Do certified cancer centers provide more cost-effective care? A health economic analysis of colon cancer care in Germany using administrative data. *Int. J. Cancer* **2021**, *149*, 1744–1754. [CrossRef]
26. Trautmann, F.; Reißfelder, C.; Pecqueux, M.; Weitz, J.; Schmitt, J. Evidence-based quality standards improve prognosis in colon cancer care. *Eur. J. Surg. Oncol.* **2018**, *44*, 1324–1330. [CrossRef]
27. Paulson, E.C.; Mitra, N.; Sonnad, S.; Armstrong, K.; Wirtalla, C.; Kelz, R.R.; Mahmoud, N.N. National Cancer Institute designation predicts improved outcomes in colorectal cancer surgery. *Ann. Surg.* **2008**, *248*, 675–686. [CrossRef]
28. Okawa, S.; Tabuchi, T.; Nakata, K.; Morishima, T.; Koyama, S.; Odani, S.; Miyashiro, I. Three-year survival from diagnosis in surgically treated patients in designated and nondesignated cancer care hospitals in Japan. *Cancer Sci.* **2021**, *112*, 2513–2521. [CrossRef]
29. Ghandourh, W.A. Palliative care in cancer: Managing patients' expectations. *J. Med. Radiat. Sci.* **2016**, *63*, 242–257. [CrossRef]
30. Bausewein, C.; Simon, S.T.; Pralong, A.; Radbruch, L.; Nauck, F.; Voltz, R. Palliative Care of Adult Patients with Cancer. *Dtsch. Arztebl. Int.* **2015**, *112*, 863–870. [CrossRef]
31. Klinkhammer-Schalke, M.; Kaiser, T.; Apfelbacher, C.; Benz, S.; Dreinhöfer, K.E.; Geraedts, M.; Hauptmann, M.; Hoffmann, F.; Hoffmann, W.; Koller, M.; et al. Manual for Methods and Use of Routine Practice Data for Knowledge Generation. *Gesundheitswesen* **2020**, *82*, 716–722. [CrossRef]
32. Stausberg, J.; Maier, B.; Bestehorn, K.; Gothe, H.; Groene, O.; Jacke, C.; Jänicke, M.; Kostuj, T.; Mathes, T.; Niemeyer, A.; et al. Memorandum Registry for Health Services Research: Update 2019. *Gesundheitswesen* **2020**, *82*, e39–e66. [CrossRef]
33. Hoffmann, F.; Kaiser, T.; Apfelbacher, C.; Benz, S.; Bierbaum, T.; Dreinhöfer, K.; Hauptmann, M.; Heidecke, C.-D.; Koller, M.; Kostuj, T.; et al. Routine Practice Data for Evaluating Intervention Effects: Part 2 of the Manual. *Gesundheitswesen* **2021**, *83*, 470–480. [CrossRef] [PubMed]
34. Lipitz Snyderman, A.N.; Fortier, E.; Li, D.G.; Chimonas, S. What do patients want to know when selecting a hospital for cancer care? *JCO* **2018**, *36*, e18810. [CrossRef]
35. Habibzadeh, F. Disparity in the selection of patients in clinical trials. *Lancet* **2022**, *399*, 1048. [CrossRef] [PubMed]
36. Kennedy-Martin, T.; Curtis, S.; Faries, D.; Robinson, S.; Johnston, J. A literature review on the representativeness of randomized controlled trial samples and implications for the external validity of trial results. *Trials* **2015**, *16*, 495. [CrossRef]
37. Diers, J.; Wagner, J.; Baum, P.; Lichthardt, S.; Kastner, C.; Matthes, N.; Löb, S.; Matthes, H.; Germer, C.-T.; Wiegering, A. Nationwide in-hospital mortality following colonic cancer resection according to hospital volume in Germany. *BJS Open* **2019**, *3*, 672–677. [CrossRef]
38. Golder, A.M.; McMillan, D.C.; Horgan, P.G.; Roxburgh, C.S.D. Determinants of emergency presentation in patients with colorectal cancer: A systematic review and meta-analysis. *Sci. Rep.* **2022**, *12*, 4366. [CrossRef]

Disclaimer/Publisher's Note: The statements, opinions and data contained in all publications are solely those of the individual author(s) and contributor(s) and not of MDPI and/or the editor(s). MDPI and/or the editor(s) disclaim responsibility for any injury to people or property resulting from any ideas, methods, instructions or products referred to in the content.

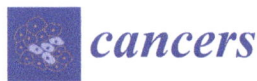

Article

Influence of Certification Program on Treatment Quality and Survival for Rectal Cancer Patients in Germany: Results of 13 Certified Centers in Collaboration with AN Institute

Mihailo Andric, Jessica Stockheim, Mirhasan Rahimli, Sara Al-Madhi, Sara Acciuffi, Maximilian Dölling, Roland Siegfried Croner and Aristotelis Perrakis *

Department of General, Visceral, Vascular and Transplant Surgery, University Hospital Magdeburg, Leipziger Str. 44, 39120 Magdeburg, Germany; mihailo.andric@med.ovgu.de (M.A.); jessica.stockheim@med.ovgu.de (J.S.); mirhasan.rahimli@med.ovgu.de (M.R.); sara.al-madhi@med.ovgu.de (S.A.-M.); sara.acciuffi@med.ovgu.de (S.A.); maximilian.doelling@med.ovgu.de (M.D.); roland.croner@med.ovgu.de (R.S.C.)
* Correspondence: aristotelis.perrakis@med.ovgu.de

Simple Summary: In the past, the German Cancer Society has implemented a certification program for colorectal cancer centers with the aims of standardizing oncological treatment, endorsing a multidisciplinary approach, and improving the outcomes. However, some critical views have argued that fulfilling the certification requirements alone would not necessarily enhance the treatment quality for colorectal cancer patients. In the present study, our objective was to investigate the treatment outcomes for patients with rectal cancer in hospitals of different medical care levels, before and after the certification process. The results of the present study indicate an improvement in terms of the treatment quality and outcomes after the official certification process. Further prospective clinical trials are necessary to investigate the influence of certification on the treatment of patients suffering from colorectal cancer.

Citation: Andric, M.; Stockheim, J.; Rahimli, M.; Al-Madhi, S.; Acciuffi, S.; Dölling, M.; Croner, R.S.; Perrakis, A. Influence of Certification Program on Treatment Quality and Survival for Rectal Cancer Patients in Germany: Results of 13 Certified Centers in Collaboration with AN Institute. *Cancers* **2024**, *16*, 1496. https://doi.org/10.3390/cancers16081496

Academic Editor: Ernest Ramsay Camp

Received: 15 February 2024
Revised: 18 March 2024
Accepted: 23 March 2024
Published: 13 April 2024

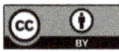

Copyright: © 2024 by the authors. Licensee MDPI, Basel, Switzerland. This article is an open access article distributed under the terms and conditions of the Creative Commons Attribution (CC BY) license (https://creativecommons.org/licenses/by/4.0/).

Abstract: Introduction: The certification of oncological units as colorectal cancer centers (CrCCs) has been proposed to standardize oncological treatment and improve the outcomes for patients with colorectal cancer (CRC). The proportion of patients with CRC in Germany that are treated by a certified center is around 53%. Lately, the effect of certification on the treatment outcomes has been critically discussed. Aim: Our aim was to investigate the treatment outcomes in patients with rectal carcinoma at certified CrCCs, in German hospitals of different medical care levels. Methods: We performed a retrospective analysis of a prospective, multicentric database (AN Institute) of adult patients who underwent surgery for rectal carcinoma between 2002 and 2016. We included 563 patients from 13 hospitals of different medical care levels (basic, priority, and maximal care) over periods of 5 years before and after certification. Results: The certified CrCCs showed a significant increase in the use of laparoscopic approach for rectal cancer surgery (5% vs. 55%, $p < 0.001$). However, we observed a significantly prolonged mean duration of surgery in certified CrCCs (161 Min. vs. 192 Min., $p < 0.001$). The overall morbidity did not improve (32% vs. 38%, $p = 0.174$), but the appearance of postoperative stool fistulas decreased significantly in certified CrCCs (2% vs. 0%, $p = 0.036$). Concerning the overall in-hospital mortality, we registered a positive trend in certified centers during the five-year period after the certification (5% vs. 3%, $p = 0.190$). The length of preoperative hospitalization (preop. LOS) was shortened significantly (4.71 vs. 4.13 days, $p < 0.001$), while the overall length of in-hospital stays was also shorter in certified CrCCs (20.32 vs. 19.54 days, $p = 0.065$). We registered a clear advantage in detailed, high-quality histopathological examinations regarding the N, L, V, and M.E.R.C.U.R.Y. statuses. In the performed subgroup analysis, a significantly longer overall survival after certification was registered for maximal medical care units ($p = 0.029$) and in patients with UICC stage IV disease ($p = 0.041$). In patients with UICC stage III disease, we registered a slightly non-significant improvement in the disease-free survival (UICC III: $p = 0.050$). Conclusions: The results of the present study indicate an improvement in terms of the treatment quality and outcomes in certified CrCCs, which is enforced by certification-specific aspects such as a more differentiated surgical approach, a lower rate of certain postoperative complications, and a multidisciplinary approach. Further prospective clinical trials are necessary to investigate the influence of certification in the treatment of CRC patients.

Keywords: rectal cancer; certification; colorectal cancer center; outcome

1. Introduction

With over 60,000 new cases and over 25,000 deaths annually, colorectal cancer is still one of the most common malignant diseases in Germany [1]. Up to 38% of these patients suffer from cancer of the rectum [1–4]. Over the last 20 years, rectal cancer treatment has evolved, and nowadays, it involves a multidisciplinary approach that includes standardized diagnostics, neoadjuvant and adjuvant therapy (if these are indicated), and interventional and supportive treatment modalities. In this setting, and in cases of a curative intent, surgery plays the most important role [5–11]. In order to standardize oncological treatment and improve the outcomes in colorectal cancer (CRC) patients, the centralization of treatment in specialized high-volume centers and the certification of oncological units as colorectal cancer centers (CrCCs) have been proposed in Germany [12].

This is a part of the certification program of the German Cancer Society, which was developed in Germany and has expanded to other member states of the European Union. The certification program for breast cancer was introduced in 2003 and the program for colorectal cancer was introduced in 2006, later being applied to centers for malignancies of diverse organ systems. The goal was to offer a treatment that is based on high quality standards at every stage of the disease [11]. Certified cancer centers form the base of this approach. The centers are required to annually demonstrate their outcomes and are obliged to meet the technical and medical requirements for the treatment of a specific tumor entity [11]. Medical guidelines (in the case of CrCCs, the "S3 guidelines for the treatment of colorectal cancer") represent the foundation for defining these quality standards [6].

However, it is not obligatory for oncological units to undergo the certification program in order to be allowed to treat specific malignances. In 2017, only 47.15% of the overall patients with colorectal cancer in Germany were treated in a CrCC, and in 2018, 53% were treated in a certified colorectal cancer center [1,12,13].

Benz et al. described an increasing proportion of rectal cancers treated in certified centers, rising from 43% to 57% during the period from 2010 to 2018 [13]. Hence, 43% of the overall rectal cancer cases in Germany are being treated in uncertified centers, with a case load of <20 operative cases per year [13].

Several recent studies have demonstrated some advantages when treatments take place in certified centers, such as a better overall survival and a lower morbidity, especially for advanced colorectal cancer patients [3,5,14–16]. On the other hand, since the introduction of the German certification program, critical views have argued that fulfilling the certification requirements alone would not necessarily enhance the treatment quality for colorectal cancer [17]. The achieved effects of centralization for CRC treatments have been described as insufficient, and a renewal of national strategies with a focus on the implementation of centralization and high-quality CrCCs was proposed [2].

Therefore, we aimed to investigate the influence of colorectal cancer center (CrCC) certification on the treatment outcomes for rectal carcinoma patients according to the database of the AN Institute of the Otto von Guericke University of Magdeburg. We evaluated data from 13 hospitals of different medical care levels on rectal cancer treatments in Germany for the period of 2002–2016.

2. Methods

2.1. Study Design

A comparative, retrospective study was conducted using data from a prospectively acquired, multicenter database of the AN Institute of the Otto von Guericke University in

Magdeburg, Germany. All of the data were acquired from the 13 associated hospitals based on standardized documentation forms, which were drafted by the scientific advisory board of the AN Institute. Since 2010 and after the implementation of the certification process by the German Cancer Society, the scientific advisory board of the AN Institute revised all of the documentation for tumor entities according to the high standards defined by the German Cancer Society.

A total of 563 patients from 13 hospitals that received treatment from five years before until five years after the official certification of the center as a CrCC (ten-year period for each observed center) were examined. The patients treated during the five-year period before the certification of a particular center were included in the group defined as "−5y" and the patients treated during the five-year period after the certification were included in the group defined as "+5y" (Figure 1). Overall, we included patients that were surgically treated during the period of 2002–2016, meaning that the certifications of all of the included centers took place between the years 2007 and 2011.

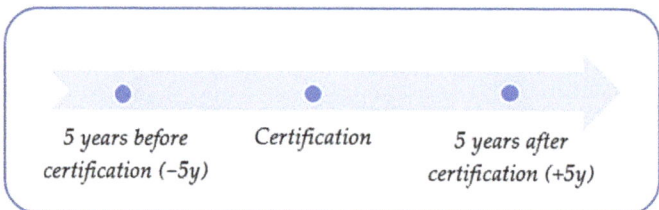

Figure 1. Presentation of time-related collective building according to the moment of the hospital's certification as a colorectal cancer center.

We performed a comparative analysis of the patient characteristics, perioperative parameters, postoperative outcomes (including morbidity and mortality), and survival data between the selected collectives from the period before and the period after the date of official certification as a colorectal cancer center (−5y vs. +5y). A subgroup analysis of survival according to the hospital care level and the UICC stage was also performed.

2.2. Inclusion Criteria

In the present study, we included adult patients (>18 years old) who underwent surgical treatment for rectal carcinoma. The patients treated during the period from 2002 to 2016 were included in the study (n = 563).

2.3. Exclusion Criteria

Patients <18 years old and patients who did not receive surgery for rectal carcinoma were excluded from the study.

2.4. Statistical Analysis

For the statistical analyses, we used SPSS 26, SPSS Inc., IBM, Armonk, New York, NY, USA.

For the data presentation, we used the means with the standard deviation or the number of cases with percentages in accordance with the type of data. The analysis and visualization of survival data were performed using a Kaplan–Meier curve. p-values of <0.05 were considered statistically significant.

3. Results

3.1. Patient Characteristics

All of the data related to demographic characteristics are presented in Table 1.

Table 1. Presentation of patient characteristics for collectives treated five years before and five years after certification.

	CrCC Certification				
	−5y		+5y		p
Parameter	N (Mean)	% (SD)	N (Mean)	% (SD)	
Number of patients	267	47.42%	296	52.58%	
Sex					
Female	109	41%	122	41%	0.925
Male	158	59%	174	59%	
Age	68	10.51	68	12.67	0.712
BMI	26	4.36	27	4.83	0.467
ASA					
ASA I	24	9%	27	9%	
ASA II	153	57%	145	49%	0.234
ASA III	87	33%	120	41%	
ASA IV	3	1%	3	1%	

A total of 563 patients were included in the study, with 267 of the patients treated during the five-year period before certification (−5y) and 296 of the patients treated after certification (+5y).

There was no significant difference between the −5y and +5y groups in the proportion of patients belonging to each sex, the mean age of the patients, the mean BMI of the patients, or the distribution of cases according to the American Society of Anesthesiologists (ASA) score.

3.2. Perioperative Parameters

All of the data related to the perioperative parameters are presented in Table 2.

Table 2. Presentation of perioperative parameters for collectives five years before and after certification.

	CrCC Certification				
	−5y		+5y		p
Parameter	N (Mean)	% (SD)	N (Mean)	% (SD)	
Number of patients	267	47.42%	296	52.57%	
Surgical approach					
Laparotomy	226	86%	114	39%	<0.001
Laparoscopy	14	5%	160	55%	<0.001
Conversion	2	6%	16	9%	0.504
Trans-anal	20	8%	3	1%	<0.001
Surgery type					
ARR	47	18%	47	17%	0.753
LARR	113	43%	112	40%	0.505
APE	43	16%	62	22%	0.084
Hartmann	3	1%	23	8%	<0.001
Anastomosis type					
Stapler	167	63%	178	61%	0.572
Intraoperative complications	14	5%	15	5,17%	0.93
Duration of surgery (Min.)	161	74.21	192	79.33	<0.001

The frequency of a minimally invasive approach (laparoscopy) for rectal surgery increased significantly after CrCC certification in comparison to the period before certification (5% vs. 55%, $p < 0.001$), without a significant increase in the conversion rate. Furthermore, the frequency of a trans-anal approach for the local excision of rectal carcinoma significantly decreased after the certification for the compared periods (8% vs. 1%, $p < 0.001$).

Regarding the type of performed surgery for rectal carcinoma, the certification process did not result in any significant changes in the proportion of anterior rectal resections (ARRs), low anterior rectal resections (LARRs), or abdominoperineal extirpations (APEs) performed between the examined periods.

On the other hand, discontinuous resections according to Hartmann increased significantly during the five years after certification (+5y) in comparison to the period before certification (−5y) (1% vs. 7%, $p < 0.001$).

The mean duration of surgery for rectal cancer showed a significant increase during the five-year period after certification (161 Min. vs. 192 Min., $p < 0.001$).

3.3. Postoperative Parameters

According to the performed analysis, the mean preoperative in-hospital stay length (preop. LOS) prior to a rectal surgery, which was mainly for completing the diagnostics, decreased significantly after certification (4.71 days vs. 4.13 days, $p < 0.001$).

On the other hand, the postoperative in-hospital stay duration (postop. LOS) shortened non-significantly after certification (16.65 days vs. 15.15 days, $p = 0.151$).

The overall length of stay (oLOS) also did not significantly change after CrCC certification (20.32 days vs. 19.54 days, $p = 0.065$), although a tendential shortening of the oLOS was observed.

Regarding the type of case dismissal following a rectal surgery (discharge, transfer to other units (such as rehab, neurology, nephrology, etc.), or death), we observed a tendency in the five-year period after certification towards more successful patient discharges (89% vs. 94%) and fewer transfers to other units (6% vs. 3%) and postoperative death cases (5% vs. 3%). Still, there was no statistical significance for this observation ($p = 0.060$).

The overall proportion of postoperative complications did not significantly change after the CrCC certification for the examined periods (23% vs. 27%, $p = 0.284$). However, the analysis of specific surgical complications showed an increase in postoperative intestinal atonia (for over 3 days) during the five-year period after certification (2% vs. 6%, $p = 0.025$) and a decrease in the occurrence of postoperative stool fistulas (small or large bowel, other than the anastomotic region; 2% vs. 0%, $p = 0.036$). Other specific surgical complications underwent no significant change after the certification process, as displayed in Table 3.

Table 3. Presentation of postoperative parameters for collectives five years before and five years after certification.

	CrCC Certification				
	−5y		+5y		p
Parameter	N (Mean)	% (SD)	N (Mean)	% (SD)	
Number of patients	267	47.42%	296	52.57%	
LOS					
Preop. LOS (days)	4.71	4.55	4.13	17.95	<0.001
Postop. LOS (days)	16.65	14.88	15.15	10.40	0.151
Overall LOS (days)	20.32	16.11	19.54	20.97	0.065
Case dismissal					
Discharge	237	89%	278	94%	
Transfer	16	6%	8	3%	0.060
Death	14	5%	9	3%	
Morbidity	85	32%	112	38%	0.174
Non-surgical complications	52	20%	52	18%	0.552
Surgical complications	61	23%	78	27%	0.284
Bleeding	5	2%	2	1%	0.208
Sepsis	6	2%	7	2%	0.904

Table 3. Cont.

Parameter	CrCC Certification				p
	−5y		+5y		
	N (Mean)	% (SD)	N (Mean)	% (SD)	
Aseptic wound healing disorder	6	2%	9	3%	0.539
Wound infection	8	3%	10	3%	0.771
Abdominal wall dehiscence	5	2%	4	1%	0.639
Ileus	5	2%	2	1%	0.208
Atonia (>3 days)	5	2%	16	6%	0.025
Abscess	2	1%	4	1%	0.475
Stool fistula	4	2%	0	0%	0.036
Presacral infection	4	2%	9	3%	0.213
Peritonitis	3	1%	1	0%	0.275
Colostomy complication	1	0%	4	1%	0.211
Multiple organ failure	2	1%	3	1%	0.725
Anastomotic leakage	21	12%	21	11%	0.940

The rate of non-surgical complications did not change significantly after CrCC certification (20% vs. 18%, $p = 0.552$). An analysis of specific non-surgical complications, such as urinary infections, non-infectious pulmonal complications, pneumonia, cardiac complications, thrombosis, lung artery embolisms, renal failure, and multiple organ failure, showed no significant changes between the two collectives.

3.4. Histopathology

The histopathological findings for the examined periods are presented in Table 4.

The number of patients with histologically verified rectal cancer prior to surgery increased significantly during the five-year period after the certification of a hospital as a colorectal cancer center (84% vs. 93%, $p = 0.001$).

Concerning the distribution of pN stages for the patients in both collectives, we registered a significant difference when the +5y period was compared to the reference period (−5y) ($p = 0.001$). Additionally, the frequency of an unclear lymph node status after the histopathological findings (pNx) was significantly reduced after certification (8% vs. 2%).

We observed a significant difference in the L status before and after certification, with a decreasing number of cases not being histologically examined for their L status (22% vs. 7%, $p < 0.001$). This resulted in an increased proportion of patients with an L0 or L+ status.

A significant difference in the V status was documented between the five-year periods before and after certification, with a decreasing number of cases not being histologically examined for their V status (24% vs. 8%, $p < 0.001$) and a subsequent increase in the number of patients with a V0 or V+ status.

A patient distribution analysis according to the UICC showed a significant difference in the distribution for the five-year periods before and after certification, with an obvious increase in the number of cases with UICC stage II or UICC stage III, but a decreasing number of UICC IV cases ($p < 0.001$).

Concerning the quality of the surgical treatment in terms of the M.E.R.C.U.R.Y. status and the coning of the specimen [18–23], a comparative analysis could not be performed because the data related to these parameters were only available after the certification. These particular values are presented in Table 4.

Table 4. Presentation of histopathological findings for collectives five years before and five years after certification.

Parameter	CrCC Certification				p
	−5y		+5y		
	N (Mean)	% (SD)	N (Mean)	% (SD)	
Number of patients	267	47.42%	296	52.57%	
Histological verification before treatment	224	84%	272	93%	0.001
pT					
pT0	4	2%	7	3%	
pT1	36	15%	28	10%	
pT2	64	26%	83	30%	0.490
pT3	117	48%	133	48%	
pT4	22	9%	26	9%	
pN					
pN0	124	48%	170	59%	
pN1	45	17%	57	20%	
pN2	58	22%	50	17%	0.001
pNX	21	8%	5	2%	
Missing	12	5%	7	2%	
L					
L0	120	46%	168	58%	
L+	83	32%	105	36%	<0.001
Not examined	56	22%	19	7%	
V					
V0	148	57%	207	71%	
V+	47	18%	63	22%	<0.001
Not examined	63	24%	22	8%	
UICC					
I	4	2%	7	2%	
II	75	29%	82	28%	
III	43	16%	65	22%	<0.001
IV	67	25%	62	21%	
Missing	53	20%	58	20%	
M.E.R.C.U.R.Y.					
I	/	/	251	94%	/
II	/	/	10	4%	/
III	/	/	5	2%	/
Coning	/	/	6	2%	/

3.5. Follow-Up and Survival

3.5.1. Survival before and after Certification for the Entire Collective and According to the Medical Care Level

Regarding the overall survival, the comparison using Kaplan–Meier curves indicated a better outcome during the five-year period after the certification (+5y) when compared to the collective treated during the five years before certification (−5y), although without reaching significant levels ($p = 0.503$).

The subgroup analysis showed a trend towards a slightly higher overall survival during the five-year period after certification for the patients from hospitals with a basic or priority level of medical care, without significance ($p = 0.750$; $p = 0.638$). A significant improvement in the overall survival was observed for the patients with rectal cancer treated in the hospitals with a maximal level of medical care during the five-year period after certification compared to the reference period ($p = 0.029$) (Figure 2).

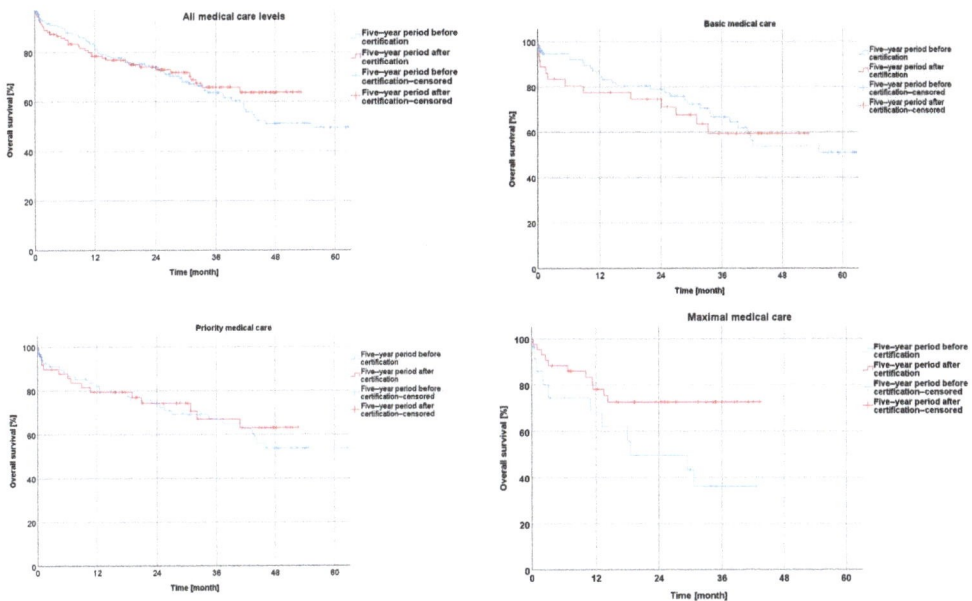

Figure 2. Presentation of overall survival five years before and five years after certification according to medical care level.

Concerning the disease-free survival during the five-year period after the certification, the Kaplan–Meier curves revealed a non-significantly better outcome after certification for the whole collective ($p = 0.163$) as well as for the subgroups from the centers with a basic, priority, or maximal care level ($p = 0.583$; $p = 0.845$; $p = 0.073$) (Figure 3).

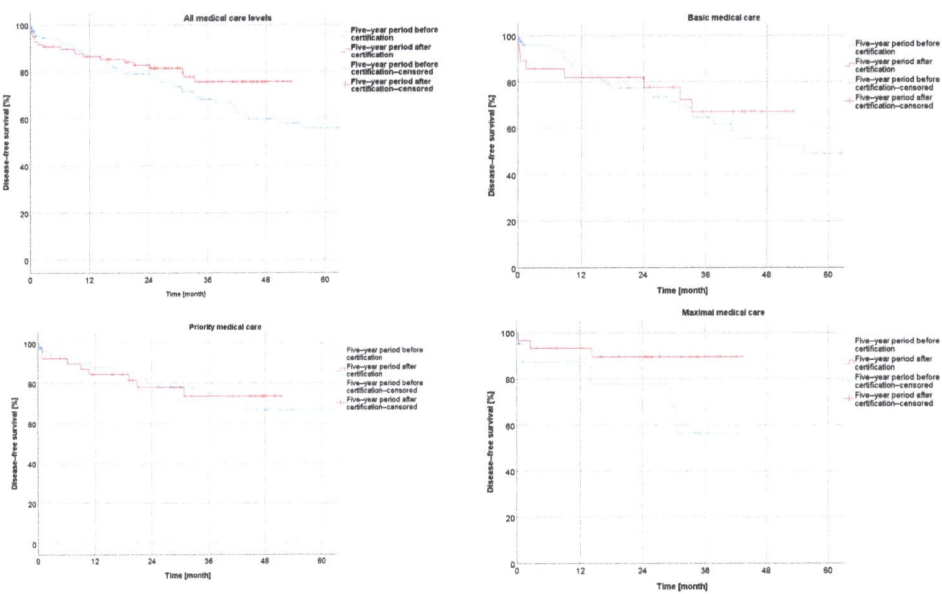

Figure 3. Presentation of disease-free survival five years before and five years after certification according to medical care level.

3.5.2. Survival According to UICC Stage

Survival before and after Certification According to UICC Stage

The Kaplan–Meier analysis according to the UICC stage of rectal cancer showed a negative correlation between the overall survival and a higher UICC stage within the −5y group (I vs. II: $p = 0.298$; I vs. III: $p < 0.001$; I vs. IV: $p < 0.001$; II vs. III: $p = 0.061$; II vs. IV: $p < 0.001$; and III vs. IV: $p < 0.001$), as well as within the +5y group (I vs. II: $p = 0.032$; I vs. III: $p = 0.001$; I vs. IV: $p < 0.001$; II vs. III: $p = 0.226$; II vs. IV: $p < 0.001$; and III vs. IV: $p = 0.015$) (Figure 4).

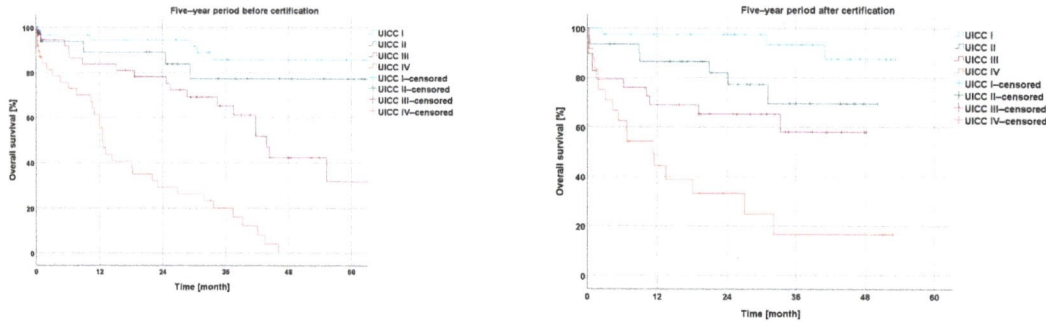

Figure 4. Presentation of overall survival five years before and five years after certification according to UICC stage.

The disease-free survival in the Kaplan–Meier curves, in relation to the UICC stage of rectal cancer, showed successively shorter values with an increasing UICC stage for the −5y collective (I vs. II: $p = 0.129$; I vs. III: $p < 0.001$; and II vs. III: $p = 0.140$) and for the +5y collective (I vs. II: $p = 0.12$; I vs. III: $p < 0.001$; and II vs. III: $p = 0.275$) (Figure 5).

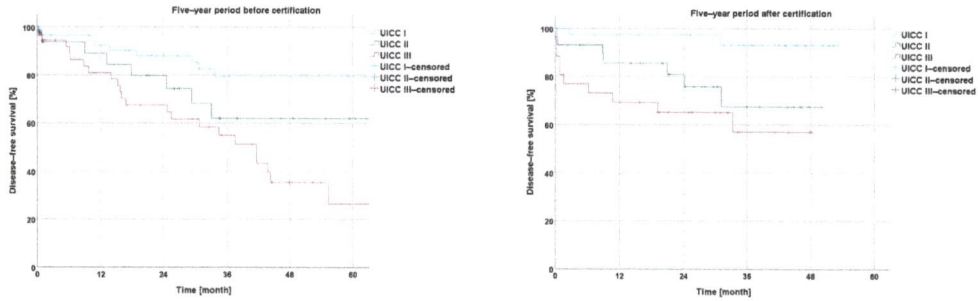

Figure 5. Presentation of disease-free survival five years before and five years after certification according to UICC stage.

Survival before and after Certification According to Particular UICC Stage

In the comparison of the UICC stages experienced by the −5y collective with those experienced by the +5y collective, the analysis showed a non-significantly longer overall survival for UICC stages I and III (I: $p = 0.347$; III: $p = 0.248$), a non-significantly shorter overall survival for UICC stage II (II: $p = 0.383$), and a significantly longer overall survival for UICC stage IV ($p = 0.041$) (Figure 6).

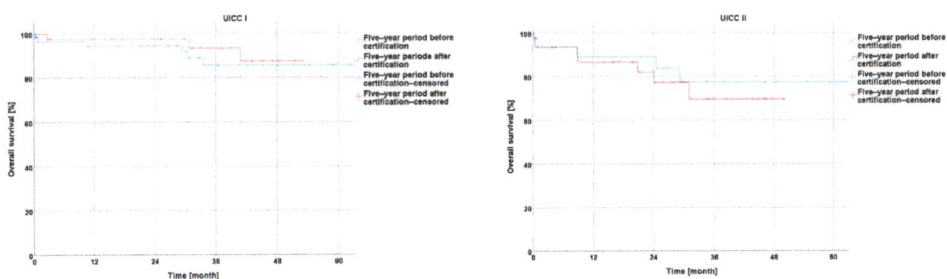

Figure 6. Presentation of overall survival five years before and five years after certification according to particular UICC stage.

An analysis of the disease-free survival showed a non-significant improvement during the five-year period after CrCC certification for UICC stages I, II, and III (I: $p = 0.188$; II: $p = 0.106$; and III: $p = 0.050$) (Figure 7).

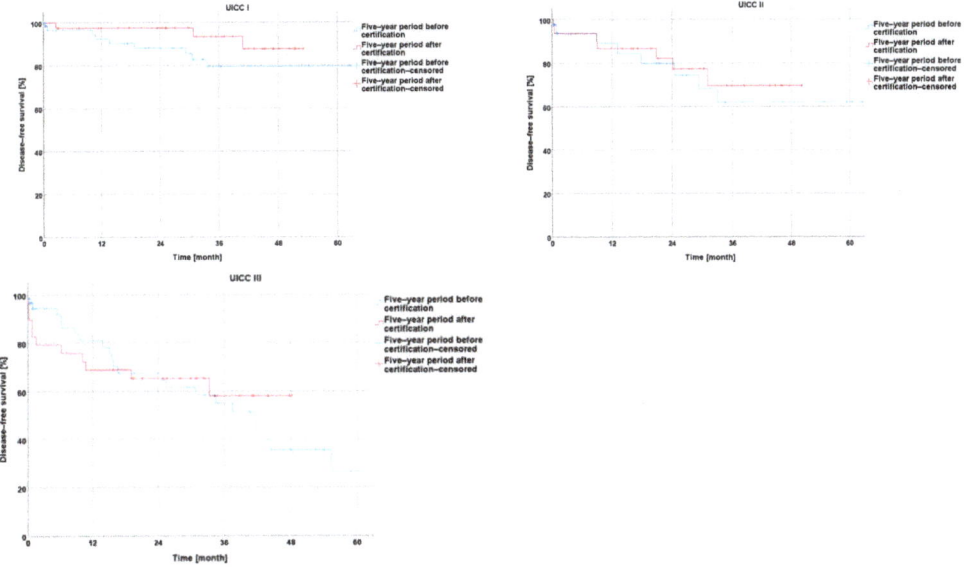

Figure 7. Presentation of disease-free survival five years before and five years after certification according to particular UICC stage.

3.5.3. Neoadjuvant and Adjuvant Treatment

Overall, we found that for all of the patients treated in the five years after certification, neoadjuvant chemoradiation (alternatively short radiation 5×5 Gy) was indicated for those with advanced rectal carcinoma (cT3/cT4 and/or cN+) in the staging imaging diagnostics (computed tomography (CT) and/or magnetic resonance imaging (MRI)). For patients with a nodal-positive status in their postoperative histopathological examination, adjuvant chemotherapy was indicated, as defined by the German S3 guidelines [6]. As for the patients treated before certification, we did not have enough data for either the neoadjuvant or the adjuvant treatment, and therefore, we could not perform a comparative analysis.

4. Discussion

Since the implementation of a certification system for oncological units in Germany, there have been divided opinions regarding whether the treatment quality and outcomes for patients with colorectal cancer would improve by meeting the criteria of the colorectal cancer centers (CrCCs) [17].

On the other hand, several studies have shown the advantages of certified, high-volume centers and the positive influence of multidisciplinary treatments on the outcomes [5,12,24,25]. For instance, a significantly better three-year overall survival for colorectal cancer was shown for patients treated in a certified center, compared to patients treated in uncertified units (71.6% vs. 63.6%, $p = 0.001$) [24]. In another study, a significant prolongation of the relative survival was observed in UICC IV rectal cancer patients treated in an experienced, certified center compared to the national average outcomes [5]. Finally, the latest WiZen study (2023) showed a longer five-year overall survival for different tumor entities, including rectal cancer (49.2% vs. 43.3%), for patients who had received an initial treatment in a certified center compared to those treated in an uncertified center [26].

Concerning the case load of oncological units and specialized surgeons, centers with a higher volume are known to achieve better outcomes with a lower morbidity and a longer overall survival [14,15,24]. Furthermore, in the study by Ghadban et al., which included an analysis of 351,028 colorectal cancer cases, a significant improvement was observed in terms of the mortality (3.8% in 2005 vs. 3.0% in 2015; $p < 0.001$), whereas the morbidity did not improve [2].

Hence, the aim of this study was to evaluate the effects of the colorectal cancer center (CrCC) certification process on the perioperative and long-term oncological outcomes for rectal cancer patients according to the database of the AN Institute of the Otto von Guericke University of Magdeburg. The main goal of this distribution was to present the advantages offered by a certification process in a dynamic fashion and while considering a timeline. Therefore, we examined the differences among 13 centers, considering the most important timeline milestone of 5 years.

Our analysis showed an increasing proportion of laparoscopic approaches from 5% to 55% during the five-year period after certification ($p < 0.001$), without an increase in the conversion rate ($p = 0.504$). Although the certification program does not directly obligate certified centers to perform a certain proportion of minimally invasive approaches for rectal surgery, an international trend of non-inferior oncological outcomes and a reduced perioperative morbidity for laparoscopies in comparison to open approaches was observed in the examined collectives after certification [6,27,28]. The proportion of laparoscopic rectal resections until 2016 in the examined collective was even higher compared to the increase from 12.3% to 48.1% reported in the German data published by Schnitzbauer et al. [29]. However, the presented trend in our data did not reach the proportion of laparoscopic colorectal surgeries performed in England within the LAPCO-program (an increase from 44% to 66%) [30]. Data concerning robotic approaches used for rectal surgeries were not available for the current analysis, as robotic colorectal surgery was developed in the included centers after the investigated period.

Furthermore, we reported a significant reduction in the number of trans-anal excisions performed after CrCC certification (8% to 1%, $p < 0.001$). The S3 guideline clearly recommends neoadjuvant chemoradiotherapy followed by a total mesorectal excision (TME) for most cases of low rectal cancers [6], and we witnessed an expansive development of endoscopic resections for adenoma and early rectal cancers in recent years [31]; therefore, we assumed that one of the above-mentioned treatment options was indicated for a greater number of patients over the studied timeline, which resulted in a decrease in the number of local surgical excisions.

The significant prolongation of the operating time after certification could be explained due to the increase in the frequency of the laparoscopic approaches. Prolonged operating times for laparoscopic approaches compared to conventional open approaches are well known and have already been reported in several studies [27].

The reported significant increase in the frequency of discontinuous resections according to Hartmann from 1% to 7% during the five-year period after certification ($p < 0.001$) was similar to that reported by Klaue et al. [17]. This observation was interpreted in the mentioned study as a possible result of the "fear of anastomotic leakage" in emergency cases, especially during the first years of a certification program [17]. After conducting thorough research and performing a statistical analysis on our collective, we did not find any significant correlation between the ASA score, age, or comorbidities and the frequency of Hartmann's resections. However, we observed a non-significant trend towards more emergency cases, as a possible explanation. The reported rate of Hartmann-reversal procedures might also be a sign of the adoption of a more careful and thoughtful approach, as reported elsewhere [32–35].

As a further aspect of improved management triggered by the certification process, several organizational advantages have been observed during the period after certification: the preoperative in-hospital length of stay was significantly reduced after certification. Furthermore, we observed a trend towards a reduction in the postoperative in-hospital length of stay. Additionally, there was a clear tendency towards a shorter overall in-hospital length of stay during the period after certification, which was comparable to other studies [36]. As reported by Aravani, the risks for a prolonged length of stay after colorectal cancer surgery are an older age (>80 years), socioeconomic deprivation, and the occurrence of a rectal cancer diagnosis [36]. The generally long in-hospital stays in the presented collective matched the data of other colorectal units in Germany in 2016 (18.6 ± 11.9 days), with a further shortening in the following years (13.8 ± 9.3 days in 2021) [37]. Although the time frames shown here represent the historic philosophy of perioperative management (diagnostics under stationary conditions, and long in-house stays until wound sutures were removed), which strongly varies from the current fast-track surgery goal [37–39], the data showed an obvious development after certification in terms of shortened in-hospital stays.

Regarding the short-term outcomes, there was a tendential shift towards an increased proportion of successful patient discharges and a decreased number of transfers to other units within the five-year period after certification. This observation could possibly be explained by the more successful and multidisciplinary handling of complicated and/or prolonged postoperative courses, involving aspects such as physiotherapy and professional nutritional support, with a reduced need to transfer patients to other specialized units. Regarding the overall in-hospital mortality, we registered a positive trend in certified centers during the five-year period after certification (decrease from 5% to 3%). These dynamics matched the significant decrease in the mortality indicated by the above-mentioned study (3.8% in 2005 vs. 3.0% in 2015; $p < 0.001$) [2].

Regarding the frequency of both surgical and non-surgical postoperative complications, we saw a significant improvement in terms of postoperative stool fistulas of the small or large bowel (other than the anastomotic region) after certification. This could possibly be an effect of the engagement of more experienced colorectal surgeons, as required by the German Cancer Society (chosen, responsible operators for the CrCC) for rectal cancer surgeries after certification.

On the other side, during the five-year period after CrCC certification, there was a significant increase in the frequency of postoperative intestinal atonia. This observation was contradictory to the results of different studies that have suggested faster postoperative bowel movements after a laparoscopic approach [40,41]. This could be the result of the standard postoperative analgetic regimen, which was mainly opioid-based in most centers associated with the AN Institute. This regimen could have led to increased intestinal atonia, as reported in several studies [42].

Histopathological findings represent a fundamental quality control after a surgical treatment of a tumor and are indispensable for further oncological treatment. Therefore, standardized histopathological reports involving all of the important tumor characteristics and the quality of the performed surgery are one of the most important requirements for the colorectal cancer center certification process [6].

Histological verification of a diagnosis is currently the gold standard before proceeding with a multidisciplinary treatment for rectal carcinoma, especially when a neoadjuvant treatment is indicated [6]. During the five-year period after certification, the number of histologically secured diagnoses before the treatment significantly increased, nearly achieving the international high-quality levels as described in the CONCORD study (94%) [3].

Although there was no relevant change in the patient distribution regarding the pathological T stage after CrCC certification, there were significant dynamics in the distribution of cases according to the pN stage within the five-year period after certification. However, the proportion of patients with an unclear postoperative lymph node status (pNx) decreased in the +5y group from 8% to 2%, indicating an increased level of engagement for full, detailed histopathological findings after certification.

Another sign of the standardization of the histopathological findings after certification was the significantly more frequent description of lymphovascular and vascular infiltration in our collective. Although the clinical relevancy of vascular infiltration (V) has not been proven, lymph vessel infiltration (L) is correlated with a higher risk of lymph node metastases [6]. Therefore, the German guideline for the treatment of colorectal cancer recommends providing a description of the L and V parameters within a TNM classification [6].

Although an analysis of surgical quality development in terms of the M.E.R.C.U.R.Y. status and the coning of surgical specimens after a total mesorectal excision (TME) could not be performed in this study, the fact that these parameters were involved in the database only after certification (+5y) showed a raised awareness of the importance of specimen quality. However, the German S3 guideline highly recommends a TME as a standard surgical technique for the treatment of rectal carcinoma, and the M.E.R.C.U.R.Y. status represents the pathological description of its quality [6,18,23]. In the study published by Sahm et al., which involved analyzing the quality of care for colorectal cancer in the federal state of Brandenburg, Germany, the reported rate of M.E.R.C.U.R.Y. I rectal resections was 96.4% in certified colorectal centers [4]. In the present study, we reported a similar rate of 94% during the five-year period after certification, suggesting at least that the recommended surgical technique was implemented after CrCC certification.

The overall survival in our collective slightly improved after certification, with a reported significance for patients with UICC stage IV disease ($p = 0.041$). This observation has also been reported by Richter et al. [5].

In terms of disease-free survival, we recorded the improvement in UICC stage III patients, only just falling short of a significant level ($p = 0.05$).

The subgroup analysis according to the medical care level (basic-, priority-, and maximal-care-level hospitals) showed a slightly superior overall survival and disease-free survival during the five-year period after certification, compared to the period before. A significant improvement in the overall survival was documented for the hospitals with a maximal level of medical care during the five-year period after certification, compared to the reference period ($p = 0.029$). We interpreted this observation as the result of a multifactorial process, including the increasing quality of the diagnostics, the selection of adequate multidisciplinary treatment modalities according to the guidelines of the German Cancer Society and the "best standard of care", the implementation of improved surgical techniques, the increased quality of histopathological documentation, and further immeasurable aspects, all indicated by the certification process.

The strength of this study lies in its comparison of rectal cancer data between defined periods before and after certification, including the survival rate in hospitals of different care levels as well as within particular stages according to the UICC classification. This comparison offers a direct view into the possible effects of certification. As mentioned before, the main goal of this distribution was to present the advantages offered by a certification process in a dynamic fashion while considering a timeline. Therefore, we offer the differences seen among 13 centers, considering the time frame of five years before and after certification. Such a comparative analysis is missing in the current literature.

Limitations

This study has several limitations. It is a retrospective analysis of a database that, while prospectively acquired, is still missing relevant data for the treatment of rectal cancer, such as neoadjuvant and adjuvant treatments, especially for patients treated prior to certification. The latter is, in our opinion, the most important limitation of the current study. There is heterogeneity as far as data collection and the quality of data are concerned. The main reason for this is a dynamic change in the gold standards for the treatment of rectal cancer, such as the use of neoadjuvant chemoradiation, the meaning of the M.E.R.C.U.R.Y. classification for surgical quality and its impact on recurrence rates, etc. The implementation of the certification process for colorectal cancer centers by the German Cancer Society was the breakthrough in terms of the data sampling quality and tumor documentation in Germany. The certification has driven centers to optimize their databases and raise their parameters. Therefore, a certification process is also important in terms of the quality of tumor documentation and treatments according to the guidelines. Although this was a multicentric study that included centers from different federal states, it only considered data up to 2016, and thus may not be representative of Germany as a whole and of the state of the art for rectal cancer treatment in 2023. Information about the case loads of certain hospitals was also not available.

Nevertheless, we firmly believe that a dynamic evolution process within the scope of a structured certification program cannot be managed only by statistical programs, because of the multivariability in the quantitative and qualitative aspects involved. Due to the latter aspect, a dynamic and continuous evaluation over a timeline is indispensable. A five-year milestone is the most important time milestone, as determined by the German Cancer Society.

5. Conclusions

The results of the present study indicate a clear trend towards improvement in terms of the treatment quality, survival, and documentation in certified colorectal cancer centers. This is demonstrated by certification-specific aspects such as more differentiated surgical approaches, a lower rate of certain complications, and a multidisciplinary approach. In our honest opinion, the qualitative aspects of a certification process (such as the need for multimodal treatment, the need to follow the guidelines and the current advancements in treatments, the need for interdisciplinary tumor boards, etc.), together with a stable volume of cases as proposed by the German Cancer Society, are the essential aspects required for improvement. Further prospective clinical trials are needed to investigate the relevance of certification in the treatment of CRC patients.

Author Contributions: Conceptualization M.A., R.S.C. and A.P.; Data extraction M.A., A.P., S.A.-M., S.A. and M.D.; Data curation M.A., A.P., J.S., M.R., S.A.-M., S.A. and M.D.; Investigation M.A., J.S., R.S.C. and A.P.; Writing—original draft M.A. and A.P.; Writing—review and editing M.A., M.R., J.S., R.S.C. and A.P. All authors have read and agreed to the published version of the manuscript.

Funding: This research received no external funding.

Institutional Review Board Statement: Ethical review and approval were waived due to the retrospective nature of this study, including patient and tumor characteristics from the years 2002–2016, as reported by the local ethical committee of the Otto von Guericke University of Magdeburg.

Informed Consent Statement: All patients gave their consent for data sampling, data extraction, data curation, and follow-up according to a standard informed consent statement, designed by the legal department of the AN Institute.

Data Availability Statement: All of the relevant data are provided in the manuscript.

Conflicts of Interest: The authors declare no conflicts of interest.

Abbreviations

CrCC	colorectal cancer center
CRC	colorectal cancer
ARR	anterior rectal resection
LARR	low anterior rectal resection
APE	abdominoperineal excision
Min.	minutes
Preop. LOS	preoperative length of stay
Postop. LOS	postoperative length of stay
oLOS	overall length of stay
UICC	Union International Contra Cancer
TME	total mesorectal excision

References

1. Erdmann, F.; Spix, C.; Katalinic, A.; Christ, M.; Folkerts, J.; Hansmann, J.; Kranzhöfer, K.; Kunz, B.; Manegold, K.; Penzkofer, A.; et al. *Robert Koch-Intitute: Cancer in Germany 2017/2018*, 13th ed.; 2022. Available online: https://edoc.rki.de/handle/176904/9042 (accessed on 15 November 2023).
2. Ghadban, T.; Reeh, M.; Bockhorn, M.; Grotelueschen, R.; Bachmann, K.; Grupp, K.; Uzunoglu, F.G.; Izbicki, J.R.; Perez, D.R. Decentralized colorectal cancer care in Germany over the last decade is associated with high in-hospital morbidity and mortality. *Cancer Manag. Res.* **2019**, *11*, 2101–2107. [CrossRef]
3. Coleman, M.P.; Quaresma, M.; Berrino, F.; Lutz, J.-M.; De Angelis, R.; Capocaccia, R.; Baili, P.; Rachet, B.; Gatta, G.; Hakulinen, T.; et al. Cancer survival in five continents: A worldwide population-based study (CONCORD). *Lancet Oncol.* **2008**, *9*, 730–756. [CrossRef] [PubMed]
4. Sahm, M.; Schneider, C.; Gretschel, S.; Kube, R.; Becker, A.; Gunther, M.; Loew, A.; Jahnke, K.; Mantke, R. Reality of care of colorectal cancer in the State of Brandenburg: With special consideration of the number of hospital cases and certification as a colorectal cancer center. *Chirurg* **2022**, *93*, 274–285. [CrossRef] [PubMed]
5. Richter, M.; Sonnow, L.; Mehdizadeh-Shrifi, A.; Richter, A.; Koch, R.; Zipprich, A. German oncology certification system for colorectal cancer—Relative survival rates of a single certified centre vs. national and international registry data. *Innov. Surg. Sci.* **2021**, *6*, 67–73. [CrossRef]
6. German S3 Guideline for Treatment of Colorectal Cancer Online. S3-Leitlinie Kolorektales Karzinom. 2019. Available online: https://register.awmf.org/assets/guidelines/021-007OLl_S3_Kolorektales-Karzinom-KRK_2019-01.pdf (accessed on 15 November 2023).
7. Hohenberger, W.; Bittorf, B.; Papadopoulos, T.; Merkel, S. Survival after surgical treatment of cancer of the rectum. *Langenbeck's Arch. Surg.* **2005**, *390*, 363–372. [CrossRef]
8. Sauer, R.; Becker, H.; Hohenberger, W.; Rodel, C.; Wittekind, C.; Fietkau, R.; Martus, P.; Tschmelitsch, J.; Hager, E.; Hess, C.F.; et al. Preoperative versus postoperative chemoradiotherapy for rectal cancer. *N. Engl. J. Med.* **2004**, *351*, 1731–1740. [CrossRef]
9. Fleischmann, M.; Diefenhardt, M.; Nicolas, A.M.; Rodel, F.; Ghadimi, M.; Hofheinz, R.D.; Greten, F.R.; Rodel, C.; Fokas, E.; German Rectal Cancer Study Group. ACO/ARO/AIO-21—Capecitabine-based chemoradiotherapy in combination with the IL-1 receptor antagonist anakinra for rectal cancer Patients: A phase I trial of the German rectal cancer study group. *Clin. Transl. Radiat. Oncol.* **2022**, *34*, 99–106. [CrossRef] [PubMed]
10. Diefenhardt, M.; Fleischmann, M.; Martin, D.; Hofheinz, R.D.; Piso, P.; Germer, C.T.; Hambsch, P.; Grutzmann, R.; Kirste, S.; Schlenska-Lange, A.; et al. Clinical outcome after total neoadjuvant treatment (CAO/ARO/AIO-12) versus intensified neoadjuvant and adjuvant treatment (CAO/ARO/AIO-04) a comparison between two multicenter randomized phase II/III trials. *Radiother. Oncol.* **2023**, *179*, 109455. [CrossRef]
11. Kowalski, C.; Graeven, U.; von Kalle, C.; Lang, H.; Beckmann, M.W.; Blohmer, J.U.; Burchardt, M.; Ehrenfeld, M.; Fichtner, J.; Grabbe, S.; et al. Shifting cancer care towards Multidisciplinarity: The cancer center certification program of the German cancer society. *BMC Cancer* **2017**, *17*, 850. [CrossRef]
12. Rückher, J.; Bokemeyer, C.; Fehm, T.; Graeven, U.; Wesselmann, S. Das Zertifizierungssystem der Deutschen Krebsgesellschaft. Nutzen und Weiterentwicklung. *Onkologe* **2021**, *27*, 969–979. [CrossRef]
13. Benz, S.; Wesselmann, S.; Seufferlein, T. Stellenwert von zertifizierten Darmkrebszentren in der Behandlung des kolorektalen Karzinoms. *Gastroenterologe* **2020**, *15*, 310–316. [CrossRef]
14. Archampong, D.; Borowski, D.; Wille-Jorgensen, P.; Iversen, L.H. Workload and surgeon's specialty for outcome after colorectal cancer surgery. *Cochrane Database Syst. Rev.* **2012**, CD005391. [CrossRef]
15. Aquina, C.T.; Probst, C.P.; Becerra, A.Z.; Iannuzzi, J.C.; Kelly, K.N.; Hensley, B.J.; Rickles, A.S.; Noyes, K.; Fleming, F.J.; Monson, J.R. High volume improves outcomes: The argument for centralization of rectal cancer surgery. *Surgery* **2016**, *159*, 736–748. [CrossRef] [PubMed]

16. Trautmann, F.; Reissfelder, C.; Pecqueux, M.; Weitz, J.; Schmitt, J. Evidence-based quality standards improve prognosis in colon cancer care. *Eur. J. Surg. Oncol.* **2018**, *44*, 1324–1330. [CrossRef] [PubMed]
17. Klaue, H.J.C. Certification of Colorectal Cancer Units—A Critical Overview on the Basis of Unsettled Aspects. *Zentralblatt Chir.* **2013**, *138*, 38–44. [CrossRef] [PubMed]
18. Hermanek, P.; Hermanek, P.; Hohenberger, W.; Klimpfinger, M.; Kockerling, F.; Papadopoulos, T. The pathological assessment of mesorectal excision: Implications for further treatment and quality management. *Int. J. Color. Dis.* **2003**, *18*, 335–341. [CrossRef] [PubMed]
19. West, N.P.; Finan, P.J.; Anderin, C.; Lindholm, J.; Holm, T.; Quirke, P. Evidence of the oncologic superiority of cylindrical abdominoperineal excision for low rectal cancer. *J. Clin. Oncol.* **2008**, *26*, 3517–3522. [CrossRef] [PubMed]
20. Leite, J.S.; Martins, S.C.; Oliveira, J.; Cunha, M.F.; Castro-Sousa, F. Clinical significance of macroscopic completeness of mesorectal resection in rectal cancer. *Color. Dis.* **2011**, *13*, 381–386. [CrossRef] [PubMed]
21. Salerno, G.; Daniels, I.R.; Moran, B.J.; Wotherspoon, A.; Brown, G. Clarifying margins in the multidisciplinary management of rectal cancer: The MERCURY experience. *Clin. Radiol.* **2006**, *61*, 916–923. [CrossRef] [PubMed]
22. Göhl, J.; Dörfer, J.; Hohenberger, W.; Merkel, S. Bedeutung der TME im operativen Therapiekonzept des Rektumkarzinoms. *Onkologe* **2007**, *13*, 365–374. [CrossRef]
23. Herzog, T.; Belyaev, O.; Chromik, A.M.; Weyhe, D.; Mueller, C.A.; Munding, J.; Tannapfel, A.; Uhl, W.; Seelig, M.H. TME quality in rectal cancer surgery. *Eur. J. Med. Res.* **2010**, *15*, 292–296. [CrossRef] [PubMed]
24. Draeger, T.; Volkel, V.; Gerken, M.; Klinkhammer-Schalke, M.; Furst, A. Long-term oncologic outcomes after laparoscopic versus open rectal cancer resection: A high-quality population-based analysis in a Southern German district. *Surg. Endosc.* **2018**, *32*, 4096–4104. [CrossRef] [PubMed]
25. Kowalski, C.; Sibert, N.T.; Breidenbach, C.; Hagemeier, A.; Roth, R.; Seufferlein, T.; Benz, S.; Post, S.; Siegel, R.; Wiegering, A.; et al. Outcome Quality After Colorectal Cancer Resection in Certified Colorectal Cancer Centers—Patient-Reported and Short-Term Clinical Outcomes. *Dtsch. Arztebl. Int.* **2022**, *119*, 821–828. [CrossRef] [PubMed]
26. Schmitt, J.; Klinkhammer-Schalke, M.; Bierbaum, V.; Gerken, M.; Bobeth, C.; Rößler, M.; Dröge, P.; Ruhnke, T.; Günster, C.; Kleihues-van Tol, K.; et al. Initial Cancer Treatment in Certified Versus Non-Certified Hospitals. *Dtsch. Ärzteblatt Int.* **2023**, *120*, 647–654. [CrossRef] [PubMed]
27. Conticchio, M.; Papagni, V.; Notarnicola, M.; Delvecchio, A.; Riccelli, U.; Ammendola, M.; Curro, G.; Pessaux, P.; Silvestris, N.; Memeo, R. Laparoscopic vs. open mesorectal excision for rectal cancer: Are these approaches still comparable? A systematic review and meta-analysis. *PLoS ONE* **2020**, *15*, e0235887. [CrossRef] [PubMed]
28. Acuna, S.A.; Chesney, T.R.; Ramjist, J.K.; Shah, P.S.; Kennedy, E.D.; Baxter, N.N. Laparoscopic Versus Open Resection for Rectal Cancer: A Noninferiority Meta-analysis of Quality of Surgical Resection Outcomes. *Ann. Surg.* **2019**, *269*, 849–855. [CrossRef] [PubMed]
29. Schnitzbauer, V.; Gerken, M.; Benz, S.; Volkel, V.; Draeger, T.; Furst, A.; Klinkhammer-Schalke, M. Laparoscopic and open surgery in rectal cancer patients in Germany: Short and long-term results of a large 10-year population-based cohort. *Surg. Endosc.* **2020**, *34*, 1132–1141. [CrossRef] [PubMed]
30. Hanna, G.B.; Mackenzie, H.; Miskovic, D.; Ni, M.; Wyles, S.; Aylin, P.; Parvaiz, A.; Cecil, T.; Gudgeon, A.; Griffith, J.; et al. Laparoscopic Colorectal Surgery Outcomes Improved After National Training Program (LAPCO) for Specialists in England. *Ann. Surg.* **2022**, *275*, 1149–1155. [CrossRef]
31. Hong, S.W.; Byeon, J.S. Endoscopic diagnosis and treatment of early colorectal cancer. *Intest. Res.* **2022**, *20*, 281–290. [CrossRef]
32. Okolica, D.; Bishawi, M.; Karas, J.R.; Reed, J.F.; Hussain, F.; Bergamaschi, R. Factors influencing postoperative adverse events after Hartmann's reversal. *Color. Dis.* **2012**, *14*, 369–373. [CrossRef]
33. Zarnescu Vasiliu, E.C.; Zarnescu, N.O.; Costea, R.; Rahau, L.; Neagu, S. Morbidity after reversal of Hartmann operation: Retrospective analysis of 56 patients. *J. Med. Life* **2015**, *8*, 488–491. [PubMed]
34. Hallam, S.; Mothe, B.S.; Tirumulaju, R. Hartmann's procedure, reversal and rate of stoma-free survival. *Ann. R. Coll. Surg. Engl.* **2018**, *100*, 301–307. [CrossRef] [PubMed]
35. Whitney, S.; Gross, B.D.; Mui, A.; Hahn, S.; Read, B.; Bauer, J. Hartmann's reversal: Factors affecting complications and outcomes. *Int. J. Color. Dis.* **2020**, *35*, 1875–1880. [CrossRef] [PubMed]
36. Aravani, A.; Samy, E.F.; Thomas, J.D.; Quirke, P.; Morris, E.J.A.; Finan, P.J. A retrospective observational study of length of stay in hospital after colorectal cancer surgery in England (1998–2010). *Medicine* **2016**, *95*, e5064. [CrossRef] [PubMed]
37. Koch, F.; Hohenstein, S.; Bollmann, A.; Kuhlen, R.; Ritz, J.P. Dissemination of fast-track concepts in Germany. *Chirurgie* **2022**, *93*, 1158–1165. [CrossRef] [PubMed]
38. Koch, F.; Green, M.; Dietrich, M.; Pontau, F.; Moikow, L.; Ulmer, S.; Dietrich, N.; Ritz, J.P. First 18 months as certified ERAS®center for colorectal cancer: Lessons learned and results of the first 261 patients. *Chirurgie* **2022**, *93*, 687–693. [CrossRef] [PubMed]
39. Koch, F.; Dietrich, M.; Green, M.; Moikow, L.; Schmidt, M.; Ristig, M.; Meier-Hellmann, A.; Ritz, J.P. The Usefulness of ERAS Concepts for Colorectal Resections—An Economic Analysis under DRG Conditions. *Zentralblatt Chir.* **2023**, *148*, 454–459. [CrossRef]
40. Harnsberger, C.R.; Maykel, J.A.; Alavi, K. Postoperative Ileus. *Clin. Colon Rectal Surg.* **2019**, *32*, 166–170. [CrossRef] [PubMed]

41. Tittel, A.; Schippers, E.; Anurov, M.; Titkova, S.; Ottinger, A.; Schumpelick, V. Shorter postoperative atony after laparoscopic-assisted colonic resection? An animal study. *Surg. Endosc.* **2001**, *15*, 508–512. [CrossRef]
42. Schwenk, E.S.; Grant, A.E.; Torjman, M.C.; McNulty, S.E.; Baratta, J.L.; Viscusi, E.R. The Efficacy of Peripheral Opioid Antagonists in Opioid-Induced Constipation and Postoperative Ileus: A Systematic Review of the Literature. *Reg. Anesth. Pain Med.* **2017**, *42*, 767–777. [CrossRef]

Disclaimer/Publisher's Note: The statements, opinions and data contained in all publications are solely those of the individual author(s) and contributor(s) and not of MDPI and/or the editor(s). MDPI and/or the editor(s) disclaim responsibility for any injury to people or property resulting from any ideas, methods, instructions or products referred to in the content.

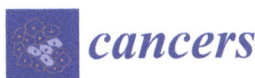

Article

Patient-Reported Sexual Function, Bladder Function and Quality of Life for Patients with Low Rectal Cancers with or without a Permanent Ostomy

Michael K. Rooney [1], Melisa Pasli [1], George J. Chang [2], Prajnan Das [1], Eugene J. Koay [1], Albert C. Koong [1], Ethan B. Ludmir [1], Bruce D. Minsky [1], Sonal S. Noticewala [1], Oliver Peacock [2], Grace L. Smith [1] and Emma B. Holliday [1,*]

[1] Department of Gastrointestinal Radiation Oncology, The University of Texas MD Anderson Cancer Center, Houston, TX 77030, USA; mkrooney@mdanderson.org (M.K.R.); paslim20@students.ecu.edu (M.P.); ssnoticewala@mdanderson.org (S.S.N.)
[2] Department of Colon and Rectal Surgery, The University of Texas MD Anderson Cancer Center, Houston, TX 77230, USA
* Correspondence: ebholliday@mdanderson.org

Simple Summary: This survey study investigates long-term patient-reported quality of life for individuals with low-lying rectal cancers, particularly focusing on the potential impact that ostomies may have on overall, sexual, and urinary quality of life. The findings suggest that patients with ostomies may experience a worse quality of life, affecting various aspects of daily life and relationships. These insights may help to inform patient counseling and shared decision making in the context of evolving rectal cancer treatment paradigms where patients have increasing multidisciplinary options.

Abstract: Background: Despite the increasing utilization of sphincter and/or organ-preservation treatment strategies, many patients with low-lying rectal cancers require abdominoperineal resection (APR), leading to permanent ostomy. Here, we aimed to characterize overall, sexual-, and bladder-related patient-reported quality of life (QOL) for individuals with low rectal cancers. We additionally aimed to explore potential differences in patient-reported outcomes between patients with and without a permanent ostomy. Methods: We distributed a comprehensive survey consisting of various patient-reported outcome measures, including the FACT-G7 survey, ICIQ MLUTS/FLUTS, IIEF-5/FSFI, and a specific questionnaire for ostomy patients. Descriptive statistics and univariate comparisons were used to compared demographics, treatments, and QOL scores between patients with and without a permanent ostomy. Results: Of the 204 patients contacted, 124 (60.8%) returned completed surveys; 22 (18%) of these had a permanent ostomy at the time of survey completion. There were 25 patients with low rectal tumors (≤5 cm from the anal verge) who did not have an ostomy at the time of survey completion, of whom 13 (52%) were managed with a non-operative approach. FACTG7 scores were numerically lower (median 20.5 vs. 22, $p = 0.12$) for individuals with an ostomy. Sexual function measures IIEF and FSFI were also lower (worse) for individuals with ostomies, but the results were not significantly different. MLUTS and FLUTS scores were both higher in individuals with ostomies (median 11 vs. 5, $p = 0.06$ and median 17 vs. 5.5, $p = 0.01$, respectively), suggesting worse urinary function. Patient-reported ostomy-specific challenges included gastrointestinal concerns (e.g., gas, odor, diarrhea) that may affect social activities and personal relationships. Conclusions: Despite a limited sample size, this study provides patient-centered, patient-derived data regarding long-term QOL in validated measures following treatment of low rectal cancers. Ostomies may have multidimensional negative impacts on QOL, and these findings warrant continued investigation in a prospective setting. These results may be used to inform shared decision making for individuals with low rectal cancers in both the settings of organ preservation and permanent ostomy.

Keywords: PROs; rectal cancer; ostomy; sexual function; bladder function; quality of life

Citation: Rooney, M.K.; Pasli, M.; Chang, G.J.; Das, P.; Koay, E.J.; Koong, A.C.; Ludmir, E.B.; Minsky, B.D.; Noticewala, S.S.; Peacock, O.; et al. Patient-Reported Sexual Function, Bladder Function and Quality of Life for Patients with Low Rectal Cancers with or without a Permanent Ostomy. *Cancers* **2024**, *16*, 153. https://doi.org/10.3390/cancers16010153

Academic Editor: Luca Roncucci

Received: 23 November 2023
Revised: 19 December 2023
Accepted: 20 December 2023
Published: 28 December 2023

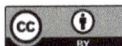

Copyright: © 2023 by the authors. Licensee MDPI, Basel, Switzerland. This article is an open access article distributed under the terms and conditions of the Creative Commons Attribution (CC BY) license (https://creativecommons.org/licenses/by/4.0/).

1. Introduction

Historically, the treatment of low rectal tumors within 5 cm of the anal verge includes abdominoperineal resection (APR) [1]. However, the widespread adoption of total mesorectal surgery techniques as well as ultralow low anterior resections have reduced the frequency with which APRs are performed [2]. Additionally, preoperative chemoradiation therapy (CRT) has proven useful to downstage low rectal tumors prior to surgery and allows for sphincter-sparing surgery (SSS) [3]. Despite these advances, it is estimated that approximately 40% of patients with rectal cancer undergo an APR and will have a permanent ostomy [4]. An ostomy refers to the exteriorization of the bowel through the abdominal wall and is a common procedure for individuals with gastrointestinal cancers requiring definitive or palliative surgery [5].

Disease-free survival is improving for patients with rectal cancer in the era of total neoadjuvant therapy (TNT) followed by surgical resection [6,7]. Aside from improved cancer cure rates, patients are increasingly interested in maintaining their quality of life (QOL) during survivorship [8]. When compared to SSS, patients undergoing APR are at increased risk for perineal wound complications, delayed healing, and increased hospital stay, which may not only delay adjuvant therapy, but may significantly impair short-term QOL [9]. Studies are mixed regarding the detrimental impact of global QOL with APR compared with SSS for low rectal cancer; some report worse QOL [10,11], others report better QOL [12,13], and most report no difference [14,15] for APR compared with SSS. Some studies suggest patients who undergo APR have more bothersome urinary symptoms than patients who undergo SSS [16], although others report no difference [14]. Data are more clear that patients who undergo APR have worse sexual function compared with those who undergo SSS; pain and body image issues related to the stoma are contributing factors as well as increased risk of autonomic pelvic nerve injury [14,17].

While not all patients may be a candidate for SSS due to tumor- or patient-specific factors, shared decision making is key for patients who do have surgical options [18]. Treatment decision making has become more complex in the era of non-operative management (NOM). The publication of the Organ Preservation in Patients with Rectal Adenocarcinoma (OPRA) trial suggested approximately 50% of well-selected patients with low rectal cancer may have a complete clinical response (cCR) to TNT and may be able to defer surgery [19]. Patient-reported functional outcomes were not published as part of the initial manuscripts, but single-institution studies suggest improved symptom-specific and QOL outcomes for patients treated with NOM compared with those who received surgery [20].

With increasing attention focused on the functional and QOL benefits of selective omission of CRT for low-risk patients [21], more data are needed regarding functional and QOL implications of utilizing CRT to either facilitate an SSS or omit surgery altogether. The aim of this brief report is to share patient-reported outcomes for patients with low rectal cancer treated at our institution with CRT followed by either APR, SSS, or NOM to evaluate for potential differences in urinary function, sexual function, and overall QOL between those with and without a permanent ostomy. Therefore, findings from this investigation could be used clinically to improve the quality of shared decision making for individuals considering various treatment strategies for low rectal tumors.

2. Materials and Methods

2.1. Survey Distribution and Data Collection

We received Institutional Review Board approval for this project (protocol 2020-0513). We contacted all consecutive patients who completed pelvic radiation for rectal adenocarcinoma at a large tertiary cancer center between 1 January 2017 and 31 December 2020 and were alive without evidence of disease recurrence. Patients eligible for this analysis had tumors ≤5 cm from the anal verge or had a permanent ostomy at the time of survey distribution. Patients all provided informed consent to participate in an online survey of validated patient-reported outcome measures (PROMs) including the Functional Assessment of Cancer Therapy-General (7-item version) (FACT-G7) survey [22], the International

Consultation on Incontinence Questionnaire (ICIQ) Male Lower Urinary Tract Symptoms (MLUTS) [23] or Female Lower Urinary Tract Symptoms (FLUTS) questionnaire [24], the International Index of Erectile Function 5-item questionnaire (IIEF-5) [25], or the Female Sexual Function Index (FSFI) questionnaire [26]. Patients with a permanent ostomy also received the City of Hope Quality of Life-Ostomy Questionnaire [27]. The survey was administered using REDCap v13.11.2(©2013 Vanderbilt University) [28], and patients who returned completed surveys received a USD 10 Amazon gift card to show appreciation for their time.

Information about oncologic treatment was obtained from the medical record. All patients were discussed at a dedicated rectal cancer multidisciplinary conference with representation by colorectal surgeons, medical oncologists, radiologists, pathologists, and radiation oncologists. Radiation dose and fractionation were chosen at the discretion of the treating radiation oncologist with input from the multidisciplinary team. During this period at our institution, preoperative short-course radiation or long-course CRT was routinely recommended for patients with T3, T4, or node-positive low rectal cancer. If a complete clinical response was confirmed by endoscopy and MRI, non-operative management was discussed. If sufficient margins could be obtained with a low coloanal anastomosis after neoadjuvant treatment, SSS would be performed. Otherwise, patients would undergo APR.

2.2. Statistical Analysis

Descriptive statistics and frequency tables were used to summarize patient demographics. Pearson's chi-square test and the Mann–Whitney U test were used to compare patient and treatment characteristics between patients treated for low rectal cancer with a permanent ostomy and those who did not receive a permanent ostomy. Descriptive statistics and frequency tables were also used to summarize FACT-G7, MLUTS or FLUTS, IIEF-5, or FSFI scores as well as answers to items on the City of Hope Quality of Life-Ostomy Questionnaire, when applicable. PROM scores were compared between patients with and without an ostomy at the time of survey completion using Pearson's chi-square tests. Statistical analysis was performed using R 4.0.3 (R Foundation for Statistical Computing, Vienna, Austria).

3. Results

Of the 204 patients contacted, 124 (60.8%) returned completed surveys; 22 (18%) of these had an ostomy at the time of survey completion. There were 25 patients with low rectal tumors ($\leq$5 cm from the anal verge) who did not have an ostomy at the time of survey completion, of whom 13 (52%) were managed with a non-operative approach. This cohort of 47 individuals was included for the primary analysis. Demographic, disease, and treatment characteristics of the study cohort are summarized in Supplemental Table S1, with results displayed separately for individuals with and without an ostomy at the time of survey completion. Overall, there were no significant differences between populations. Most respondents were non-Hispanic (80.9%) white (85.1%) men (66%). Most patients were treated with long course radiotherapy (78.7%) using a 3DCRT technique (61.7%). The median (first quartile Q1–third quartile Q3) time from completion of radiotherapy to survey completion was 34.2 months (20.3–49.5 months).

Distributions of PROs are summarized in Table 1, with results stratified by presence of an ostomy. Composite and subscore distributions of the FACT G7 score are displayed in Figure 1. Overall, individuals with an ostomy reported numerically worse FACT G7 composite scores, although differences were not statistically significant ($p = 0.12$). There were no differences in FACTG7 scores by sex (mean score for females and males were 20.7 and 20.6, respectively; $p = 0.8$). Sexual (IIEF, FSFI) and urinary-related (MLUTS, FLUTS) PROs are summarized in Supplemental Figure S1, with results stratified by ostomy status. Composite IIEF and FSFI were numerically greater (indicating better sexual function) for men and women without an ostomy, although results were not significantly different

(p = 0.18 and 0.83, respectively). MLUTS and FLUTS scores were higher for men and women with an ostomy (p = 0.06 and 0.01, respectively), indicative of worse urinary symptoms.

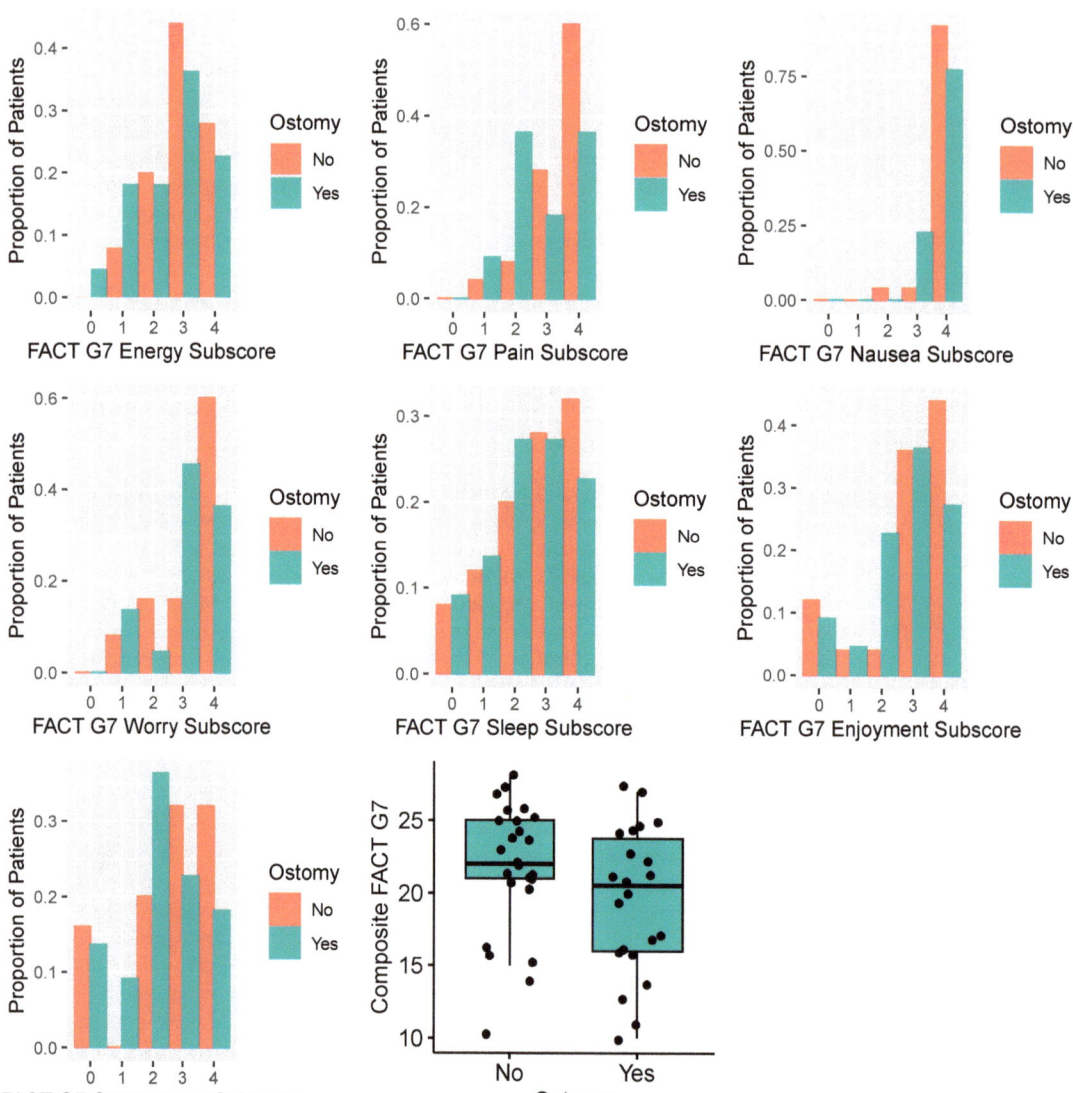

Figure 1. Distribution of Functional Assessment of Cancer Therapy General 7 (FACTG7) question instrument scores with results displayed separately by presence of an ostomy at survey completion. Higher scores reflect better quality of life.

Survey responses related directly to ostomy and function and the impact on quality of life are summarized in Figure 2. Most patients reported significant impacts of the ostomy across myriad domains, including gastrointestinal concerns such as gas, odor, diarrhea, constipation, and pouch leakage. Many patients also responded that the ostomy had significant negative impacts on personal relationships and sex life. Further, most patients reported the ostomy negatively affecting their ability to participate in social and recreational activities.

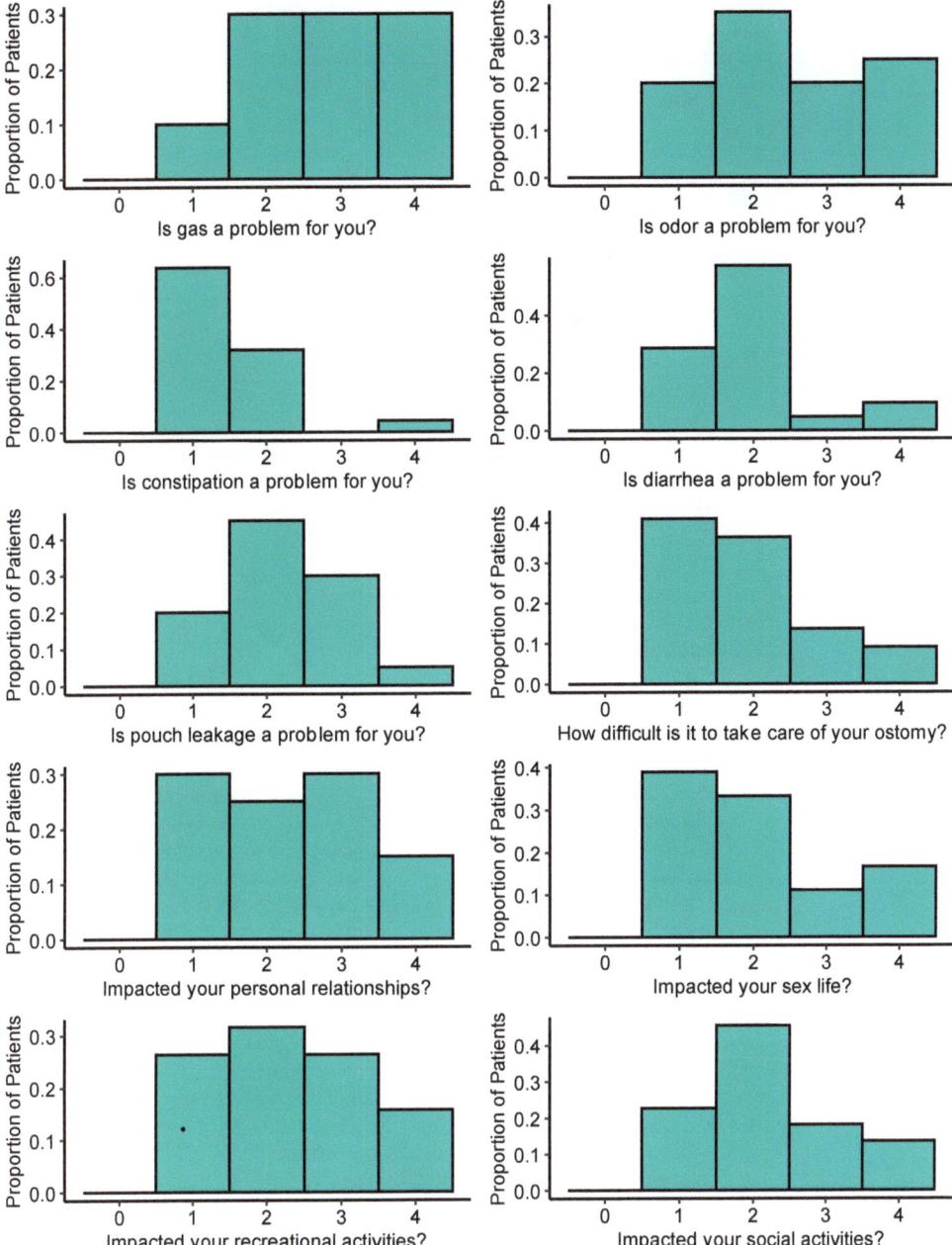

Figure 2. Distribution of survey responses related to ostomy function and impact on quality-of-life based on the City of Hope Quality of Life-Ostomy Questionnaire. Higher scores reflect greater symptom burden or impact on quality of life.

Table 1. Patient-reported outcomes with results displayed separately by presence of an ostomy at survey completion.

Score	Presence of a Permanent Ostomy			p-Value
	No	Yes	Overall	
FACTG7	n = 25	n = 22	n = 47	
Mean (SD)	21.8 (4.54)	19.5 (4.99)	20.7 (4.84)	0.12
Median [Q1, Q3]	22 [20.5, 25]	20.5 [16, 24]	21 [16, 25]	
IIEF	n = 17	n = 12	n = 29	
Mean (SD)	15.5 (6.37)	11.9 (7.33)	14 (6.89)	0.18
Median [Q1, Q3]	16 [9, 22]	8.5 [6.5, 19.5]	14 [7.5, 21]	
FSFI	n = 4	n = 6	n = 10	
Mean (SD)	18.3 (9.19)	15.1 (5.78)	16.4 (7.02)	0.83
Median [Q1, Q3]	18.6 [10.4, 26.15]	14.2 [10.5, 16.6]	14.2 [10.5, 25.4]	
MLUTS	n = 18	n = 12	n = 30	
Mean (SD)	6.50 (4.66)	14.3 (13.7)	9.60 (9.92)	0.06
Median [Q1, Q3]	5.50 [3, 8]	11.0 [4.5, 17]	6.50 [3, 13]	
FLUTS	n = 6	n = 9	n = 15	
Mean (SD)	5.33 (3.27)	15.8 (7.92)	11.6 (8.23)	0.01
Median [Q1, Q3]	5.50 [3, 7]	17 [8.5, 22]	10 [4, 18]	

Abbreviations: FACTG7 = Functional Assessment of Cancer Therapy—General 7 Question Survey; IIEF = International Index of Erectile Function; FSFI = Female Sexual Function Index; MLUTS = Male Lower Urinary Tract Symptom score; FLUTS = Female Lower Urinary Tract Symptom Score.

4. Discussion

In this observational survey-based study, we investigated long-term patient-reported QOL for individuals with low rectal cancers treated with multimodality therapy, focusing particularly on the impact of permanent ostomies on function and QOL during long-term survivorship. We found that QOL was numerically worse for individuals with ostomies compared to those without, as measured by various instruments assessing general QOL, sexual function, and bladder function. Furthermore, patients with ostomies reported that the ostomies themselves often had a significant impact on their relationships and daily lives, including worry about odor and gas, and that they can be difficult to manage. The results of this study can be used to improve patient education and shared decision making for patients with low rectal cancers who may be candidates for various treatment options.

QOL following treatment of rectal cancer has been studied extensively. Most early reports focused on the impact of multimodality therapy on bowel, urinary, and sexual function, suggesting a multifaceted negative effect of treatment [29]. However, the treatment paradigm for rectal cancer has evolved significantly over the past decade with randomized evidence suggesting that select individuals may benefit from treatment de-escalation via omission of various modalities including radiotherapy and surgery [19,30]. These strategies may lead to improved patient QOL, and thus, efforts to compare long-term outcomes across approaches are critically needed. Initial reports from the PROSPECT trial (Alliance N1048) suggest important differences in QOL for those receiving neoadjuvant therapy consisting of CRT with fluorouracil compared with fluorouracil and oxaliplatin alone [21]. However, there are limited data to date comparing the impact that omission of surgery may have on QOL, and even fewer studies exist aiming specifically to understand the impact that ostomy placement may have on patient experience. As such, this investigation fills an unmet need by comparing outcomes for individuals with low rectal tumors that may be candidates for various de-escalation strategies including organ-preservation to avoid ostomy. Our center is a large tertiary referral center and thus is uniquely positioned to provide needed data in this understudied area.

The FACT G7 instrument has been utilized to study patient-reported QOL for individuals with cancer for over a decade and has been validated across numerous cancer types [31,32]. It includes seven broadly spanning questions related to daily functional and physical well-being with composite scores ranging from 0–28, with higher scores indicating better QOL. Prior research surveying over 400 patients with colorectal cancers showed a mean score of approximately 20, with more advanced disease status being associated with lower (worse) scores [33]. These results closely resemble the results from our study cohort (Table 1). Among respondents, those with ostomies tended to have lower scores overall, indicative of worse overall QOL, although results were not statistically significant ($p = 0.12$), possibly indicative of a limited sample size to detect differences across groups. Studies evaluating QOL after ostomy for patients with colorectal cancer found that living with a permanent ostomy impacts QOL negatively due to sexual problems, depressive feelings, gas, constipation, dissatisfaction with appearance, change in clothing, travel difficulties, feeling tired, and worry about noises [34–37]. Alternatively, our results may support published studies which suggest that the presence of a permanent ostomy does not have an adverse impact on overall QOL [38,39].

When assessing patient-reported sexual and urinary function via the IIEF and FSFI, and MLUTS and FLUTS, respectively, we found similar results, wherein individuals with ostomies tended to report worse function and QOL. IIEF scores range from 5 to 25 and FSFI scores range from 2 to 36, with higher scores reflecting better sexual function. In this study population, the median overall IIEF score was 14, with numerically higher scores in men without an ostomy; similarly, the median overall FSFI was 16.4 with lower scores in women with an ostomy, suggesting worse sexual function in both sexes. Unfortunately, not all individuals were sexually active when they completed the survey, and there were relatively few women in the study population. We were unable to show a statistically significant difference between groups as a result, likely due to this inadequate sample size, but these results are in line with other published results suggesting worse sexual function following permanent ostomy placement [40,41].

Patient-reported urinary dysfunction was less common in this cohort, with median MLUTS and FLUTS of 9.6 and 11.6, respectively. For reference, cutoff values of 12 or higher have been proposed to define moderate to severe urinary dysfunction [42]. Despite the small sample size, women with ostomies had significantly higher FLUTS scores (median 17 vs. 5.5, $p = 0.01$), indicating worse urinary dysfunction. Similarly, MLUTS scores were higher for men with ostomies (median 11 vs. 5.5, $p = 0.06$), but the results did not reach statistical significance despite a large numeric difference between the groups, likely owing to limited power. Taken together, these results corroborate prior research showing that urinary dysfunction is quite common for individuals with rectal cancers [43] and importantly suggest that permanent ostomy placement is a risk factor for worse urinary function.

Our results also provide valuable data regarding the real-world impact that an ostomy may have on daily lifestyle and activity based upon responses from the City of Hope Quality of Life-Ostomy Questionnaire. Many patients reported concern about gastrointestinal symptoms including worry about odor, gas, and diarrhea (Figure 2). Further, many individuals felt that their relationships with others and their ability to participate in recreational activities were affected by their ostomy. These data are critical to consider during the shared decision making and informed consent process for rectal cancer treatment [44]. NOM is becoming increasingly possible for select individuals [45], and our data lend support to studies such as the Dutch Watch-and-Wait Consortium which show some functional issues after definitive chemoradiation, but overall better QOL scores compared with those requiring total mesorectal excision [46].

Although this study draws strength from rigorous survey methodology to assess a holistic battery of patient-reported outcomes, it is limited by several factors related to experimental design. First, only a relatively small portion of the responding population had ostomies at the time of survey completion, and thus the study sample size was quite low, which limits our ability to detect differences between groups. Furthermore, because many patients received follow-up care at outside institutions, we were unable to perform a pre-specified power calculation to determine an ideal survey sample size for individuals with a permanent ostomy. Second, we did not have the ability to measure baseline data, so we may be incompletely capturing the true impact that an ostomy has on primary outcomes. Additionally, it is important to recognize that there are various approaches to ostomy placement that may impact patient-reported experience and QOL. For example, perineal colostomy refers to a procedure wherein the ostomy is connected to the perineum as opposed to the abdominal wall; prior research has suggested improved QOL with this approach [47]. In the present study, we did not attempt to investigate the impact of various ostomy procedures and thus our results may not be generalizable across all patients. Last, although we were unable to find any significant baseline differences between individuals with and without ostomies and had limited power to perform a matching approach across groups, it is possible that there were unaccounted factors that might affect the necessity for an ostomy and thus introduce potential confounding with survey responses. Nonetheless, these data raise important questions and contribute valuable information [47] in a relatively understudied area.

5. Conclusions

For individuals with low-lying rectal cancers, patient-reported QOL tended to be worse for individuals with ostomies compared to those without, as measured using various instruments assessing general QOL, sexual function, and bladder function. Ostomies themselves can be difficult to take care of and may affect a person's relationships with others and his or her ability to participate in normal activities. The results of this study may be used to counsel patients who require an APR and may also be used to improve shared decision making for patients with low-lying rectal tumors who could be potential candidates at the time of treatment decision making for various treatment options, including organ preservation vs. permanent ostomy. In future studies, more data are needed, ideally collected in a multicenter prospective manner, to specifically compare relative functional and QOL issues between selective omission of radiation and definitive surgery versus the use of definitive chemoradiation and selective omission of surgery.

Supplementary Materials: The following supporting information can be downloaded at: https://www.mdpi.com/article/10.3390/cancers16010153/s1, Supplemental Table S1: Characteristics of the study population. Supplemental Figure S1: Sexual (IIEF, FSFI) and urinary (MLUTS, FLUTS) patient-reported outcomes, with results displayed separately according to presence of an ostomy.

Author Contributions: Conceptualization, M.K.R., M.P. and E.B.H.; methodology, M.K.R., M.P. and E.B.H.; formal analysis, M.K.R. and E.B.H.; investigation, M.K.R. and E.B.H.; writing—original draft preparation, M.K.R., M.P. and E.B.H.; writing—review and editing, all authors; supervision, E.B.H.; project administration, E.B.H.; funding acquisition, E.B.H. All authors have read and agreed to the published version of the manuscript.

Funding: This research received no external funding.

Institutional Review Board Statement: The study was conducted in accordance with the Declaration of Helsinki, and approved by the Institutional Review Board of MD Anderson Cancer Center (protocol 2020-0513).

Informed Consent Statement: Informed consent was obtained from all subjects involved in the study.

Data Availability Statement: Data will be made available upon reasonable request to the study authors.

Acknowledgments: We would like to thank all patients for their participation in the survey.

Conflicts of Interest: The authors declare no conflicts of interest.

Abbreviations

APR	abdominoperineal resection
CRT	chemoradiation
FACTG7	Functional Assessment of Cancer Therapy—General 7 Question Survey
FLUTS	Female Lower Urinary Tract Symptom Score
FSFI	Female Sexual Function Index
IIEF	International Index of Erectile Function
MLUTS	Male Lower Urinary Tract Symptom Score
NOM	non-operative management
PROM	patient-reported outcome measure
QOL	quality of life
SSS	sphincter-sparing surgery
TNT	total neoadjuvant therapy

References

1. Hawkins, A.T.; Albutt, K.; Wise, P.E.; Alavi, K.; Sudan, R.; Kaiser, A.M.; Bordeianou, L.; Continuing Education Committee of the SSAT. Abdominoperineal Resection for Rectal Cancer in the Twenty-First Century: Indications, Techniques, and Outcomes. *J. Gastrointest. Surg.* **2018**, *22*, 1477–1487. [CrossRef] [PubMed]
2. Bordeianou, L.; Maguire, L.H.; Alavi, K.; Sudan, R.; Wise, P.E.; Kaiser, A.M. Sphincter-Sparing Surgery in Patients with Low-Lying Rectal Cancer: Techniques, Oncologic Outcomes, and Functional Results. *J. Gastrointest. Surg.* **2014**, *18*, 1358–1372. [CrossRef] [PubMed]
3. Sauer, R.; Liersch, T.; Merkel, S.; Fietkau, R.; Hohenberger, W.; Hess, C.; Becker, H.; Raab, H.-R.; Villanueva, M.-T.; Witzigmann, H.; et al. Preoperative versus Postoperative Chemoradiotherapy for Locally Advanced Rectal Cancer: Results of the German CAO/ARO/AIO-94 Randomized Phase III Trial after a Median Follow-up of 11 Years. *J. Clin. Oncol.* **2012**, *30*, 1926–1933. [CrossRef] [PubMed]
4. Garcia-Henriquez, N.; Galante, D.J.; Monson, J.R.T. Selection and Outcomes in Abdominoperineal Resection. *Front. Oncol.* **2020**, *10*, 1339. [CrossRef] [PubMed]
5. Mulita, F.; Lotfollahzadeh, S. Intestinal Stoma. In *StatPearls*; StatPearls Publishing: Treasure Island, FL, USA, 2023.
6. Conroy, T.; Bosset, J.-F.; Etienne, P.-L.; Rio, E.; François, É.; Mesgouez-Nebout, N.; Vendrely, V.; Artignan, X.; Bouché, O.; Gargot, D.; et al. Neoadjuvant Chemotherapy with FOLFIRINOX and Preoperative Chemoradiotherapy for Patients with Locally Advanced Rectal Cancer (UNICANCER-PRODIGE 23): A Multicentre, Randomised, Open-Label, Phase 3 Trial. *Lancet Oncol.* **2021**, *22*, 702–715. [CrossRef] [PubMed]
7. Bahadoer, R.R.; Dijkstra, E.A.; van Etten, B.; Marijnen, C.A.M.; Putter, H.; Kranenbarg, E.M.-K.; Roodvoets, A.G.H.; Nagtegaal, I.D.; Beets-Tan, R.G.H.; Blomqvist, L.K.; et al. Short-Course Radiotherapy Followed by Chemotherapy before Total Mesorectal Excision (TME) versus Preoperative Chemoradiotherapy, TME, and Optional Adjuvant Chemotherapy in Locally Advanced Rectal Cancer (RAPIDO): A Randomised, Open-Label, Phase 3 Trial. *Lancet Oncol.* **2021**, *22*, 29–42. [CrossRef] [PubMed]
8. McMullen, C.K.; Bulkley, J.E.; Altschuler, A.; Wendel, C.S.; Grant, M.; Hornbrook, M.C.; Sun, V.; Krouse, R.S. Greatest Challenges of Rectal Cancer Survivors: Results of a Population-Based Survey. *Dis. Colon Rectum* **2016**, *59*, 1019–1027. [CrossRef]
9. Wiatrek, R.L.; Thomas, J.S.; Papaconstantinou, H.T. Perineal Wound Complications after Abdominoperineal Resection. *Clin. Colon Rectal Surg.* **2008**, *21*, 76–85. [CrossRef]
10. Du, P.; Wang, S.-Y.; Zheng, P.-F.; Mao, J.; Hu, H.; Cheng, Z.-B. Comparison of Overall Survival and Quality of Life between Patients Undergoing Anal Reconstruction and Patients Undergoing Traditional Lower Abdominal Stoma after Radical Resection. *Clin. Transl. Oncol.* **2019**, *21*, 1390–1397. [CrossRef]
11. Engel, J.; Kerr, J.; Schlesinger-Raab, A.; Eckel, R.; Sauer, H.; Hölzel, D. Quality of Life in Rectal Cancer Patients: A Four-Year Prospective Study. *Ann. Surg.* **2003**, *238*, 203–213. [CrossRef]
12. Grumann, M.M.; Noack, E.M.; Hoffmann, I.A.; Schlag, P.M. Comparison of Quality of Life in Patients Undergoing Abdominoperineal Extirpation or Anterior Resection for Rectal Cancer. *Ann. Surg.* **2001**, *233*, 149–156. [CrossRef] [PubMed]
13. Feddern, M.-L.; Emmertsen, K.J.; Laurberg, S. Quality of Life with or without Sphincter Preservation for Rectal Cancer. *Color. Dis.* **2019**, *21*, 1051–1057. [CrossRef] [PubMed]
14. Konanz, J.; Herrle, F.; Weiss, C.; Post, S.; Kienle, P. Quality of Life of Patients after Low Anterior, Intersphincteric, and Abdominoperineal Resection for Rectal Cancer--a Matched-Pair Analysis. *Int. J. Color. Dis.* **2013**, *28*, 679–688. [CrossRef] [PubMed]
15. Bong, J.W.; Lim, S.-B.; Lee, J.L.; Kim, C.W.; Yoon, Y.S.; Park, I.J.; Yu, C.S.; Kim, J.C. Comparison of Anthropometric Parameters after Ultralow Anterior Resection and Abdominoperineal Resection in Very Low-Lying Rectal Cancers. *Gastroenterol. Res. Pract.* **2018**, *2018*, 9274618. [CrossRef] [PubMed]
16. Wani, R.A.; Bhat, I.-U.-A.; Parray, F.Q.; Chowdri, N.A. Quality of Life After "Total Mesorectal Excision (TME)" for Rectal Carcinoma: A Study from a Tertiary Care Hospital in Northern India. *Indian J. Surg. Oncol.* **2017**, *8*, 499–505. [CrossRef]
17. Näsvall, P.; Dahlstrand, U.; Löwenmark, T.; Rutegård, J.; Gunnarsson, U.; Strigård, K. Quality of Life in Patients with a Permanent Stoma after Rectal Cancer Surgery. *Qual. Life Res.* **2017**, *26*, 55–64. [CrossRef] [PubMed]

18. Herrinton, L.J.; Altschuler, A.; McMullen, C.K.; Bulkley, J.E.; Hornbrook, M.C.; Sun, V.; Wendel, C.S.; Grant, M.; Baldwin, C.M.; Demark-Wahnefried, W.; et al. Conversations for Providers Caring for Patients with Rectal Cancer: Comparison of Long-Term Patient-Centered Outcomes for Patients with Low Rectal Cancer Facing Ostomy or Sphincter-Sparing Surgery. *CA Cancer J. Clin.* **2016**, *66*, 387–397. [CrossRef] [PubMed]
19. Verheij, F.S.; Omer, D.M.; Williams, H.; Lin, S.T.; Qin, L.-X.; Buckley, J.T.; Thompson, H.M.; Yuval, J.B.; Kim, J.K.; Dunne, R.F.; et al. Long-Term Results of Organ Preservation in Patients with Rectal Adenocarcinoma Treated with Total Neoadjuvant Therapy: The Randomized Phase II OPRA Trial. *J. Clin. Oncol.* **2023**, JCO2301208. [CrossRef]
20. Rooney, M.K.; De, B.; Corrigan, K.; Smith, G.L.; Taniguchi, C.; Minsky, B.D.; Ludmir, E.B.; Koay, E.J.; Das, P.; Koong, A.C.; et al. Patient-Reported Bowel Function and Bowel-Related Quality of Life After Pelvic Radiation for Rectal Adenocarcinoma: The Impact of Radiation Fractionation and Surgical Resection. *Clin. Color. Cancer* **2023**, *22*, 211–221. [CrossRef]
21. Basch, E.; Dueck, A.C.; Mitchell, S.A.; Mamon, H.; Weiser, M.; Saltz, L.; Gollub, M.; Rogak, L.; Ginos, B.; Mazza, G.L.; et al. Patient-Reported Outcomes During and After Treatment for Locally Advanced Rectal Cancer in the PROSPECT Trial (Alliance N1048). *J. Clin. Oncol.* **2023**, *41*, 3724–3734. [CrossRef]
22. Yanez, B.; Pearman, T.; Lis, C.G.; Beaumont, J.L.; Cella, D. The FACT-G7: A Rapid Version of the Functional Assessment of Cancer Therapy-General (FACT-G) for Monitoring Symptoms and Concerns in Oncology Practice and Research. *Ann. Oncol.* **2013**, *24*, 1073–1078. [CrossRef] [PubMed]
23. Donovan, J.L.; Peters, T.J.; Abrams, P.; Brookes, S.T.; de aa Rosette, J.J.; Schäfer, W. Scoring the Short Form ICSmaleSF Questionnaire. International Continence Society. *J. Urol.* **2000**, *164*, 1948–1955. [CrossRef] [PubMed]
24. Brookes, S.T.; Donovan, J.L.; Wright, M.; Jackson, S.; Abrams, P. A Scored Form of the Bristol Female Lower Urinary Tract Symptoms Questionnaire: Data from a Randomized Controlled Trial of Surgery for Women with Stress Incontinence. *Am. J. Obs. Gynecol.* **2004**, *191*, 73–82. [CrossRef] [PubMed]
25. Rosen, R.C.; Cappelleri, J.C.; Smith, M.D.; Lipsky, J.; Peña, B.M. Development and Evaluation of an Abridged, 5-Item Version of the International Index of Erectile Function (IIEF-5) as a Diagnostic Tool for Erectile Dysfunction. *Int. J. Impot. Res.* **1999**, *11*, 319–326. [CrossRef] [PubMed]
26. Wiegel, M.; Meston, C.; Rosen, R. The Female Sexual Function Index (FSFI): Cross-Validation and Development of Clinical Cutoff Scores. *J. Sex Marital. Ther.* **2005**, *31*, 1–20. [CrossRef] [PubMed]
27. Krouse, R.; Grant, M.; Ferrell, B.; Dean, G.; Nelson, R.; Chu, D. Quality of Life Outcomes in 599 Cancer and Non-Cancer Patients with Colostomies. *J. Surg. Res.* **2007**, *138*, 79–87. [CrossRef] [PubMed]
28. Harris, P.A.; Taylor, R.; Thielke, R.; Payne, J.; Gonzalez, N.; Conde, J.G. Research Electronic Data Capture (REDCap)--a Metadata-Driven Methodology and Workflow Process for Providing Translational Research Informatics Support. *J. Biomed. Inf.* **2009**, *42*, 377–381. [CrossRef] [PubMed]
29. Thaysen, H.V.; Jess, P.; Laurberg, S. Health-related Quality of Life after Surgery for Primary Advanced Rectal Cancer and Recurrent Rectal Cancer: A Review. *Color. Dis.* **2012**, *14*, 797–803. [CrossRef]
30. Schrag, D.; Shi, Q.; Weiser, M.R.; Gollub, M.J.; Saltz, L.B.; Musher, B.L.; Goldberg, J.; Al Baghdadi, T.; Goodman, K.A.; McWilliams, R.R.; et al. Preoperative Treatment of Locally Advanced Rectal Cancer. *N. Engl. J. Med.* **2023**, *389*, 322–334. [CrossRef]
31. Du, X.; Mao, L.; Leng, Y.; Chen, F. Validation of the FACT-G7 in Patients with Hematologic Malignancies. *Front. Oncol.* **2023**, *13*, 1183632. [CrossRef]
32. Mah, K.; Swami, N.; Le, L.W.; Chow, R.; Hannon, B.L.; Rodin, G.; Zimmermann, C. Validation of the 7-item Functional Assessment of Cancer Therapy-General (FACT-G7) as a Short Measure of Quality of Life in Patients with Advanced Cancer. *Cancer* **2020**, *126*, 3750–3757. [CrossRef]
33. Pearman, T.; Yanez, B.; Peipert, J.; Wortman, K.; Beaumont, J.; Cella, D. Ambulatory Cancer and US General Population Reference Values and Cutoff Scores for the Functional Assessment of Cancer Therapy. *Cancer* **2014**, *120*, 2902–2909. [CrossRef] [PubMed]
34. Robitaille, S.; Maalouf, M.F.; Penta, R.; Joshua, T.G.; Liberman, A.S.; Fiore, J.F.; Feldman, L.S.; Lee, L. The Impact of Restorative Proctectomy versus Permanent Colostomy on Health-Related Quality of Life after Rectal Cancer Surgery Using the Patient-Generated Index. *Surgery* **2023**, *174*, 813–818. [CrossRef] [PubMed]
35. Vonk-Klaassen, S.M.; de Vocht, H.M.; den Ouden, M.E.M.; Eddes, E.H.; Schuurmans, M.J. Ostomy-Related Problems and Their Impact on Quality of Life of Colorectal Cancer Ostomates: A Systematic Review. *Qual. Life Res.* **2016**, *25*, 125–133. [CrossRef] [PubMed]
36. Maguire, B.; Clancy, C.; Connelly, T.M.; Mehigan, B.J.; McCormick, P.; Altomare, D.F.; Gosselink, M.P.; Larkin, J.O. Quality of Life Meta-Analysis Following Coloanal Anastomosis versus Abdominoperineal Resection for Low Rectal Cancer. *Color. Dis.* **2022**, *24*, 811–820. [CrossRef] [PubMed]
37. Fucini, C.; Gattai, R.; Urena, C.; Bandettini, L.; Elbetti, C. Quality of Life among Five-Year Survivors after Treatment for Very Low Rectal Cancer with or without a Permanent Abdominal Stoma. *Ann. Surg. Oncol.* **2008**, *15*, 1099–1106. [CrossRef]
38. Orsini, R.G.; Thong, M.S.Y.; van de Poll-Franse, L.V.; Slooter, G.D.; Nieuwenhuijzen, G.a.P.; Rutten, H.J.T.; de Hingh, I.H.J.T. Quality of Life of Older Rectal Cancer Patients Is Not Impaired by a Permanent Stoma. *Eur. J. Surg. Oncol.* **2013**, *39*, 164–170. [CrossRef]
39. Allal, A.S.; Bieri, S.; Pelloni, A.; Spataro, V.; Anchisi, S.; Ambrosetti, P.; Sprangers, M.A.; Kurtz, J.M.; Gertsch, P. Sphincter-Sparing Surgery after Preoperative Radiotherapy for Low Rectal Cancers: Feasibility, Oncologic Results and Quality of Life Outcomes. *Br. J. Cancer* **2000**, *82*, 1131–1137. [CrossRef]

40. Tschann, P.; Weigl, M.; Brock, T.; Frick, J.; Sturm, O.; Presl, J.; Jäger, T.; Weitzendorfer, M.; Schredl, P.; Clemens, P.; et al. Identification of Risk Factors for Sexual Dysfunction after Multimodal Therapy of Locally Advanced Rectal Cancer and Their Impact on Quality of Life: A Single-Center Trial. *Cancers* **2022**, *14*, 5796. [CrossRef]
41. Li, K.; He, X.; Tong, S.; Zheng, Y. Risk Factors for Sexual Dysfunction after Rectal Cancer Surgery in 948 Consecutive Patients: A Prospective Cohort Study. *Eur. J. Surg. Oncol.* **2021**, *47*, 2087–2092. [CrossRef]
42. Guzelsoy, M.; Erkan, A.; Ozturk, M.; Zengin, S.; Coban, S.; Turkoglu, A.R.; Koc, A. Comparison of Three Questionnaire Forms Used in the Diagnosis of Lower Urinary Tract Symptoms: A Prospective Study. *Prostate Int.* **2022**, *10*, 218–223. [CrossRef] [PubMed]
43. Karlsson, L.; Bock, D.; Asplund, D.; Ohlsson, B.; Rosenberg, J.; Angenete, E. Urinary Dysfunction in Patients with Rectal Cancer: A Prospective Cohort Study. *Color. Dis.* **2020**, *22*, 18–28. [CrossRef] [PubMed]
44. Hrabe, J.E.; Kapadia, M.R. Guiding Patients Through a "Watch-and-Wait" Approach for Rectal Cancer-Understanding the Functional Outcomes. *JAMA Surg.* **2023**, *158*, e230165. [CrossRef] [PubMed]
45. Loria, A.; Tejani, M.A.; Temple, L.K.; Justiniano, C.F.; Melucci, A.D.; Becerra, A.Z.; Monson, J.R.T.; Aquina, C.T.; Fleming, F.J. Practice Patterns for Organ Preservation in US Patients With Rectal Cancer, 2006–2020. *JAMA Oncol.* **2023**. [CrossRef]
46. Custers, P.A.; van der Sande, M.E.; Grotenhuis, B.A.; Peters, F.P.; van Kuijk, S.M.J.; Beets, G.L.; Breukink, S.O.; Dutch Watch-and-Wait Consortium. Long-Term Quality of Life and Functional Outcome of Patients with Rectal Cancer Following a Watch-and-Wait Approach. *JAMA Surg.* **2023**, *158*, e230146. [CrossRef]
47. Mulita, F.; Tepetes, K.; Verras, G.-I.; Liolis, E.; Tchabashvili, L.; Kaplanis, C.; Perdikaris, I.; Velissaris, D.; Maroulis, I. Perineal Colostomy: Advantages and Disadvantages. *Gastroenterol. Rev.* **2022**, *17*, 89–95. [CrossRef]

Disclaimer/Publisher's Note: The statements, opinions and data contained in all publications are solely those of the individual author(s) and contributor(s) and not of MDPI and/or the editor(s). MDPI and/or the editor(s) disclaim responsibility for any injury to people or property resulting from any ideas, methods, instructions or products referred to in the content.

MDPI AG
Grosspeteranlage 5
4052 Basel
Switzerland
Tel.: +41 61 683 77 34

Cancers Editorial Office
E-mail: cancers@mdpi.com
www.mdpi.com/journal/cancers

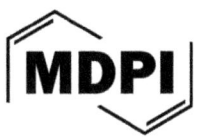

Disclaimer/Publisher's Note: The statements, opinions and data contained in all publications are solely those of the individual author(s) and contributor(s) and not of MDPI and/or the editor(s). MDPI and/or the editor(s) disclaim responsibility for any injury to people or property resulting from any ideas, methods, instructions or products referred to in the content.

www.ingramcontent.com/pod-product-compliance
Lightning Source LLC
LaVergne TN
LVHW070630100526
838202LV00012B/770